PEDIATRIC TRAUMA

INITIAL ASSESSMENT AND MANAGEMENT

EDWARD G. FORD, MD, FACS, FAAP, FACN
Associate Professor of Surgery and Clinical Pediatrics
Director, Division of Pediatric Surgery
Tulane University School of Medicine
New Orleans, Louisiana

RICHARD J. ANDRASSY, MD, FACS, FAAP, FACN
A.G. McNeese Professor of Surgery and Pediatrics
University of Texas Medical School at Houston
Chief of Pediatric Surgery
M.D. Anderson Cancer Center, Hermann Children's Hospital,
and Lyndon B. Johnson Hospital
Houston, Texas

W.B. SAUNDERS COMPANY
A Division of Harcourt Brace & Company

Philadelphia   London   Toronto   Montreal   Sydney   Tokyo

W.B. SAUNDERS COMPANY

A Division of
Harcourt Brace and Company

The Curtis Center
Independence Square West
Philadelphia, PA 19106

Library of Congress Cataloging-in-Publication Data

Pediatric trauma : initial assessment and management / [edited by]
 Edward G. Ford, Richard J. Andrassy.
  p.   cm.
 ISBN 0-7216-2913-X
 1. Children—Wounds and injuries—Treatment. I. Ford, Edward G.
II. Andrassy, Richard.
 [DNLM: 1. Wounds and Injuries—in infancy & childhood.
2. Emergencies—in infancy & childhood.   WO 700 1994]
 RD93.5.C4P445 1994
 617.1'0083—dc20
 DNLM/DLC   94-6679

PEDIATRIC TRAUMA: INITIAL ASSESSMENT   ISBN   0-7216-2913-X
AND MANAGEMENT

Printed in the United States of America

Last digit is the print number: 9   8   7   6   5   4   3   2   1

*For those children we had the privilege
and pleasure to care for.*

Acknowledgment

I have slowly learned that any major new undertaking hides within itself innumerable joys and frustrations. The editing of a textbook is no exception. We have tried to produce a text that is most usable to those who are most likely to be the first caregivers to victims of pediatric trauma. This book targets the emergency room physicians and staff, family practitioners, general practitioners, community pediatricians, and internists. It is not the definitive treatise on pediatric trauma but rather provides a framework for the *initial* assessment and management of pediatric victims of traumatic disease. We have attempted to provide a straightforward and factual representation of ideology, and where controversy exists, the literature on both sides of the issues are presented.

Writing such a text is a formidable undertaking that requires enormous professional emotional support. I will always be thankful to Richard Andrassy for teaching me to write and stimulating an enormous interest in pediatric surgery. Ms. Heide Dyer is my administrative assistant who has put in countless hours for the past year in chapter revisions, re-revisions, and editing. Ave McCracken is the senior medical editor for W.B. Saunders, whose fresh enthusiasm was a stimulus to push on to completion. Each of the contributing authors were purposely chosen but may not be the world's expert on a given clinical situation. Instead, we have chosen authors with a great deal of practical experience who can appreciate the clinical issues that may face the initial health care provider. The chapters are outstanding representations of subspecialty expertise, and the literature for each is absolutely complete to date. Additionally, each of the chapters is fully illustrated with line drawings and photographs to make the text an even more useful ready reference.

Edward G. Ford, M.D.

Preface

The pediatric population accounts for an enormous number of private practice and hospital emergency room visits each year. The number one disease process in this patient population is characteristically associated with accidental injury. There are currently several large, well-written, and authoritative texts which deal with pediatric trauma. These works discuss in considerable detail everything from methods for establishing emergency medical systems, data bases for accidental injury reporting and trending, and lengthy discussions of the tertiary care of injured pediatric patients. We found those texts to be wonderful references for subspecialty physicians such as pediatric intensivists and pediatric surgeons; however, the information is a bit voluminous for easy reference in a private practice office or emergency room setting. We have limited the scope of our book to the *initial* assessment of the pediatric patient with accidental injury and the initial management of that patient. Our target audience is those health care providers and physicians who have the initial interface with the injured child. We have attempted to include a large number of graphic illustrations, roentgenograms, tabular data, and practice hints for care so that any provider may feel comfortable dealing with the injured child in an emergency setting. We hope our ideas and approach will enhance the care given to this special patient population in those essential first critical hours following injury.

Edward G. Ford
Richard J. Andrassy

Contributors

Richard J. Andrassy, MD, FACS, FAAP, FACN
A. G. McNeese Professor of Surgery and Pediatrics, University of Texas Medical School at Houston; Chief of Pediatric Surgery, M. D. Anderson Cancer Center, Hermann Children's Hospital, and Lyndon B. Johnson Hospital, Houston, Texas
Considerations Unique to Children

Daniel A. Beals, MD
Chief, Pediatric Surgery, Keesler Medical Center, Biloxi, Mississippi
Head and Neck Trauma

Joseph N. Corriere, Jr., MD
Professor of Surgery and Urology, University of Texas Medical School at Houston; Staff Physician, Hermann Children's Hospital, Lyndon B. Johnson Hospital, M. D. Anderson Cancer Center, Shriner's Hospital for Crippled Children, and The Institute for Rehabilitation and Research, Houston, Texas
Urinary Tract Injuries

Chris Cribari, MD, FACS
Clinical Assistant Professor of Surgery, Uniformed Services University of the Health Sciences, Bethesda, Maryland; Staff Surgeon, Pondre Valley Hospital, Fort Collins, Colorado
Vascular Trauma

Edward G. Ford, MD, FACS, FAAP, FACN
Associate Professor of Surgery and Clinical Pediatrics; Director, Division of Pediatric Surgery, Tulane University School of Medicine, New Orleans, Louisiana
Trauma Triage; Abdominal Injury; Burn Injury; Nutritional Support

James E. Foster, II, MD, FACS

Clinical Assistant Professor of Surgery, Uniformed Services University of the Health Sciences, Bethesda, Maryland; Chief, General Surgery and Director, General Surgery Residency Training, Keesler Medical Center, Biloxi, Mississippi
Burn Injury

Kevin D. Halow, MD

Chief Resident in Surgery, Keesler Medical Center, Biloxi, Mississippi
Abdominal Injury

Jeffrey R. Horwitz, MD, MPH

Pediatric Surgery Fellow, University of Texas Medical School at Houston; Staff Physician, Hermann Children's Hospital and Lyndon B. Johnson Hospital, Houston, Texas
Considerations Unique to Children

Kent P. Hymel, MD

Director, Ambulatory Pediatrics; Medical Director, Family Advocacy Program, Keesler Medical Center, Biloxi, Mississippi
Child Abuse

Bruce P. Jaufmann, MD

Staff Neurosurgeon, Cape Fear Valley Medical Center and Highsmith Rainey Hospital, Fayetteville, North Carolina
Central Nervous System Injuries

Sue C. Kaste, DO

Assistant Professor, Department of Radiology, University of Tennessee at Memphis, College of Medicine; Assistant Member, Department of Diagnostic Imaging, St. Jude Children's Research Hospital; Consultant, Department of Radiology, LeBonheur Children's Medical Center, Memphis, Tennessee
Emergency Pediatric Imaging

Matthew L. Lukens, MD

Attending Vascular Surgeon, Keesler Medical Center; Consulting Vascular Surgeon, Veterans Administration Medical Center, Biloxi, Mississippi
Vascular Trauma

Jay S. Miller, MD

Clinical Assistant Professor of Surgery, Uniformed Services University of the Health Sciences, Bethesda, Maryland; Chief of Vascular Surgery and Director, Intensive Care Unit, Keesler Medical Center; Consulting Vascular Surgeon, Veterans Administration Medical Center, Biloxi, Mississippi

Vascular Trauma

Carol Mary Medins, BS, RD, LD

Clinical Manager and Clinical Dietitian, Nutrition Support Team Dietitian, Keesler Medical Center, Biloxi, Mississippi

Nutritional Support

Michael W. Paluzzi, MD

Clinical Assistant Professor of Surgery, Uniformed Services University of the Health Sciences, Bethesda, Maryland; Staff Surgeon, Keesler Medical Center; Consultant in Laparoscopic Surgery, Veterans Administration Medical Center, Biloxi, Mississippi

Alkali and Chemical Injuries of the Esophagus

Douglas E. Paull, MD, FACS

Staff Thoracic Surgeon, Cardinal Cushing Hospital and Brockton Hospital, Brockton, Massachusetts; Goddard Memorial Hospital, Stockton, Massachusetts; Milton Hospital, Milton, Massachusetts; Carney Hospital, Boston, Massachusetts; Quincy Hospital, Quincy, Massachusetts

Thoracic Injury in Children

Harry C. Sax, MD

Assistant Professor of Surgery, University of Rochester School of Medicine and Dentistry; Medical Director, Adult Nutritional Support Service, Strong Memorial Hospital, Rochester, New York

Metabolic Responses to Injury

Thomas E. Scott, MD, MPH

Associate Professor of Clinical Surgery, Uniformed Services University of the Health Sciences, Bethesda, Maryland; Chairman, Department of Surgery, Keesler Medical Center, Biloxi, Mississippi

Decision Making in Pediatric Trauma Care

Contents

UNIT
I

INTRODUCTORY TOPICS

Considerations Unique to Children

Jeffrey R. Horwitz
Richard J. Andrassy

Trauma is the leading cause of death for children over 1 year of age, and among children ages 1 to 19, injuries cause more deaths than all other diseases combined. Injury is the leading cause of disability in this age group. Each year childhood injuries are responsible for over 150,000 deaths, approximately 600,000 hospital admissions, and more than 80,000 permanent disabling conditions. Costs from these injuries are estimated to exceed $7.5 billion each year. An estimated $8 billion cost is expected from future productivity losses.[1] The most common causes of childhood injury include motor vehicle accidents, homicide, assault and abuse, suicide and suicide attempts, drowning and near-drowning, pedestrian injuries, and fire and burns.

MOTOR VEHICLE OCCUPANT ACCIDENTS

One half of all injury deaths in children are due to motor vehicle accidents. This is the major cause of childhood injury death in the United States. Among all pediatric injuries, motor vehicle accidents account for the third highest hospitalization rate and the third highest emergency room visit rate.[2,3] The cost of motor vehicle injuries exceeds all other pediatric injuries. Age and sex are important risk factors in the epidemiology of vehicular injuries. Fatality rates for 15- to 19-year-olds are 10 times higher than those of children under 10 years of age. The death rate for males is twice that for females, and alcohol is involved in nearly 50% of adolescent motor vehicle fatalities.[4]

HOMICIDE, ASSAULT, AND ABUSE

In the past quarter century, homicide rates for all childhood age groups have at least doubled. Currently homicide is the second leading cause of injury deaths among children. Most homicide deaths are among males, and nearly two thirds of these deaths are among 15-19 year old persons. Homicide rates for black children are nearly five times higher than for white children. The circumstances of injury vary with the age of the child. Among children up to 4 years of age about half of homicides are due to physical violence and 10% are the result of firearms. Firearm injuries increase to nearly 70% among children ages 15 to 19 years.

Abuse and neglect affect an estimated 1.6 million children yearly. Physical abuse or neglect accounts for more than 50% of these incidents.[6] The skin and soft tissue are the most common sites of manifestations of child abuse. Bruising may be evident at multiple body sites, and often there are distinctive patterns characteristic of the offending instrument (e.g., handprints, burn marks). Physical abuse rates increase with age. Older adolescents are abused twice as often as those in younger age groups.

SUICIDE AND ATTEMPTED SUICIDE

During the last three decades suicide rates for persons aged 10 to 19 years have more than doubled. Among this same age group, 80% of suicide victims were male and whites outnumbered nonwhites by nearly 3 to 1.[7] Firearms are involved in 60% of cases involving 15- to 19-year-old persons. Suicide attempts represent another significant social and medical problem. Unsuccessful suicide attempts are estimated to be up to eight times more common than successful ones. Twenty percent of those attempting suicide end up hospitalized at a cost of $8 million in direct medical care.[7]

DROWNING AND NEAR-DROWNING

Childhood drowning is most common among males 15 to 19 years of age and children 4 years of age and younger.[8-10] In some states (California, Florida, and Arizona) drowning is the leading cause of fatal injury among young children. Up to 90% of drownings in the younger age groups occur in residential swimming pools. Cases involving adolescent males occur in a variety of environments and in 40% to 50% of cases are associated with alcohol use. The number of emergency department visits for near-drowning is believed to be nearly 30,000 a year. An estimated 20% of hospitalized survivors of near-drowning are left with a permanent neurologic disability, which carries an estimated cost for direct care exceeding $200 million a year.[8]

PEDESTRIAN INJURIES

Pedestrian injuries are the fifth leading cause of injury-related deaths in children. Pedestrian injuries are the leading cause of death among children 5 to 9 years of age.[11] The risk of pedestrian injury appears to be inversely related to socioeconomic status; children from poor families have two or three times the risk of other children.[12] Males outnumber females, and fatality rates for nonwhite children are 1.5 times the rates for whites.[11] In children less than 5 years of age, nontraffic pedestrian injuries typically occur when a young child is backed over in the driveway at home by a vehicle driven by a family member. Usually the vehicle is a light truck or van, which may make it more difficult to see a small child moving around the back of the vehicle. Among older children, injuries usually result from darting out into traffic or crossing the street in the middle of a block.[11,13]

FIRES AND BURNS

Each year nearly 400,000 children are treated in emergency departments, clinics, or physicians' offices for burn injuries. Fires and burns are the leading cause of accidental death in the home for children under the age of 14 years. House fires account for approximately 80% of fire and burn deaths, and electrical and scald burn injuries make up the remainder. Children 10 years of age and younger represent 75% of all pediatric burn deaths. Black children account for 34% of pediatric fire and burn deaths, although represent only 15% of the pediatric population. Older children are more frequently injured as a result of flame burns, whereas infants and toddlers are frequently the victim of scald injuries.[14] The impact on society is appreciated when it is noted that 50% of burned children require up to a 1-month hospital stay and 25% require up to 2 months of inpatient medical care. The cost of caring for fire and burn injuries is estimated at $3.6 billion a year.[15]

INITIAL EVALUATION AND TRIAGE
Classification Systems

Numerous scoring systems (e.g., Trauma Score, Injury Severity Score, Trauma Score–Injury Severity Score, Pediatric Trauma Score) have been developed and used as predictors of injury severity and projected outcome in trauma patients. These scoring systems are used to determine appropriate triage in the field, assess the effectiveness of overall patient care, and compare patient populations in scientific and epidemiologic research. These systems and their applications in the care of the pediatric trauma patient are discussed in detail in Chapter 4.

Resuscitation Techniques Unique to Children

Although the principles of resuscitation of injured children are similar to those of adults, appreciation of anatomic and physiologic features specific to pediatric patients is essential for successful initial therapy and eventual outcome.

Airway and breathing. Multiple anatomic differences between the pediatric and the adult airway affect patient management and may make the airways of infants and children more difficult to evaluate and manage.[16] Small amounts of airway edema produce a disproportionate increase in resistance and decrease in cross-sectional area in the infant airway (Fig. 1–1). The mouth, pharynx, and trachea form a more acute angle in the infant and young child than in an adult. Placing the child in the "sniffing" position creates the optimal alignment of these structures for unobstructed air flow. The neck should be slightly flexed on the chest and the head slightly extended on the neck (Fig. 1–2). Because of compliance of the pediatric trachea, overextension of the head on the neck may result in upper airway obstruction.[17,18]

Endotracheal intubation in a child may present even the experienced clinician with several challenges. The child's larynx is both more anterior and more cephalad than the adult's, and the vocal cords are angled more posteriorly. The relatively large tongue and hypertrophied tonsils may impede visual examination of the vocal cords. In addition, the child's epiglottis is omega shaped and protrudes farther into the pharynx than an adult's. Lifting the epiglottis with the blade of a straight laryngoscope should allow a clearer view of the airway in infants and young children than a curved blade would. The anterior position of the airway in the hypopharynx and the high vascularity of the adenoidal tissue with its risk for significant bleeding combine to make nasotracheal intubation a difficult procedure that is not recommended. A needle cricothyroid-

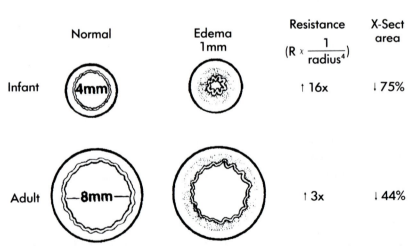

Figure 1–1. Comparison of the effects of edema on airway resistance and cross-sectional area in the infant and adult patient. (From Cotes CJ, Todres ID: The pediatric airway. In Ryan JF, Todres ID, Cotes CJ, et al: *A practice of anesthesia for infants and children,* New York, 1986, Grune & Stratton, p 39.)

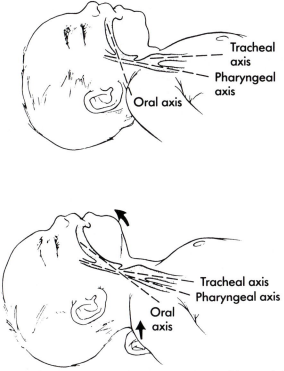

Figure 1–2. Airway alignment in the infant. (Reproduced with permission. *Textbook of Pediatric Advanced Life Support*, 1988, 1990. Copyright American Heart Association.)

otomy with a 12- or 14-gauge angiocatheter may be necessary in cases of severe upper airway obstruction. The adapter from a 3.0 or 3.5 mm endotracheal tube is attached to the catheter, and manual ventilation is carried out with an Ambu bag. Another technique is to attach a Y-connector to the endotracheal tube adapter and connect a pressurized oxygen source (25 to 50 psi) to one limb of the Y. Ventilation is accomplished by periodic occlusion of the open port with the thumb. This should be considered only a temporizing measure and must be converted to a formal surgical airway because significant levels of carbon dioxide will build up within 30 to 40 minutes.

The proper size of the endotracheal tube for a pediatric patient can be rapidly estimated by measuring the width of the patient's little finger or by using the equation 16 + age (yr)/4 = internal diameter (mm) of the tube. Cuffed endotracheal tubes should rarely be used before 8 years of age because young children have an area of subglottic narrowing formed by the developing cricoid cartilage that creates the narrowest point in the pediatric airway.[19] A cuffed tube may produce subglottic edema, ulceration, and eventual stenosis. This differs from older children and adults, whose airway is narrowest at the level of the vocal cords.

Circulation. After confirmation of adequate ventilation and oxygenation, ensuring oxygen delivery to the tissues is the next priority in trauma resuscitation. Children may not show obvious signs of shock until they have lost approximately 25% of their blood volume. Not uncommonly, signs of shock develop when the heart rate increases and vasoconstriction occurs in an effort to maintain a normal blood pressure. Early signs of hypoperfusion include tachycardia, sluggish capillary refill, alteration of mental status, cool clammy skin, and poor urine output. The practitioner must be familiar with the normal vital signs for a child's age (Table 1–1) so that abnormalities can be recognized and rapidly corrected with aggressive fluid replacement. Peripheral access with large-bore intravenous catheters is the preferred management technique, but an alternative approach is intraosseous cannulation, which has proved effective for infusion of drugs and fluids with flow rates greater than 100 ml/hr. The proximal tibial plateau is the most often used site, but the distal femur, distal tibia, sternum, clavicle, and humerus may be used. An initial fluid bolus of an isotonic crystalloid solution, 20 ml/kg, should be administered immediately to any child with evidence of hypovolemia or shock. If no improvement is seen after the initial infusion, a second 20 ml/kg bolus should follow. If the child still fails to respond, significant internal bleeding is likely and an infusion of 10 ml/kg of packed red blood cells should be started.[20]

Cervical spine. Cervical spine injuries are less common in children than in adults. In children under 12 years of age, cervical spine injuries are mainly soft tissue injuries rather than true fractures because of the greater mobility and elasticity of the cervical spine and the supporting ligaments.[21] In a young child or infant the larger relative mass of the head and the lack of muscle strength in the neck create greater stress to the cervical spine during acceleration-deceleration injuries than occurs in adults. This difference explains why 60% to 70% of pediatric cervical spine fractures occur in the C1 or C2 region whereas only 16% of adult fractures are seen there.

Table 1–1. Normal Vital Signs

	Pulse	Blood Pressure	Respiration
Infant	160	80	40
Preschooler	140	90	30
Adolescent	120	100	20

From American College of Surgeons, Committee on Trauma: *Advanced trauma life support course,* Chicago, 1984, American College of Surgeons, p 293.

The diagnosis of injury to the spinal cord should not be based on radiologic data alone because in up to 67% of children with such an injury no radiologic abnormality is seen.[22] Clues to the diagnosis include transient paresthesia, numbness, or paralysis after an injury. When multiple trauma is present or the mechanism of an injury is known to produce cervical spine injury, the child should be assumed to have such as injury and should be adequately immobilized during transport. Immobilization must be maintained until cervical spine injury is ruled out. Children in car seats who are involved in motor vehicle accidents should remain in the car seat during transport to reduce the risk of cervical spine manipulation.

Thermoregulation. Infants lack a well-developed homeostatic thermoregulatory response and do not tolerate cold environments well. Because they have a larger body surface area relative to their weight, less insulating fat, and less muscle mass available for shivering and heat generation than adults, they are more susceptible to heat loss. Blankets, hats, radiant warmers, and warmed intravenous fluids should be used to help maintain a core temperature of 36° to 37°C.[23]

INJURY PATTERNS UNIQUE TO CHILDREN
Head Injuries

In pediatric trauma victims the most common cause of death is head injury. At least 80% of children dying with multiple trauma have significant head injuries, compared with 50% of adults. Several factors are responsible for this difference: children have a larger head/body ratio, a less myelinated and more easily injured brain, and thinner, more compliant cranial bones that afford less protection to the brain.[24] The compliance of the skull and the fact that the fontanelles and sutures remain open until an average age of 16 months allow an infant to better tolerate an increase in intracranial pressure and may delay the early warning signs of intracranial hypertension.

Thoracic Injuries

The patterns of thoracic injury in children are the result of specific differences in the chest wall and mediastinum between children and adults. The greater elasticity of the bony and cartilaginous chest wall structures makes fractures of the ribs and sternum and flail chest less common than in adults. This elasticity causes kinetic energy to be more readily transmitted to the underlying parenchyma. This is reflected in the higher incidence of pulmonary contusion than rib fractures and flail chest in children.[25] A child's ability to compensate for a serious thoracic injury is limited by (1) a larger oxygen consumption, which increases the susceptibility to hypoxia; (2) less pulmonary but more chest wall compliance, and (3) an increased dependence on diaphragmatic musculature for the majority of the work of breathing.[26] The complaint mediastinum found in children also decreases the tolerance to a pneumothorax. Wide deviations in mediastinal structures not only decrease venous return and cardiac output by angulating the vena cava but also impair pulmonary function by compressing the contralateral lung.

Abdominal Injuries

The majority of abdominal trauma in children occurs as the result of motor vehicle, pedestrian, and bicycle accidents. Solid organ injury predominates with an approximately equal division between liver and spleen injuries. Abdominal injuries are usually seen in patients with multiple injuries and nonoperative management is successful in the majority of cases of blunt trauma. The abdomen is at greater risk for injury in a child than in an adult for a number of reasons. The smaller size of the abdomen predisposes the child to multiple rather than single injuries as energy from the impacting force is dissipated. The large solid organs, which are most often injured, are covered with only a very flexible rib cage and a less developed abdominal musculature, which provide little protection.

Penetrating abdominal trauma in a child is managed similarly to that in an adult. Blunt trauma, however, is evaluated differently in children and in adults. The spleen is the most commonly injured organ. Both the spleen and the liver frequently stop bleeding without surgical intervention. Fear of postsplenectomy sepsis and the child's stronger splenic capsule, which holds suture material well, have made splenic repair the procedure of choice for children with splenic injuries who require surgery. Among stable patients, serial clinical examinations in a pediatric intensive care unit combined with CT scanning provides the most useful diagnostic approach when a patient is to be managed nonoperatively.

Extremity Injuries

Fractures are more common in children than adults and are more likely to result from seemingly minimal trauma. Pediatric cortical bone is highly porous and is easily disrupted. In contrast, the periosteum is more resilient, elastic, and vascular. These characteristics result in higher percentages of both incomplete and complete but nondisplaced, fractures, making a diagnosis based on conventional radiography less straightforward.[26] Other distinguishing features of pediatric skeletal trauma are (1) a rapid rate of healing and rare incidence of nonunion, (2) remodeling in the plane of the fracture, (3) a high incidence of ischemic vascular injuries, especially for fractures around the elbow, and (4) a low incidence of associated ligamentous injuries. Injuries near the growth plate may be complicated by significant long-term growth disturbances. The treatment of most closed pediatric fractures involves nonoperative management. Rehabilitation needs are generally minimal, and allowing the child to resume normal activity if home exercises to increase range of motion are performed is usually sufficient.

METABOLIC RESPONSE TO INJURY

Response to the stress of surgery and injury in adults is well documented and, in contrast to starvation, is characterized by increased metabolic rate and energy requirements to support the reparative process. The metabolic and endocrine responses include increases in plasma levels of cortisol, catecholamines, glucagon, prolactin, and growth hormone while insulin secretion in suppressed. These changes result in increasing protein breakdown, glycogenolysis, gluconeogenesis, and lipolysis. This response is not always beneficial and may increase morbidity and mortality rates in critically ill adult patients.

Much less is known of the metabolic responses to stress during infancy and childhood. Anand and associates[27] studied the stress responses to surgery in 33 term and preterm neonates. They found that newborn infants do mount a substantial endocrine and metabolic response to surgical stress. The main feature of the stress response was an increase in plasma levels of glucose and lactic acid mediated by an increase in catecholamine release. Insulin release was markedly reduced during the early postoperative period, probably because of direct inhibition by epinephrine. By 12 hours postoperatively, however, insulin levels were found to be significantly increased, restoring blood glucose to normal levels. Compared with term infants, preterm infants had significantly greater increases in serum lactate and significantly lower increases in insulin release. Surgical stress produces marked changes in lymphocyte numbers, subsets, and function in these children.[28] These catabolic responses were of a greater magnitude and shorter duration in children than in adults. In all groups evaluated the magnitude of the metabolic and endocrine response correlated with the severity of the surgical stress.[29] Although clearly a measurable stress response occurs in infants and older pediatric patients, further detailed studies are necessary to define specific regimens that will alter these responses and thus improve both postinjury and postoperative outcomes in critically ill children.

TRANSPORTATION OF THE INJURED CHILD

Survival of critically ill and seriously injured pediatric patients is more likely when they are treated in regional pediatric centers rather than in localized community hospitals.[30] Although large volumes of literature are available regarding the transport of neonates and adults, little research has been conducted on the transportation of older infants and children. Pediatric transport teams, a relatively new concept, have the responsibility of delivering skilled pediatric care at the referral hospital and providing safe transport to the receiving facility.[31]

Beyond the usual differences between adult and pediatric medicine, pediatric transport teams must respond quickly. Although most emergency centers can comfortably stabilize a seriously injured adult patient until transport can be arranged, many children are being initially evaluated in hospitals that, because of physician inexperience or inadequate equipment, offer nothing more than the most basic stabilization techniques for pediatric patients. These patients need to be transferred to an appropriate tertiary care center but may be considered too unstable for transport by a standard emergency medical services team.

Recently the American Academy of Pediatrics Committee on Hospital Care published its guidelines for air and ground transportation of pediatric patients,[32] and a national leadership conference on pediatric interhospital transport was held.[33] General recommendations were made for air and ground transport systems, including guidelines for transport team composition, education, and experience. Although consensus opinions had been put forward, McCloskey and Johnston[34] in a 1988 survey study found that there was no uniform provision of care for pediatric critical care transport. Only 60% of the major pediatric hospitals responding to the questionnaire had a pediatric critical care transport team. Of those, only 28% complied with the recommendation that the transport physician always be a PL-3 level resident or higher and only 17% of the transport teams could mobilize consistently in 15 minutes or less. The authors recommended (1) that each team carry out minimum number of transports in a given period to maintain expertise, (2) that team members be based in a critical care unit, (3) that in-house personnel be used, (4) that all methods of transport (helicopters, ambulances and fixed-wing aircraft) be available, and (5) that all transport vehicles be equipped as mobile critical care units to give the best possible care available to the patient.[34]

Studies have supported the use of physicians as members of air transport teams that serve adults.[35] Currently pediatric critical care transport teams are operating successfully with a variety of staffing systems (nurse-paramedic, nurse–respiratory therapist, physician-nurse). The question of the necessity to include a physician on the pediatric transport team has also been addressed. In a retrospective study of the interventions performed by physicians in 191 transfers by their pediatric critical care transport team, McClosky, King, and Byron[36] found that sending a physician as a member of the team may not always be necessary. In only 9% of their transports was a procedure performed that required a physician. In 66% no medications requiring a physician were used, and in almost half the cases the physician believed that his or her presence during the transport was not needed. A related study by McClosky and Johnson[37] attempted to predict the need for a physician during interhospital transports. Transport physicians were asked both before and after a transport to make a determination of their need. An accurate prediction occurred in 73% of the cases. In cases where the presumed need changed, 25% of the respondents indicated a decrease in their presumed need for a physician after completion of the transport. A significant increase over the prediction for the need of a physician occurred in only 2% of the cases. Thus it may be possible to select in advance situations in which a physician is not required as a member of the pediatric transport team, although constant communication with a physician experienced in pediatric critical care or emergency medicine is strongly recommended.

The method of transport depends on a number of decisions made at the scene of the injury. Ground transportation is by far the most commonly used mode of transport for trauma patients. During the Korean and Vietnam wars, aeromedical transport reached fairly sophisticated levels. Transportation of injured patients by helicopter or fixed-wing aircraft offers advantages in time, avoidance of driving through densely populated urban areas, and regionalization of specialized care. Disadvantages of air transport include the need for a designated landing area, the need for an additional patient transfer, limited range owing to fuel restrictions, noise and vibration that may interfere with patient monitoring, lack of pressurization techniques (in helicopter transport), and high maintenance costs.[32]

CARE IN THE EMERGENCY CENTER

More than 90% of pediatric emergency room visits are to general emergency departments where on the average 10 adult patients are treated for every child. This makes it unlikely that the staff can achieve significant expertise in pediatric trauma by emergency department experience alone. As previously emphasized, children are not miniature adults and their responses to trauma differ significantly from those in adults. Equipment, medications, and training need to be specifically focused on providing care to the injured child.

Equipment

Resuscitative equipment designed for children is essential in any emergency center dedicated to caring for pediatric trauma patients. Components for airway management, intravenous access, gastric and pleural decompression, spinal immobilization, urinary catheterization, and electrocardiographic monitoring sized appropriately for use in children are necessary. Blood pressure cuffs of appropriate size are needed to obtain accurate readings, and a Doppler ultrasound is useful in cases when a pressure cannot be adequately auscultated even with the appropriate size cuff. Radiant warmers are essential in the emergency room to prevent significant morbidity and mortality from hypothermia. A list of suggested equipment appears in Table 1–2.

Table 1–2. Suggested Equipment for Emergency Department

	Standard Supply	Minimum Quantity
Medication		
Albuterol sulfate 0.5%	20 ml bottle	1
Atropine sulfate	0.1 mg/ml in 10 ml prefilled syringe	2
Dextrose 25%	12.5 g in 10 ml prefilled syringe	2
Dextrose 50%	25 g in 50 ml prefilled syringe	2
Diazepam	5 mg/ml in 2 ml vial	1
Diphenhydramine HCl	50 mg/ml in 1 ml vial	1
Epinephrine 1 : 1,000	1 mg/ml in 1 ml ampule	2
Epinephrine 1 : 10,000	0.1 mg/ml in 10 ml prefilled syringe	3
Glucagon	1 mg in vials (mixing required)	1
Lidocaine HCl	10 mg/ml in 10 ml prefilled syringe	2
Metaproterenol sulfate 5%	10 ml or 30 ml bottle	1
Naloxone HCl	1 mg/ml in 2 ml ampule	2
Normal saline	500 or 1000 ml bag	3
Sodium bicarbonate 4.2%	1 mEq/ml in 10 ml prefilled syringe	2
Sodium bicarbonate 8.4%	1 mEq/ml in 50 ml prefilled syringe	1
Sodium chloride injection 0.9%	10 ml vial	4
Airway		
Laryngoscope handle	Penlite size	1
Miller blades	#0, #1, #2, #3	1 each
Macintosh blades	#2, #3	1 each
Stylets	6F and 14F	1 each
Oropharyngeal airways	00-5	1 each
Nasopharyngeal airways	5.5, 6.0, 7.0, 8.0	1 each
Endotracheal tubes (uncuffed)	2.5, 3.0, 3.5, 4.0, 4.5, 5.0, 5.5	2 each
Endotracheal tubes (cuffed)	6.0, 7.0, 8.0	2 each
Nasogastric tubes	5F, 8F, 10F, and 14F	1 each
Suction catheters	6F, 7F, 10F, 12F, and 14F	1 each
Magill forceps	Pediatric size	1
Magill forceps	Adult size	1
Oxygen supply tubing		1
High-concentration mask	Pediatric size	1
Nebulizer		1
Bag-valve-mask resuscitator	Child and infant size	1 each
Transparent ventilation masks	Premature, newborn, infant, child, and small adult sizes	1 each
Bulb syringe		1
Syringes		
1 cc		3
3 cc		3
5 cc		5
10 cc		5

Modified from Burg JM, O'Malley P, Vinci R, et al: *Medic IV emergency medical services project: paramedic treatment protocols for pediatric patients and suggested pediatric equipment and medications,* Burlington, Mass, 1990, Metropolitan Boston Hospital Council.

Table 1–2. Suggested Equipment for Emergency Department *Continued*

	Standard Supply	Minimum Quantity
Needles—Straight Metal		
23 gauge		5
21 gauge		5
19 gauge		5
Needles—Butterfly		
25 gauge		2
23 gauge		2
Intraosseous Needle		
Jamshidi/Kormed disposable bone marrow needle (sternal/iliac aspiration needle), 15 gauge		2
Intravenous Catheters		
24 gauge		2
22 gauge		2
20 gauge		2
18 gauge		2
16 gauge		2
14 gauge		2
Miscellaneous		
Pediatric defibrillator paddles		1 set
Child size sphygmomanometer		1
Baby No Neck, pediatric, short Stifneck extrication collars		1 each
		1
Stockinette cap		6
Pediatric monitoring electrodes		2
Minidrip administration set		2
Maxidrip administration set		2
Intravenous extension set		
Alcohol prep pads		
Band Aids		
Tape, 1 inch and ½ inch		
Arm boards		
Topical antiseptic ointment (single use)		
Isolation masks		
Venous constricting bands (Penrose drain, elastic band)		
Spare AA batteries		
Spare laryngoscope bulb		
22 gauge		
20 gauge		
18 gauge		
16 gauge		
14 gauge		

Medications

Successful resuscitation of pediatric trauma patients requires a knowledge of drug therapy with dosages adjusted to the estimation of the child's weight. Pediatric dosages of the drugs most commonly used during resuscitation are listed in Table 1–3.

Staff Training

A fundamental part of a successful pediatric trauma program is the education of team members. Prehospital emergency medical services providers, emergency room physicians, pediatricians, nurses, and surgeons involved in the care of trauma patients need specific training focused on the care of children. Such courses as the Advanced Trauma Life Support (ATLS) prepared by the American College of Surgeons, Pediatric Advanced Life Support (PALS) instituted by the American Academy of Pediatrics, and the Pediatric Emergency Medical Services Training Program (PEMSTP) developed in part by the Children's National Medical Center in Washington, D.C., were introduced to provide standardized treatment protocols and to establish a systematic approach to childhood trauma victims. The curriculum of these courses includes overviews of the physiologic and anatomic differences between children and adults, in-

Table 1–3. Pediatric Dosages of Common Drugs Used During Resuscitation

Drug	Dosage
Drugs for Tracheal Intubation	
Thiopental	4.0–6.0 mg/kg
Ketamine	0.5–2.0 mg/kg
Diazepam	0.5–1.0 mg/kg
Succinylcholine	1.0–3.5 mg/kg
Pancuronium	0.1–0.2 mg/kg
Cardiovascular Drugs	
Calcium chloride (10%)	10.0–20.0 mg/kg
Calcium gluconate (10%)	15.0–60.0 mg/kg
Epinephrine	1.0–10.0 mg/kg/min
Initial	0.1–2.0 mg/kg min
Maintenance	0.1–2.0 mg/kg min
Isoproterenol	1.0–20.0 mg/kg/min
Dopamine	0.5–1.0 mg/kg
Furosemide	1.0–4.0 mEq/kg
Sodium bicarbonate	Dependent on base deficit

Modified from Holbrook PR, Mickel J, Pollack MM, Fields AI: *Crit Care Med* 8:588, 1980.

cluding their responses to trauma; instruction on the primary trauma survey; management of specific injuries; and training in the special skills and management techniques necessary for treating childhood victims of trauma.[19]

FUTURE OF PEDIATRIC TRAUMA CARE

Even with the many recent advances in trauma care, trauma remains the leading cause of death among children over the age of 1 year in North America.[38] Because only 25% of trauma victims seen in large centers are children, it is not feasible, based on available resources, to treat seriously injured pediatric trauma victims in every major medical center across the country. The care of these patients will likely become based in large regionalized institutions that specialize in treating critically injured children. These centralized institutions will have beds available for the medically neediest patients. The more rural and isolated institutions will be called upon to see more patients initially and to provide stabilization for severely ill children before transport to the regional center. To lessen the burden on the referral hospitals, larger urban centers can treat injured children who do not require a specialized approach. Trauma registries will be used to document the magnitude of the injury problem in different regions, as well as to determine the best strategies for defining community needs, allocating resources, and measuring the effectiveness of the system.[2] These components, in combination with injury control research, community intervention programs, and public awareness regarding the significant health care costs and loss of human potential associated with pediatric trauma, are needed to control this major health care problem.

REFERENCES

1. Malek M, Chang B, Gallagher S, Guyer B: The cost of medical care for injuries to children, *Ann Emerg Med* 20:997–1005, 1991.
2. Division of Injury Control, Center for Environmental Health and Injury Control, Centers for Disease Control: Childhood injuries in the United States, *Am J Dis Child* 144:627–652, 1990.
3. Agram P, Castillo D, Winn D: The causes, impact and preventability of childhood injuries in the United States: childhood motor vehicle occupant injuries, *Am J Dis Child* 144:653–662, 1990.
4. Guyer B, Ellers B: The causes, impact and preventability of childhood injuries in the United States: the magnitude of childhood injuries—an overview, *Am J Dis Child* 144:649–652, 1990.
5. O'Carroll PW, Smith JC: Suicide and homicide. In Wallace HM, Ryan GM, Oglesby AC, eds: *Maternal and child health practices*, ed 3, Oakland, Calif, 1988, Third Party Publishing, pp 583–597.
6. Christoffell KK: The causes, impact and preventability of childhood injuries in the United States: childhood assaults in the United States, *Am J Dis Child* 144:697–706, 1990.

7. Hollinger PC: The causes, impact and preventability of childhood injuries in the United States, *Am J Dis Child* 144:670–676, 1990.
8. Wintemute GJ: The causes, impact and prevention of childhood injuries in the United States, *Am J Dis Child* 144:663–669, 1990.
9. Pearn J, Wong RYC, Brown J, et al: Drowning and near drowning in children: a five-year total population study from the city and county of Honolulu, *Am J Public Health* 69:450–454, 1979.
10. Spyker DA: Submersion injury, *Pediatr Clin North Am* 32:113–125, 1985.
11. Rivara FP: The causes, impact and prevention of childhood injuries in the United States: childhood pedestrian injuries in the United States, *Am J Dis Child* 144:692–696, 1990.
12. Rivara FP, Barber M: Demographic analysis of childhood pedestrian injuries, *Pediatrics* 76:375–381, 1985.
13. Brison R, Wickland K, Mueller B: Fatal pedestrian injuries to young children: a different pattern of injury, *Am J Public Health* 78:793–795, 1988.
14. McLoughlin E, Mcguire A: The causes, impact and preventability of childhood injuries in the United States: childhood burn injuries in the United States, *Am J Dis Child* 144:677–683, 1990.
15. Herndon D, Rutan R, Allison W, Cox C: Management of burn injuries. In Eichelberger M, ed: *Pediatric trauma: prevention, acute care, rehabilitation,* St Louis, 1993, Mosby, pp 568–590.
16. Kissoon N, Dreyer J, Walia M: Pediatric trauma: differences in pathophysiology, injury pattern and treatment compared with adult trauma, *Can Med Assoc J* 142(1):27–39, 1990.
17. Orlowski JP: Cardiopulmonary resuscitation in children, *Pediatr Clin North Am,* 27:495–512, 1980.
18. Rosenberg N: Pediatric cardiac arrest, *Emerg Clin North Am* 1:609–617, 1983.
19. Advanced Trauma Life Support Program: *American College of Surgeons instructions manual,* Chicago, 1989, Committee on Trauma, American College of Surgeons, p 231.
20. Schwartzberg SD, Bergman KS, Harris BH: A pediatric trauma model of continuous hemorrhage, *J Pediatric Surg* 23:605, 1988.
21. Henrys P, Lyne ED, Lufton C, et al: Clinical review of cervical spine injuries in children, *Clin Orthop* 129:172–177, 1977.
22. Pang D, Wilberger JE: Spinal cord injuries without radiographic abnormalities in children, *J Neurosurg* 57:114–129, 1982.
23. Oliver TK: Temperature regulation and heat production in the newborn, *Pediatr Clin North Am* 12:765–779, 1965.
24. Walker ML, Storrs BB, Mayer TA: Head injuries. In Mayer TA, ed: *Emergency management of pediatric trauma,* Philadelphia, 1985, WB Saunders, pp 272–286.
25. Eichelberger MR, Randolph JG: Thoracic trauma in children, *Surg Clin North Am* 61:1181–1197, 1981.
26. Rockwood CA, Wilkins, KE, King RE, eds: *Fractures in children,* ed 4, Philadelphia, 1991, JB Lippincott.
27. Anand KJS, Brown MJ, Causon RC, et al: Can the human neonate mount an endocrine and metabolic response to surgery? *J Pediatr Surg* 20:41–48, 1985.
28. Ward Platt MP, Lovat PE, Watson JG, et al: The effects of anesthesia and surgery on lymphocyte populations and function in infants and children, *J Pediatr Surg* 24:884–887, 1989.

29. Anand KJS, Aynsley-Green A: Measuring the severity of surgical stress in newborn infants, *J Pediatr Surg* 23:297–305, 1988.
30. Pollack MM, Alexander SR, Clarke N, et al: Comparison of tertiary and nontertiary intensive care: a statewide comparison (abstract), *Pediatr Res* 23:234A, 1988.
31. Dobrin RS, Black B, Gilman JI, Massaro TA: The development of a pediatric emergency transport system, *Pediatr Clin North Am* 27:633, 1980.
32. American Academy of Pediatrics, Committee on Hospital Care: Guidelines for air and ground transportation of pediatric patients, *Pediatrics* 78:943–950, 1986.
33. Day S, McCloskey K, Orr R, et al: Pediatric interhospital critical care transport: consensus of a national leadership conference, *Pediatrics* 88:696–704, 1991.
34. McCloskey K, Johnston C: Pediatric critical care transport survey: team composition and training, mobilization time, and mode of transportation, *Pediatric Emerg Care* 6:1–3, 1990.
35. Rhee KT, Burney RE, MacKenzie JR: Is the flight physician needed in helicopter emergency medical services? *J Trauma* 24:680, 1984.
36. McCloskey K, King W, Byron L: Pediatric critical care transport: is a physician always needed on the team? *Ann Emerg Med* 18:247–249, 1989.
37. McCloskey K, Johnston C: Critical care interhospital transports: predictability of the need for a pediatrician, *Pediatr Emerg Care* 6:89–92, 1990.
38. Greensher J: Recent advances in injury prevention, *Pediatr Rev* 10:171–177, 1988.

2

Decision Making in Pediatric Trauma

Thomas E. Scott

The unexamined life is not worth living.
Thoreau

Life is short,
Art is long,
The moment fleeting,
And judgement is hard . . .
Hippocrates

Rampant health care expenditures consumed 12% of the Gross National Product in the early 1990s and have possibly become the gravest threat to the United States' economic viability.[1] In December 1992, President-elect Bill Clinton asserted, before a distinguished panel of business leaders and economists, that the cost of health care "is going to bankrupt this country."[2]

The challenge to health care providers as caretakers of important public resources is to preserve the quality of health care while controlling its costs. Health care spending is determined largely by the myriad of diagnostic and therapeutic decisions implemented by providers seeking solutions to their patients' health-related problems. Making and executing decisions are the essence of clinical management. The clinical strategies pursued should be those that most efficiently and effectively solve the patient's health problem. Good clinical decision making involves critical use of the best information available to provide the highest quality of care under conditions of uncertainty, to the largest number of patients, at the least resource cost.

This chapter examines the clinical decision-making process and advocates structured, explicit, systematic problem-solving strategies. The important components of analytic decision making, with specific applications to trauma care, are explored in detail, especially those mechanisms that deal with uncertainty.

The techniques of clinical decision analysis espoused by Weinstein, Fineberg, and others[3-6] are particularly helpful. These techniques facilitate problem solving by drawing conclusions from conceptual models (decision trees) that forecast the likelihood of potential consequences (outcomes) and aggregate costs (dollars spent, work hours expended, pain and suffering) that might be incurred in the pursuit of various alternate strategies (treatment plans or other courses of action). In this sense, successful modeling is the essence of good decision making.

PROBLEM-SOLVING AND DECISION-MAKING MODES

Decision making in clinical medicine is directed at disposing of the root causes of, or at least mitigating the effects of, patients' physical, mental, or emotional impairment. The underlying causes of these problems must therefore be understood as completely as possible. The traditional basic tools of clinical problem solving are the patient's symptoms, physical findings, ancillary data, and the problem solver's fund of knowledge and experience.

How are the tools of problem solving used? The traditional method of clinical problem solving and decision making is intuitive/gestaltist. The venerable practice of obtaining a complete history from the patient to characterize the problems as accurately and precisely as possible and then performing a thorough physical examination, gleaning whatever physical evidence is readily available, is the starting point for hypothesis formulation. This is the stage of problem solving in which the clinician conjectures about the causes of the patient's problems. Hypotheses are tested and either verified or discarded until the root causes are deduced and the solution(s) suggested. Cognitive processes involved in this mode of problem solving are complex and poorly understood or characterized.

Some authors have suggested that the most effective problem solvers rapidly develop "rules of thumb" to narrow down potential causes (a heuristic approach to hypothesis refinement).[4] They quickly generate a brief list of accurate hypotheses and move insightfully to narrow the list. Learning, experience, and habit all greatly influence this process. Most medical disciplines depend on varying periods of apprenticeship with intense behavior modeling and proctoring to convey facility with these intuitive methods. Problem solving through heuristics is a process of trial and error aided at best by cumulative individual or group experience and is a process that has many potential sources of error. The reader is referred to the excellent treatment by Sox and associates[4] for specifics.

When the heuristic approach is used, the process connecting causes, effects, and solutions is usually obscured in hypothesis formulation and testing. The impact of uncertainty is poorly accounted for, the available information is frequently not used efficiently, and high-quality, reliable information is poorly discriminated from that which is potentially misleading. An alternative approach involves systematic analysis with creation of explicit constructs to specify all reasonable courses of action, and then forecasting of expected outcomes associated with each construct. This highly structured approach has been criticized as too time consuming and impractical for the daily press of clinical practice, but it offers these advantages:

- Explicit, unambiguous; focuses or refines problem definition
- Facilitates the quantitative management of uncertainty
- Deals with the quality and expected value of information
- Facilitates communication about available options between members of the health care team and the patients

CLINICAL DECISION ANALYSIS

Clinical decision analysis is a structured systems approach to making clinical decisions. A model, or conceptual-symbolic representation of reality, is created to allow forecasting of the results of alternative actions in sequence by iteration with systematic alteration of important variables about which the clinician is uncertain.

The stepwise process for clinical decision analysis is represented in Figure 2–1. The first and often most difficult step is framing the problem. This requires careful specification of the situation at hand: clinical states involved at different points of time, information currently known about the problem, information that can reasonably be obtained, and various alternative actions and their effects. The problem is then structured over time by creation of a decision tree. A decision tree is a conceptual, graphic or schematic model or a "map" of a decision problem in proper temporal sequence.

Use of Models

The generic form of a decision tree is shown in Figure 2–2. By convention, decision trees read from left to right and begin with specification of the initial or index circumstances. In the case of a clinical problem this might be the patient's symptoms when first examined. The initiation node is followed by a sequential array of specific alternative actions (preceded by a *choice* node, indicating that an array of controllable or volitional actions follow). Next come the potential effects of the choices (preceded by a *chance* node, indicating that an array of events follow that are nonvolitional and probabilistically determined). These in turn are followed by further possible actions and so forth until the termini of the various "paths" are reached and no further actions or chance events are reasonably possible. The resulting states are defined as "outcomes." Choice nodes are indicated in the schematic "tree" by a small box and chance nodes by a small circle. The alternative actions or choices and their subsequent effects (chances) are referred to as "branches." Branches emanating from a choice

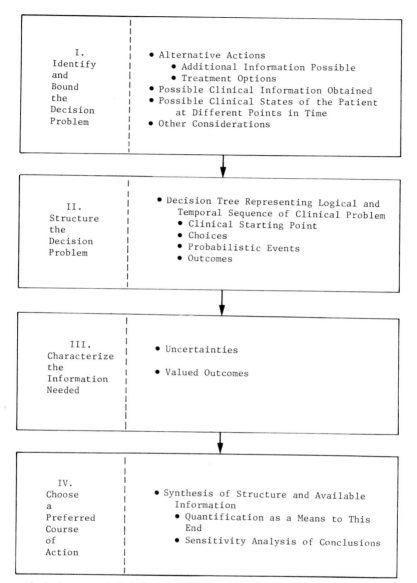

Figure 2–1. Process of clinical decision analysis. (From Weinstein MC, Fineberg NV (eds): *Clinical decision analysis,* Philadelphia, WB Saunders, 1980.)

node are always associated with a probability that specifies the likelihood of occurrence of the effect associated with the branch. A series of associated branches constitutes a "path."

After the decision tree is developed, the mathematics of probability is applied to the model to calculate the likelihood that the various health states at

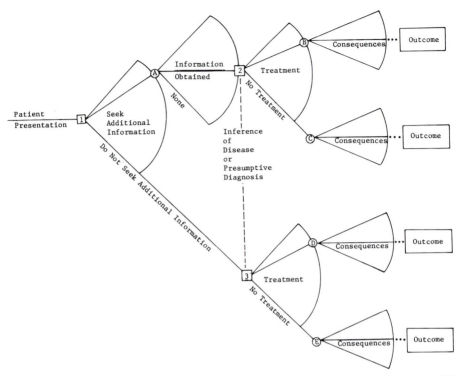

Figure 2–2. Generalized clinical decision tree. (From Weinstein MC, Fineberg HV (eds): *Clinical decision analysis,* Philadelphia, WB Saunders, 1980.)

the path termini (outcomes) will be achieved, relative valuations of these health states are made, and "expected values" of the various alternative courses of action are determined. These terms are defined more fully later in the chapter. A preferred course of action is then chosen in concert with the patient and parents, and a course of action pursued.

The method for clinical decision analysis may be illustrated by the situation facing the surgeon treating a 10-year-old boy who has fallen 10 feet from a tree branch to the ground, landing on his left side. The child, who was previously in good health, has remained conscious and now complains of pain in the left upper abdomen, along the left costal margin, and in the lower anterolateral chest. Abdominal examination shows moderate tenderness but no peritoneal irritation. Laboratory data are within normal limits, and chest x-ray examination shows no abnormalities. The problem might be structured as shown in Figure 2–3. The initial options might be to send the patient home, admit him for observation, perform exploratory laparotomy, or seek more information. Various consequences of each of these options would unfold until a final outcome

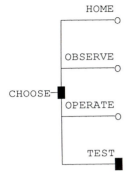

Figure 2–3. Possible alternative actions for clinical problem of patient who has fallen from tree.

is achieved, as exemplified in Figure 2–4 following the choice to pursue more information.

The surgeon might, for example, choose to obtain a computed tomography (CT) scan or perform peritoneal lavage. The CT scan could be either positive or negative. If the CT scan is positive, the surgeon might consider operative intervention. If the scan is negative or shows a contained subcapsular hematoma, continued observation would probably be the alternative chosen. If operation

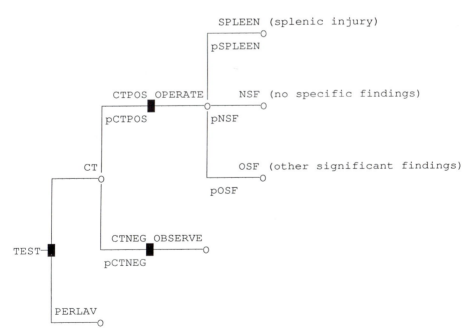

Figure 2–4. Possible consequences if seeking more information is the option selected.

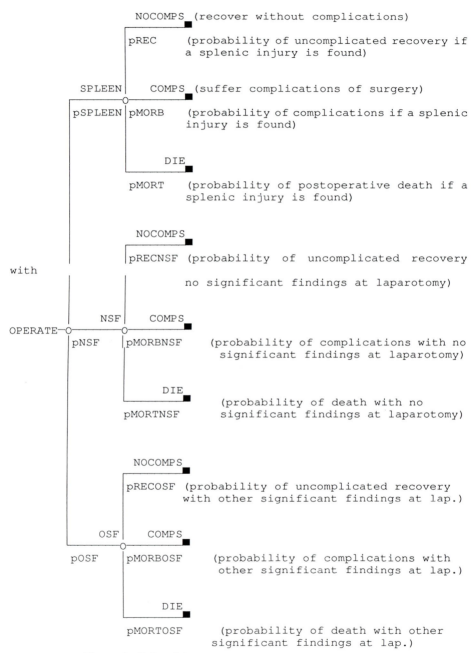

Figure 2–5. Possible consequences if surgeon decides to operate.

is pursued, the subsequent course might unfold as depicted in Figure 2–5. If peritoneal lavage is performed, events might follow as shown in Figure 2–6.

The decision tree could be structured in a number of ways depending on how the problem is "bound" in the first place and the focus of the analysis. The thinking process involved in binding the problem often reveals surprising details, options, or outcomes that would be missed in a less analytic approach. Such is the challenge as well as the reward of accurate and effective problem identification. The process outlined in Figure 2–1 is cyclic and reiterative, rather than linear, with many steps that occur simultaneously and feed into each other as the decision tree is refined. For example, the surgeon might be interested in handling the test result in other than a binary fashion. The decision tree might then be structured as in Figure 2–7. Such a structure would allow scrutiny of the decision to operate or continue to observe if results of the CT scan are equivocal.

Quantitative Management of Uncertainty

Uncertainty abounds in clinical medicine. Many factors contributing to the consequences of clinical actions are beyond the clinician's control. A patient's true condition usually is not directly observable but must be inferred on the basis of various cues such as physical findings and diagnostic tests. These cues seldom provide information that is completely accurate and reliable, and interpretation of the cues is often subjective ("operator dependent").

Reference to the decision trees in Figures 2–3 to 2–7 reveals many points where there is uncertainty. For example, how likely is the CT scan to be positive given the patient's signs and symptoms? How likely would be the finding of splenic injury if the CT scan were moderately abnormal? How likely would be the finding of ruptured spleen with a positive peritoneal lavage?

Such events are "probabilistic," involving an element of chance and plenty of room for confusion. An understanding of the laws of chance, the mathematics of probability, and the quantitative management of uncertainty is fundamental to clinical decision analysis. The probability of a future event is an expression of the likelihood that it will occur. A probability may be a statement of belief or an observation of the frequency of the event's occurrence in the past (empiric data obtained from organized trials or estimates from the literature), accompanied by the speculation that the event will occur as frequently in the future. The notation for the probability of an event (E) is p[E].

Probability is usually expressed by a number between 0 and 1. An event unlikely to occur has a probability closer to zero; a most likely event will have a probability closer to 1. Another way to express probability is by specifying the "odds," or the ratio between the times an event is expected to occur and

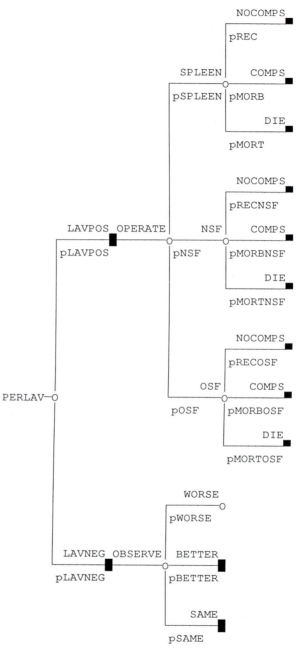

Figure 2–6. Possible consequences if peritoneal lavage is clinical option chosen.

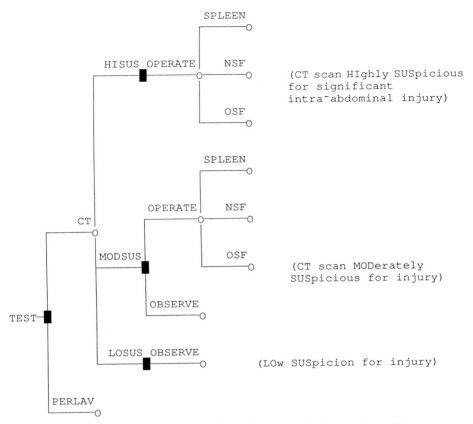

Figure 2–7. Alternatives if CT scan information is stratified rather than dichotomous.

the number of times it is not expected to occur in a finite number of trials. The odds are related to the probability of an event by the formula

(1) $$\text{Odds } [E] = p[E]/1 - p[E]$$

The sum of all possible variations or outcomes of a chance event must equal 1 (*something* is certain to happen!). Examples of an exhaustive list of outcomes of an event would be a "heads" or "tails" on the toss of a fair coin or a "positive" or "negative" result on some tests. These are binary events; the probability of an event and its complement must sum to 1. If the probability of a positive result (p) is .25, the probability of a negative must be .75 (1 − p). The general case is

(2) $$\sum_{n=1}^{\infty} p[E_n] = 1$$

where E_n represents the nth outcome of event E. All of the probabilities at a chance node must therefore equal 1 (a sanity check on tree design).

Some events, such as serial tosses of a fair coin, are independent, and events that precede or follow have no impact on their probability. Event A is said to be independent of some other event B if the probability of A occurring given that B has occurred is the probability of A alone:

$$(3) \qquad p[A \mid B] = p[A]$$

This is further denied notationally by showing that the probability of two events occurring jointly is equal to the product of their respective individual probabilities:

$$(4) \qquad p[A \text{ and } B] \ (p[A,B]) = p[A] \times p[B]$$

Other events are dependent, with probabilities that are determined in part by what has preceded (conditional probability). Prior odds or probabilities refer to the likelihood of an event occurring before some other event (or observation) occurs on which the eventuality under consideration depends. The likelihood of an event considering the antecedents is known as the posterior odds or probabilities. (These concepts are useful for understanding the value of diagnostic information in refining estimates of the likelihood of clinical events and guiding decision making. Briefly, in the absence of perfect knowledge, tests of great value are associated with a large increase in certainty with minimal cost to the patient or system.)

The relationship between joint and conditional probability for dependent events is specified by the formula

$$(5) \qquad p[A,B] = p[A \mid B] \times p[B]$$

This states that the probability of events A and B both occurring equals the product of the probability of A occurring given that B has occurred and the probability of B alone occurring. The summation principle for joint probabilities is crucial to clinical decision analysis and states that the probability of any event E is the sum of the joint probabilities of E and all possible related events

$$(6) \qquad p[E] = p[E,F_0] + p[E,F_1] + \ldots p[E,F_n] = \Sigma \, p[E,F_n]$$

providing that events F_0, $F_1 \ldots F_n$ are independent (mutually exclusive) of one another. Applying the relationship between joint and conditional probability for dependent events, the decision maker obtains

$$(7) \quad p[E] = (p[E|F_0] \times p[F_0]) + \ldots (p[E|F_n] \times p[F_n]) = \Sigma \, p[E|F_n] \times p[F_n]$$

For example, by reference to the tree in Figure 2–4,

$$p[CT^+] = p[CT^+, SPLEEN] + p[CT^+, OSF] + p[CT^+, NSF]$$

This means that, if the CT scan is positive, the patient *must* subsequently have a ruptured spleen, some other significant finding (OSF), or no significant finding (NSF). Any other conceivable outcome subsequent to the CT scan that the model does not account for would invalidate the summation principle of joint probabilities and possibly lead to faulty conclusions from the analysis.

The path probability of a consecutive series of events is the product of probabilities in the sequence and arises from the relationship between the joint probabilities for independent events (Eq. 4) and joint and conditional probabilities for dependent events (Eq. 5).

Outcomes

The health state achieved at the terminus of a given path is referred to as an outcome. An outcome may have a single or multiple attributes of interest to the patient and other decision makers, such as life expectancy; different kinds of morbidity, including pain and suffering; and economic characteristics, such as workdays lost. Some relative value (utility) must be placed on these attributes to allow the decision makers to choose strategies that provide the highest possibility of achieving desired states and avoiding less desired outcomes.

Some attributes such as mortality rates have inherently scaled discrete numerical utilities; nominal scales may be related to a simple linear numerical scale. Generally, the least desired outcome (such as death) is placed at one extreme and valued at 0 and the most desired outcome (recovery without complication) is valued at 1. Intermediate states are then arranged on the scale. Various mathematical mechanisms, such as the standard reference gamble, exist to aid in the relative scaling and the elicitation of preferences. The reader is referred to standard texts[3,4] for a full discussion of these concepts.

The utilities of health states with multiple attributes are handled expediently by definition of a composite index such as the Health Status Index, the Sickness Impact Profile, the Injury Severity Score, and APACHE II (see Chapter 3).[7-10] Another method of summarizing multiple attributes of a health state is to express years of life in the state of concern as quality-adjusted life years (QALY).[3] Quality adjustment acknowledges that a period of time spent on dialysis, for example, does not have the same quality as that time spent in enjoyment of perfect health. Assigning monetary values to health states also may be useful. A substantial body of literature exists concerning life and limb valuations.[11-14] Utilities should be assigned according to the preferences of the individuals most affected by the decision, usually the patient or, in the case of a child, the patient's parents or guardians acting as proxy.

In the case of the decision facing the parents of the boy who is operated on after a fall from a tree, relative values would have to be attached to recovery without complications, recovery with complications, and death. A simple utility scale could be used:

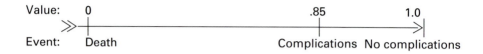

The tree then appears as shown in Figure 2–8.

It is possible to assign utilities in terms of dollar costs aggregated along the path (Fig. 2–9). The dollar cost of death is often approximated by the worth of the patient's lost net productivity, which is the difference between projected lifetime economic production and lifetime consumption. This approach has a geriatric and gender bias favoring young male children. Econometric measurements of health status, and decisions based on analysis involving econometric measurements, are more valid for groups of individuals than for specific individuals.

At any rate, in clinical decision analysis the definition of quality in health care requires strategies that result in the highest probability of achieving favored outcomes, measured in terms of utilities, and that minimize the probability of disfavored outcomes, measured in terms of disutilities.

Expected Value Decision Making

One strength of decision analysis is that the method allows choices to be based on explicitly approximated expected values of alternatives. The expected value of an alternative is the sum of the products of the path probabilities of chance events that follow that choice, and the utilities of the health states achieved at the path termini. This represents a "weighted average" of the possible values of the strategy or choice and is represented by the formula

(8) $$EV(x) = \sum_{n=1}^{\infty} p[O_n] \times \mu_n$$

where $EV(x)$ is the expected value of option x, $p[O_n]$ is the path probability for the nth outcome, and μ_n is the utility of the nth outcome.

As noted previously, path probability is the product of probabilities in a sequence of chance events. A 30% chance of a 30% chance of achieving some state is a net 9% chance ($.30 \times .30 = .09$). If the probability of finding a splenic injury (p[SPLEEN]) by pursuing the OPERATE strategy as modeled in Figure 2–5 is .25 and the probability of subsequent recovery without complication (p[NOCOMPS|SPLEEN]) is .85, the path probability is $.25 \times .85 = .2125$. This means that 21 patients of every 100 who are operated

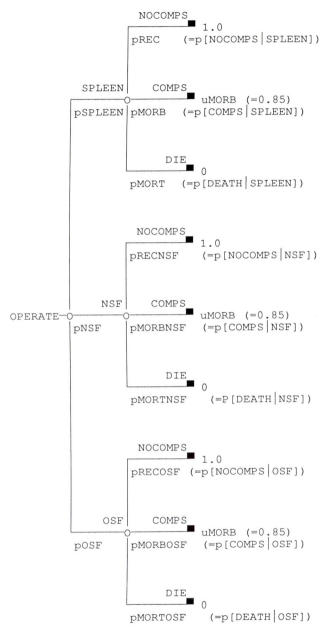

Figure 2–8. Decision tree with morbidity and mortality utilities assigned to outcomes following the decision to operate.

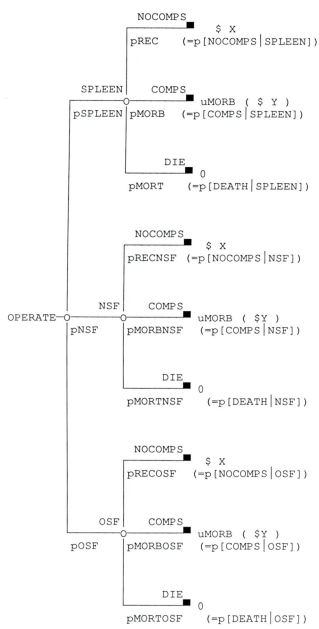

Figure 2–9. Decision tree with resource cost utilities assigned to outcome states following the decision to operate.

on initially would be expected to have a splenic injury repaired and to recover without complication (if the probabilities are accurate). The path probability is also the weight to apply to the utility of the state NOCOMPS in calculating the net long run probable value of the strategy OPERATE.

Another strength of clinical decision analysis is that it can be used to examine the impact of systematically altering assumptions in the model (probabilities, utilities, tree construction) on the expected values of the various choices or strategies. This is known as sensitivity analysis. Such analysis may reveal a threshold for some variable at which point the best choice changes. Identifying decision thresholds of key variables is a useful way to summarize the findings of an analysis.

ANALYZING THE VALUE OF INFORMATION
Test Characteristics

The a priori probability of a state ($p[S]$) frequently is known or can be determined epidemiologically as the prevalence of the state in a population. A state may be a disease process, a neuropsychiatric condition, or any physical state. The probability of a test being positive in persons with a disease can be determined by performing the test on a defined population of those known to have the disease according to some accepted "gold standard." The posterior (posttest) probability of the state ($p[S^+|T^+]$) is the more critical variable in clinical decision analysis and can be estimated by the application of Bayes' theorem and the sensitivity and specificity of the test. The relationships among probability statements, sensitivity, specificity, and other test results are shown in Table 2–1.

Table 2–1. The Relationships Among Sensitivity, Specificity and Probability Statements

Probability Statement	Test Result
$p[T^+|S^+]$ (probability of test positive given the state present)	True positive rate (TPR) = TP/(TP + FN), sensitivity
$p[T^-|S^+]$ (probability of test negative given the state present)	False negative rate (FNR) = FN/(TP + FN)
$p[T^+|S^-]$ (probability of test positive given the state absent)	False positive rate (FPR) = FP/(TN + FP)
$p[T^-|S^-]$ (probability of test negative given the state absent)	True negative rate (TNR) = TN/(TN + FP), specificity
$p[S^+]$ (probability of state present)	TP + FN/(TP + FP + TN + FN)
$p[S^-]$ (probability of state absent)	TP + FP/(TP + FP + TN + FN)

TP, number of true positives; *FP,* false positives; *TN,* true negatives; *FN,* false negatives.

Bayes' theorem allows calculation of $p[S^+|T^+]$ as

(10)
$$p[T^+|S^+] = \frac{p[T^+|S^+] \times p[S^-]}{p[S^+] + p[T^+|S^-]} \times p[S^-]$$

Probability Revision

Expected value decision making in assessing the usefulness of diagnostic information amounts to analysis of the expected value of the decision to "seek additional information" in the generic case (see Fig. 2–2). The objective of expected value analysis is to refine the assessment of the probabilities of downstream events. The efficiency and accuracy of probability revision are important measures of the value of additional information. Comparing the expected values of alternatives with and without the additional information is one way to assess the value of additional information. The likely impact of the information, its probable effect on subsequent choices, is another important feature.

The ratio between the probability of disease given a positive test result and the a priori probability of disease (prevalence in the population of which the patient is a member)

(11)
$$p[D|T^+] \div p[D]$$

is another index of the power of a test in revising probability. The power of a test depends on test sensitivity and specificity and on the prior probability of the state in the population.

Test results are often not simply positive or negative but have frequency distributions for patients with or without the state of concern on a numerically discrete continuous scale described by a central tendency (or mean) and spread (standard deviation). The task facing the decision maker is to choose a reasonable cut-off point separating the distributions that define "positive" from "negative." Difficulty arises when the distributions of test values for patients with and without the state of concern are close or overlap, which unfortunately is the usual circumstance. An excellent discussion of these considerations can be found in Weinstein and Fineberg's text.[4]

ANALYZING THE VALUE OF CHOICES
Risk-Benefit Analysis

Risk-benefit analysis defines strategies that minimize morbidity and mortality apart from resource cost considerations and generally deal with trade-offs between different morbidities or between morbidity and mortality. From these analyses the decision maker recommends choices that maximize the probability of spending the longest time in the highest quality health state.

Cost-Effectiveness Analysis and Cost-Benefit Analysis

An expansion of the definition of quality given previously requires weighing health benefits against resource costs. This is the province of cost-effectiveness analysis (CEA) and cost-benefit analysis (CBA).[5,15,16] The decision analysis methods described previously yield an estimate of the likelihood of achieving various health states as a consequence of choices pursuing various diagnostic or therapeutic strategies. These outcomes are all valued in some fashion (i.e., preferences are elicited to define utilities and disutilities). The resource costs of these various diagnostic and treatment decisions are aggregated and compared to outcomes.

In CEA, ratios between costs and health benefits are determined (Eq. 12); therefore benefits need not be valued in the same way as resource costs. Health benefits might include increased longevity, risks (morbidity or mortality) avoided, lives spared, or gains in any number of components of health status. Resource costs are generally dollar denominated either directly or by conversion. Typically, CEA results are expressed as dollars per quality-adjusted life year (QALY) gained, dollars per survival month or year, or dollars per marginal or extra case found (a common way to express the value of diagnostic tests).

(12) Cost-effectiveness Ratio = Cost (\$) ÷ Marginal Utility Gain

Benefits as well as costs must be expressed in economic terms in CBA:

(13) $\Delta C = BEN\$ - RES\$$

where BEN\$ is the economic value of all health benefit(s) and RES\$ is the aggregate value of all resources consumed to provide health benefit(s). Any strategy that results in a net excess of the economic value of benefits over resource costs is potentially worth pursuing. Choices are made on the basis of the magnitude of excess benefits.

Applications

The relative value of CT scan versus diagnostic peritoneal lavage may be estimated by calculating the expected values of the options CT and PERLAV in Figures 2–4 and 2–6 with the baseline assumptions in Table 2–2. Utilities are assigned according to the following scale:

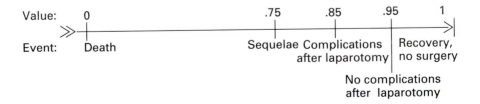

Table 2–2. Baseline Assumptions for Analysis of "Test"

Variable	Assumption
pBETTER	.85
pSAME	.05
pWORSE	.10
pMORB	.10
pMORT	.05
pMORBNSF	.02
pMORTNSF	.005
pMORBOSF	.15
pMORTOSF	.05
pSPLEEN	.10
pOSF	$.33 \times$ pSPLEEN
pNSF	$1 - (\text{pOSF} + \text{pSPLEEN})$
sensCT	.95
sensPL	.98

The values of pSPLEEN and therefore of pOSF and pNSF were allowed to vary over a reasonable range during multiple iterations of a risk-benefit analysis. Calculations were performed with a computer program for decision analysis called SMLTREE, a proprietary product developed by Jim Hollenberg. Expected values in this analysis represent the average long-run probability of reaching a health state as favored as "recovery without laparotomy and without complication" (found at the terminus of the option HOME) as a consequence of how the utilities were defined. No thresholds were detected for sensCT and sensPL, and therefore no sensitivity analyses were performed for these variables. Figure 2–10 shows the results of sensitivity analysis on the variable pSPLEEN. The expected values of the options CT and peritoneal lavage (PERLAV) are graphed against the value of pSPLEEN. There are very slight differences between these TEST options favoring CT except at relatively high values for the probability of a splenic (or other significant) injury. The threshold for pSPLEEN that favors peritoneal lavage is .441.

The least resource-costly strategy should be pursued because the differences in risk-benefit between CT and peritoneal lavage are small in this analysis. The aggregate cost per patient or per theoretical cohort could be estimated and compared per probability unit (per thousand) difference in the expected value of CT or peritoneal lavage.

The most compelling applications of clinical decision analysis will arise because this technique is a powerful instrument for critical path analysis, which is central to the new drive toward continuous quality improvement in health care.[17] With urging from the federal government, many health care organizations

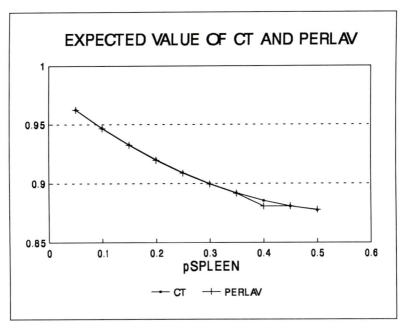

Figure 2–10. Results of clinical decision analysis for the variable pSPLEEN.

are adopting highly prescriptive clinical practice guidelines as a method of controlling health care delivery costs. Clinical decision analysis provides a rigorous and explicit approach to the development and promulgation of practice guidelines. High-quality decision models will be flexible and readily allow the incorporation of new strategies or the refinement of data. Decision analysis could reveal areas for focusing research efforts to refine the knowledge base and settle issues that will truly determine the best choices in health care.

REFERENCES

1. Peebles RJ, Schneidman DS, eds: *Socio-economic factbook for surgery, 1991–92,* Chicago, 1992, American College of Surgeons.
2. *USA Today,* Dec 16, 1992.
3. Weinstein MC, Fineberg HV, eds: *Clinical decision analysis,* Philadelphia, 1980, WB Saunders.
4. Sox HC, Blatt MA, Higgins MC, Marton KI: *Medical decision making,* Boston, 1988, Butterworths.
5. Eddy DM: Medicine, money, and mathematics, *ACS Bull* 77(6):36–49, 1992.
6. Weinstein MC, Stason WB: Foundations of cost-effectiveness analysis for health and medical practices, *N Engl J Med* 296(13):716–721, 1977.
7. Boyle MH, Torrance GW: Developing multiattribute health indices, *Med Care* 22(11):1045–1057, 1984.

8. Pliskin JS, Shepard DS, Weinstein MC: Utility functions for life years and health status, *Op Res* 28(1):206–224, 1980.
9. Torrance GW, Boyle MH, Horwood SP: Application of multi-attribute utility theory to measure social preferences for health states, *Op Res* 30(6):1043–1069, 1982.
10. Bergner M, Bobbitt RA, Carter WB, Gilson BS: The sickness impact profile: development and final revision of a health status measurement, *Med Care* 19(8):787–806, 1981.
11. Graham JD, Vaupel JW: Value of a life: what difference does it make? *Risk Analysis* 1(1):89–95, 1981.
12. Viscusi WK: Labor market valuations of life and limb: empirical evidence and policy implications, *Public Policy* 26(3):359–386, 1978.
13. Mishan EJ: Evaluation of life and limb: a theoretical approach, *J Pol Ec* 79:687–705, 1971.
14. Acton JP: *Measuring the value of lifesaving programs,* pub no P-5675, Santa Monica, Calif, 1976, Rand Corp.
15. Weinstein MC, Stason WB: Foundations of cost-effectiveness analysis for health and medical practices, *N Engl J Med* 296(13):716–721, 1977.
16. Shepard DS, Thompson MS: First principles of cost-effectiveness analysis in health, *Pub Health Rep* 94(6):535–543, 1979.
17. Ballinger WF, Hepner JO: Total quality management and continuous quality improvement: an introduction for surgeons, *Surgery* 113(3):250–254, 1993.

CHAPTER

3

Child Abuse

Kent P. Hymel

If the medical provider manages pediatric trauma, he or she cares for victims of child abuse. For clinicians helping such injured children the challenge is to recognize even the subtle presentations of inflicted trauma.[1-4] Early intervention in the cycle of family violence may be lifesaving.

The diverse spectrum of child abuse is divided into four broad categories: physical abuse, sexual abuse, neglect, and psychologic abuse. The focus of this chapter is the recognition and management of the acute, traumatic injuries of physical and sexual abuse. First, however, the scope and variety of child abuse are briefly summarized.

EPIDEMIC OF CHILD ABUSE
Child Abuse Fatalities

According to estimates in the Annual Fifty State Survey,[5] more than 2.9 million reports of child abuse were received in the United States during 1992. More than 1.1 million (40%) of the case reports were eventually substantiated, including 1261 deaths from child abuse or neglect. In 1992 more than three children died from child maltreatment each day in the United States. Of these deaths, 87% occurred in children less than 5 years of age and an alarming 46% were in children less than 1 year of age. With the emergence of child death review teams[6] and the development of standards for investigating child deaths,[7] it is likely that a much higher number of child fatalities from abuse will be recognized.

Patterns

The 1992 Annual Fifty State Survey[5] revealed the following case percentages among substantiated cases of child abuse: physical abuse 24%, sexual abuse 19%, neglect 43%, and psychologic abuse 10%.

41

Prevalence

Reports of child abuse have increased an average of 6% a year over the past 7 years. In 1992, 45 of every 1000 children were reported to be victims of child abuse. Less than 1% of cases involved foster or day care settings. Economic stress, parental substance abuse, and greater public awareness were the principal factors contributing to the increase in reports of child maltreatment in 1992.[5]

ETIOLOGIES[8]
Sociocultural Values

Societal acceptance of corporal punishment, glorification of violence in the media, unwillingness of family or neighbors to intervene, and devaluation of children may all contribute to parents' use of physical force to discipline their children.

Parental Factors

More specific parental factors believed to increase the likelihood of abuse include personal acceptance of corporal punishment for disciplining children, history of being abused as a child, low self-esteem, ignorance of childrearing and child development, unwillingness to seek outside help, unrealistic expectations regarding child behavior, depression, substance abuse, marital discord and violence, being a single or working parent, and the stresses of poverty and unemployment.

Child Factors

Any child the parent perceives to be physically, mentally, behaviorally, or temperamentally different in some manner is at increased risk for abuse.

Triggering Event

When the preceding risk factors are present, an episode of child abuse usually occurs as an out-of-control response to a simple triggering event, such as incessant crying, school difficulty, a toileting mishap, or any other new family stress.

NEGLECT
Definition

The National Center on Child Abuse and Neglect (NCCAN) defines neglect as "acts of omission: specifically, the failure of a parent or other person legally responsible for a child's welfare to provide for the child's basic needs and proper level of care with respect to food, clothing, shelter, hygiene, medical attention, or supervision."

Scope

Examples of child neglect include nutritional failure-to-thrive (Fig. 3–1), failure to seek medical treatment, and inadequate supervision or safety measures. In situations of poverty, unemployment, single working parent, cognitively deficient parents, or lack of adequate affordable day care, a clear determination of child neglect may be difficult. Helfer[9] has eloquently described the "muddy waters" of the child neglect diagnostic arena.

Impact

Neglect represents the largest single category of substantiated child abuse in the United States.[5] Physical neglect appears to be related to low income.[10] Hospitalization is indicated for failure-to-thrive when the infant's or child's

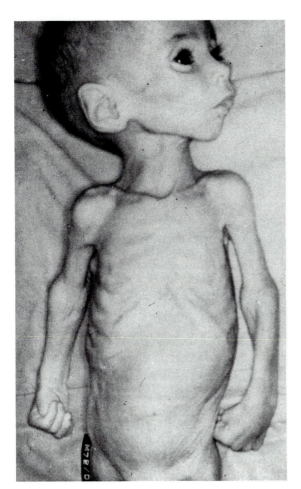

Figure 3–1. Failure-to-thrive. Infant with severe nutritional neglect. Weight less than 70% of predicted weight-for-height is indication for intensive inpatient nutritional intervention. (Courtesy Dr. Carole Jenny.)

weight is less than 70% of the predicted weight for height. Long-term consequences of nutritional neglect may include immune suppression and developmental delays.[11] More than one third of deaths from child maltreatment in 1992 in the United States were due to child neglect.[5] Pediatric clinicians should remember the potential deadly outcome of child neglect, even in the absence of physical abuse or trauma.

PSYCHOLOGIC ABUSE
Definition

The NCCAN defines psychologic abuse as "child abuse which results in impaired psychological growth and development. [It] frequently occurs as verbal abuse or excessive demands on a child's performance and results in a negative self-image on the part of the child and disturbed child behavior."

Scope and Impact

Psychologic abuse of children usually accompanies the other forms of abuse. Therefore psychologic abuse is probably the most prevalent form of child abuse. Persistent verbal aggression that parents direct toward their children has been associated with higher rates of physical aggression, delinquency, and interpersonal problems.[12]

UNUSUAL MANIFESTATIONS OF CHILD ABUSE
Munchausen Syndrome by Proxy

Munchausen syndrome by proxy is a bizarre form of child abuse in which parents fabricate or create illness in their child. Unlike persons with hypochondriasis, disturbed parents actively cause childhood illness in an effort to seek secondary gain or attention. The most common reported examples of induced illness in children include bleeding, seizures, central nervous system depression, diarrhea, vomiting, fever, and rash.

Children with Munchausen syndrome by proxy present a difficult diagnostic dilemma until the cause is suspected. Children so victimized often undergo multiple diagnostic procedures and suffer long-term medical and psychologic consequences. The reported mortality is as high as 9%.[13] In an unusual recent variation at our institution, unexplained gastrointestinal bleeding in an infant was eventually determined to be induced by the parental addition of ground glass to the powdered formula.

Microwave Oven Burns

Burns inflicted in a microwave oven demonstrate a characteristic histologic pattern on biopsy (Fig. 3–2), in which tissue levels of higher water content (muscle) heat to a greater degree than tissues of lower water content (fat).

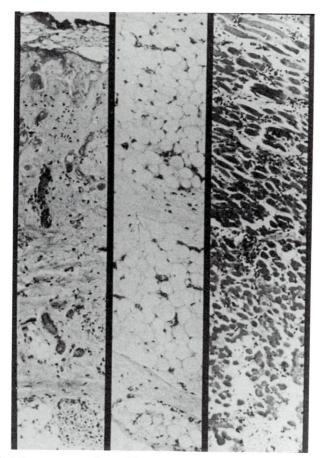

Figure 3–2. Microwave oven burn. Photomicrograph of debrided skin of right foot, 5 days after burn. *Left,* There is full-thickness coagulation necrosis of epidermis and dermis; *center,* subcutaneous fat is spared; *right,* skeletal muscle shows coagulation necrosis with infiltration by polymorphonuclear cells. (Hematoxylin and eosin; original magnification x100.) (From Alexander RC et al: *Pediatrics* 79:255–260, 1987. Reproduced with permission of *Pediatrics.*)

Children with a microwave oven burn may therefore have sharply demarcated burn areas with relative sparing of specific deeper tissue layers.[14]

Other Unusual Examples of Child Abuse

Unusual medical presentations of child abuse include illicit drug ingestions,[15] hypernatremic dehydration from water restriction[16] or salt intoxication,[17] and fatal asphyxia from forced aspiration of pepper poured down the child's throat as punishment.[18] Examples of unusual inflicted traumatic injury are hypovolemic shock from massive subcutaneous bleeding following paddling,[19] cutaneous "stun gun" injuries,[20] and small bowel evisceration.[21] Child abuse should be suspected when children present with highly unusual medical illness or traumatic injury.[22]

CHALLENGE OF RECOGNIZING CHILD ABUSE

Family dysfunction and stress cause child abuse and neglect. To stop abuse, medical professionals need to intervene in the private lives of families, one family at a time. This requires courage.

However, the initial challenge for medical personnel treating pediatric trauma patients is simply to recognize child abuse. Only by first recognizing child abuse can health care practitioners prevent recurrences through a multidisciplinary family intervention approach. To this end, the remaining sections of the chapter focus on the recognition and management of child abuse masquerading as accidental pediatric trauma.

CHILD SEXUAL ABUSE
Definition

The NCCAN defines child sexual abuse as "contact or interaction between a child and an adult, when the child is being used for the sexual stimulation of that adult or another person. Sexual abuse may also be committed by another minor, when that person is either significantly older than the victim, or when the abuser is in a position of power or control over that child."

Prevalence

In a recent anonymous national telephone survey, 27% of female and 16% of male adult respondents disclosed that they were sexually victimized during childhood.[23] Although disclosure of child sexual abuse is increasing, careful analysis of prevalence surveys suggests that the actual prevalence of child sexual abuse has remained generally constant over the past 40 years.[24]

Scope

Child sexual abuse may occur in a variety of circumstances. The perpetrator often is a trusted family acquaintance or a family member or infrequently is a stranger. The abusive act may involve inappropriate looking, fondling, or penetration of the oral, vaginal, or rectal orifices. It may occur as an isolated single event or as an ongoing sexual relationship. It may evolve from the coercion or seduction of a single child or may involve many victims in a group setting such as a day care center. The perpetrator may be an impulsive adolescent or a pedophile desiring a silent, long-term, sexually gratifying partnership. Promotion of child prostitution and child pornography also falls into the realm of sexual abuse of children. The causes, dynamics, and outcomes for each of these manifestations of child sexual abuse vary, necessitating individualized interventions.

Impact

Sexual abuse has been more correctly described as sexual misuse of a relationship.[25] The majority of perpetrators of child sexual abuse are trusted authority figures known to the victim.[23] Sexual victimization is initially seductive and later coercive to maintain the child's cooperation.[26,27] The long-term psychologic trauma from child sexual abuse can be devastating and may include sexual dysfunction, anxiety, mental disorders, depression, and self-destructive behaviors.[28–31]

Timing of Medical Examination

Most sexually abusive acts against children do not result in severe genital injury. Abnormalities on genital examination are usually absent, even in legally proven cases of child sexual abuse.[32] Disclosure of child sexual abuse may be delayed for weeks, months, or even years. For all of these reasons the medical evaluation of nonacute child sexual abuse can usually be delayed until the appropriate time, setting, and expertise are available. Interested readers are directed to several excellent reviews on the medical evaluation of suspected child sexual abuse.[25,33–40]

Acute Rape Examination

Indication. According to an American Academy of Pediatrics (1990) policy statement, "When the alleged sexual abuse has occurred *within 72 hours,* and the child provides a history of sexual abuse including ejaculation, the exam should be performed immediately."[41]

Protocol. Most hospitals use a rape kit for the examination, which provides simple, easy-to-follow instructions for the examining physician. Proper labeling of specimens and careful maintenance of the chain of evidence are crucial. The general components of a medical examination for acute sexual assault are outlined in Table 3–1. For detailed discussion the reader is referred to references by Enos[42] and Heger.[35]

An experienced clinician should examine the patient in a caring, supportive manner. The victim's clothing should be removed over a sheet. Both clothing and sheet should thereafter be submitted in a brown paper bag. Loose material or pubic hair should be submitted in provided envelopes, as should specimens of the patient's head and pubic hair.

Wood's lamp examination for the presence of semen allows collection of semen onto moistened cotton swabs, which should thereafter be air dried and

Table 3–1. Acute Child Sexual Assault Medical Examination

1. Ensure thorough and accurate documentation and proper "chain of custody" of medical evidence.
2. Remove clothing over sheet. Submit both in paper bag.
3. Submit loose material and pubic hair in provided envelopes.
4. Submit specimen of patient's head hair and pubic hair in provided envelopes.
5. Perform Wood's lamp examination for dried semen.
6. Collect semen onto moistened cotton swabs, air dry, and submit in provided envelope.
7. Obtain vaginal, oral, and rectal aspirates and washings for microscopic slide examination for spermatozoa.
8. Obtain throat, rectal, and vaginal cultures for *Neisseria gonorrhoeae* and *Chlamydia trachomatis*.
9. Obtain other cultures for sexually transmitted diseases if appropriate by Hx/PE.
10. Examine Gram's stain of vaginal smear for clue cells.
11. Examine wet mount of vaginal smear for trichomonads.
12. Examine potassium hydroxide preparation of vaginal smear for *Candida*.
13. Consider pregnancy test if postmenarcheal.
14. Consider postcoital pregnancy prophylaxis.
15. Consider antibiotic prophylaxis for sexually transmitted diseases.
16. Consider testing for human immunodeficiency virus and rapid plasma reagin.
17. Refer to proper social service, legal, and investigative authorities on child protection team.
18. Accomplish colposcopic examination and photography of external genitalia and rectum.
19. Consider examination under anesthesia in consultation with gynecologist if vaginal bleeding present.

placed in the provided envelopes. Vaginal, oral, and rectal aspirates or washings should be collected for microscopic slide examination for the presence of spermatozoa.

At a minimum, specimens for cultures to grow *Neisseria gonorrhoeae* and *Chlamydia trachomatis* should be obtained from the rectum, throat, and vagina. Microscopic evaluation of Gram-stained vaginal smear and wet mounts for clue cells and trichomonads should be accomplished. A potassium hydroxide preparation of a vaginal smear can be examined microscopically for *Candida*.

Ideally, colposcopic examination[43] and photography of the genitalia by an experienced clinician should occur as soon as possible after sexual assault on a child. Although most accidental straddle injuries to the perineum cause trauma to the pubic, clitoral, and anterior and lateral labial structures (Fig. 3–3), forceful sexual assault with attempted vaginal penetration is more likely to cause injury posteriorly in the areas of the fossa navicularis, posterior fourchette, posterior

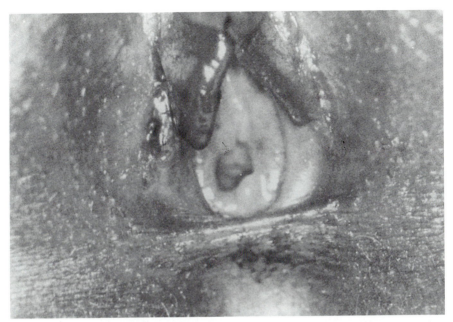

Figure 3–3. Acute straddle injury. Injury was sustained when 5-year-old fell on monkey bars. A 2 to 3 mm laceration of right labium minus is seen. (From Chadwick DL et al: *Color atlas of child sexual abuse,* Chicago, 1989, Year Book.)

hymen, and possibly the perineum (Fig. 3–4). If genital or vaginal bleeding is present, careful history taking and inspection are needed to determine if conservative therapy or examination under anesthesia in cooperation with the gynecologist is required.

Additional evaluation and treatment considerations for victims of sexual assault or rape include pregnancy test for all postmenarchal girls before a decision regarding postcoital pregnancy prophylaxis, consideration of prophylactic antibiotic therapy for sexually transmitted diseases, testing for human immunodeficiency virus, and the rapid plasma reagent test for syphilis. Medical evaluation of child sexual abuse is complete only when proper referral to investigative and social support agencies is accomplished.

Acute Genital Injury

Evaluation and therapy. Pokorny and associates[44] recommend that the clinician dealing with an acute genital injury (1) first consider what object allegedly caused the injury and (2) determine if the anatomic features of symmetry and hymenal transection are present.

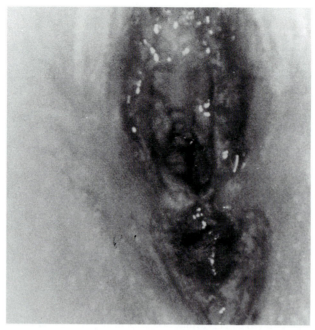

Figure 3–4. Acute traumatic rape. This 7-year-old Hispanic girl stated she had been raped by her stepfather. Examination revealed marked introital erythema and gaping vaginal opening with laceration at 6 o'clock position, exposing perineal musculature. Injury extended posteriorly past posterior fourchette and internally past hymenal orifice. (From Chadwick DL et al: *Color atlas of child sexual abuse,* Chicago, 1989, Year Book.)

If the object is of the penetrating type, especially in the presence of a symmetric injury and hymenal transection, the possibility of higher internal injury is great. Even if the child is having minimal bleeding and is in no apparent distress, examination under anesthesia is recommended.

Conversely, if the object is too small or too wide to penetrate higher, more conservative management may be indicated even when the child is screaming and has significant bleeding. Such management consists of reassuring the child and keeping the child quiet and supine.

Applying ice and pressure packs to the perineum often decreases swelling and pain sufficiently to gain the child's cooperation. Thereafter, wound lavage and examination adequate to determine the full extent of the injury may be accomplished without general anesthesia. If the injury is found to be asymmetric and the hymen remains intact, the child should be restricted to quiet and supine activities, given frequent tub or sitz baths, and closely followed up over the next few days.

PHYSICAL ABUSE
Bruises

Accidental versus inflicted bruising. Bruises are an expected part of the everyday life of healthy, active children. Accidental bruising occurs primarily on the knees, shins, forehead, and elbows of crawling or ambulatory children. Accidental bruising is unusual before the age of 9 months.

Bruises are the most common manifestation of inflicted child maltreatment, occurring in 39% of 313 children reported for abuse in 1987 by Children's Hospital of Columbus, Ohio.[1] Bruising patterns that should prompt suspicion of inflicted injury are described in the following sections.

Pinch marks. Infants who are crying uncontrollably may be force fed in an attempt to quiet them. A stressed parent may pinch the cheeks on the sides of the infant's mouth in an effort to get the child to accept the bottle, leaving oval bruises on each side of the face (Fig. 3–5). In this circumstance, force feeding may also result in a torn frenulum or swollen lip.

Paired oval bruises or pinch marks caused by the offender's thumb and forefinger may occur when a child is pinched on the arm, earlobe, or elsewhere

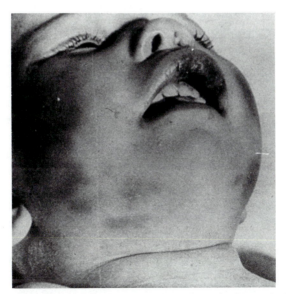

Figure 3–5. Pinch marks on infant's cheeks from force feeding. Lip is swollen and bruised. (From Schmitt BD: *The visual diagnosis of non-accidental trauma and failure to thrive,* Elk Grove Village, IL, 1978, American Academy of Pediatrics and the National Center for the Prevention and Treatment of Child Abuse and Neglect. Used with permission of the American Academy of Pediatrics.)

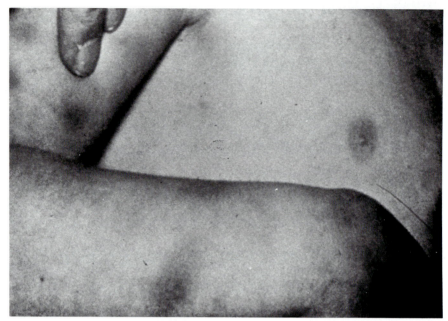

Figure 3–6. Paired, oval pinch marks on upper and lower arm. (From Schmitt BD: *The visual diagnosis of non-accidental trauma and failure to thrive,* Elk Grove Village, IL, 1978, American Academy of Pediatrics and the National Center for the Prevention and Treatment of Child Abuse and Neglect. Used with permission of the American Academy of Pediatrics.)

(Fig. 3–6). When a caretaker also pulls the child by the ear, bruising may occur at the attachment of the pinna, where capillaries have stretched and torn because of the traction applied.

In exasperation a parent may lift an infant or child by the trunk with both hands and shake the child forcefully back and forth. Oval pinch marks called trunk encirclement bruises may result. When infant shaking is violent, this pattern of bruising may be associated with shaken infant syndrome, posterior rib fractures, and vertebral compression fractures (see later discussion).

Linear bruises. The child who has been slapped across the cheek, buttocks, or elsewhere may bear characteristic parallel linear bruises finger width apart, which occur where capillary stretching and tearing are maximal between the fingers of the offender's hand. The slapped cheek bruise (Fig. 3–7) is present on the child's left if the perpetrator is right handed, and vice versa.

When a child is spanked excessively with a belt or paddle, the buttocks and sometimes the posterior thighs and trunk often bear a pattern of linear bruises that are generally oriented in one primary direction. If a belt was used, the linear bruising wraps around body surfaces and closely resembles the shape of the belt (Fig. 3–8).

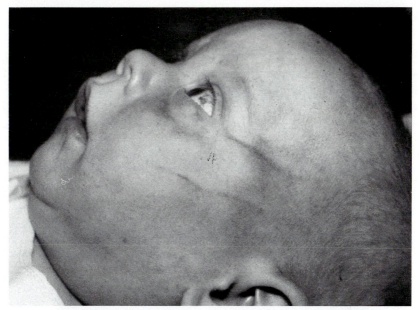

Figure 3–7. Parallel linear bruises of slapped cheek. (From Jenny C, Hay TC: *The visual diagnosis of child physical abuse,* Elk Grove Village, IL, 1993, American Academy of Pediatrics and C Henry Kempe Center. Used with permission of the American Academy of Pediatrics.)

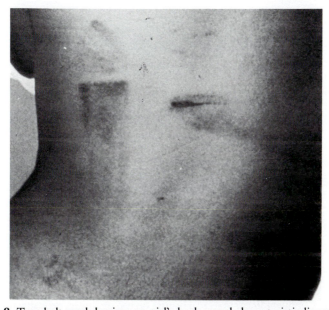

Figure 3–8. Two belt mark bruises on girl's back reveal characteristic linear bruises of uniform width that wrap around body surfaces. Tapered end of belt left bruise that extends upward. (From Schmitt BD: *The visual diagnosis of non-accidental trauma and failure to thrive,* Elk Grove Village, IL, 1978, American Academy of Pediatrics and National Center for the Prevention and Treatment of Child Abuse and Neglect. Used with permission of the American Academy of Pediatrics.)

Linear bruises along the posterior and superior edges of the pinnae (Fig. 3–9) or vertically oriented along either side of the gluteal cleft (Fig. 3–10) have recently been linked to abuse.[45] These specific linear bruises probably resulted from maximal deformation of the skin along these lines at the time of severe slapping or spanking. Linear bruises of the pinnae might be anticipated as a finding in the tin ear syndrome (see later discussion).

Electric cord marks. If an electric cord or similar object is used to whip a child, characteristic loop marks occur (Fig. 3–11). Because capillary tearing

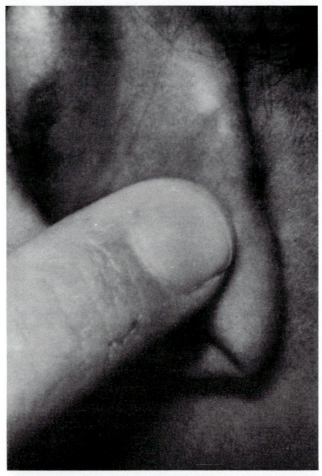

Figure 3–9. Confluent linear petechial bruises on top of pinnae, probably result of blow to head resulting in capillary injury causing rim of petechiae. Look for these bruises in cases of subdural hematoma and tin ear syndrome. (From Feldman KW: *Pediatrics* 90:633–636, 1992. Reproduced with permission of *Pediatrics*.)

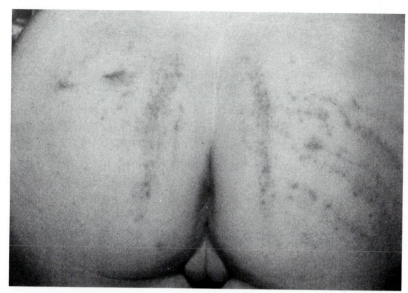

Figure 3–10. Vertical gluteal cleft bruises in 3½-year-old girl are probably due to exaggerated skin deformation in these locations during spanking. Parallel linear horizontal bruises on buttocks suggest finger marks from spanking. (From Feldman KW: *Pediatrics* 90:633–636, 1992. Reproduced with permission of *Pediatrics*.)

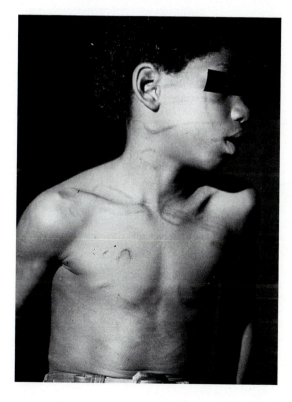

Figure 3–11. Looped and C-shaped injuries and scars from beatings with electrical cord. (Courtesy Dr. E. Thomas Sproles III.)

55

occurs along the edges of the cord where skin stretching is maximal, an electric cord characteristically leaves parallel lines of bruising in the shape of a loop. Such bruises often wrap around body surfaces. If the cord is narrow, the skin may be abraded or cut, particularly at the closed end of the loop mark. Repetitive abuse with electric cords is common and often leaves linear or C-shaped scars.[46]

Ligature marks and gag marks. In children whose ankles or wrists have been bound by rope or cord in an effort to restrict mobility, abrasions, friction burns (Fig. 3–12), or cuts may develop if the cord is narrow (Fig. 3–13). The child who is gagged in a desperate effort to silence him or her typically has abrasions or cuts extending from the corners of the mouth (Fig. 3–14). Children restricted in these ways commonly manifest other signs of nutritional neglect and abuse.

Bite marks. In unusual circumstances (such as parental mental illness) an adult may bite a child (Fig. 3–15). These bruises may be difficult to differentiate from other oval or circular dermatologic conditions.[47] The examining medical provider may distinguish between bite marks left by a child and those left by an adult by measuring the maxillary intercanine distance. If the distance is greater

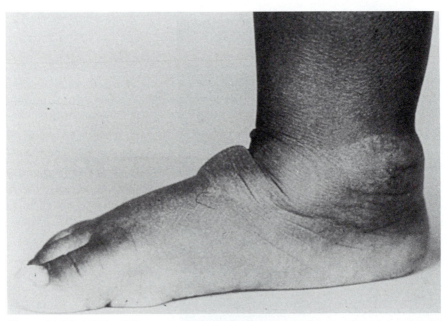

Figure 3–12. Friction blisters on ankle caused by rope or sheet used to tie or restrain child. (From Schmitt BD: *The visual diagnosis of non-accidental trauma and failure to thrive*, Elk Grove Village, IL, 1978, American Academy of Pediatrics and National Center for the Prevention and Treatment of Child Abuse and Neglect. Used with permission of the American Academy of Pediatrics.)

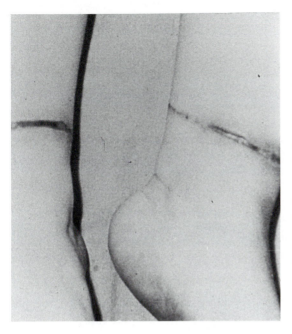

Figure 3–13. While mother went out for the evening, child was tied to bed by narrow cord or rope. (From Schmitt BD: *The visual diagnosis of non-accidental trauma and failure to thrive,* Elk Grove Village, IL, 1978, American Academy of Pediatrics and National Center for the Prevention and Treatment of Child Abuse and Neglect. Used with permission of the American Academy of Pediatrics.)

Figure 3–14. Gag mark in a 3-year-old child. Gag was applied to control excessive screaming and yelling. (From Schmitt BD: *The visual diagnosis of non-accidental trauma and failure to thrive,* Elk Grove Village, IL, 1978, American Academy of Pediatrics and National Center for the Prevention and Treatment of Child Abuse and Neglect. Used with permission of the American Academy of Pediatrics.)

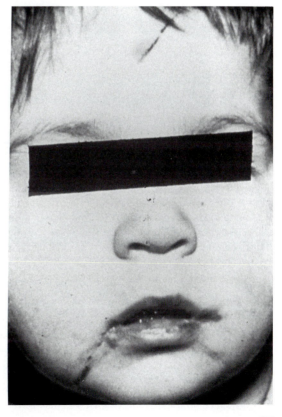

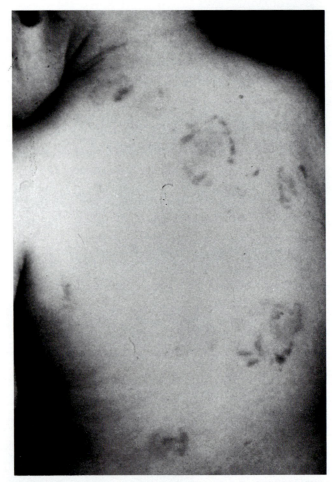

Figure 3–15. Ringlike bruising pattern of human bites with individual teeth marks visible. Bites may appear as paired, crescent-shaped bruises as well. (From Schmitt BD: *The visual diagnosis of non-accidental trauma and failure to thrive,* Elk Grove Village, IL, 1978, American Academy of Pediatrics and National Center for the Prevention and Treatment of Child Abuse and Neglect. Used with permission of the American Academy of Pediatrics.)

than 3 cm, the bite was inflicted by an adult. If a particular adult perpetrator is suspected, dental impressions can be used to definitively match the bruise pattern to that individual. A saline-moistened swab of the fresh bite (even if the skin remained intact) may be useful for identifying the perpetrator by using salivary ABO blood group testing.[48] Copious irrigation of human bites and careful assessment for possible secondary infection risk are indicated.

Bizarre shapes. A child with a bruise of distinct or unusual pattern should be closely examined for evidence of physical child abuse. Usually the specific shape of the bruise closely resembles the object used (Fig. 3–16).

Age of bruises. The age of a given bruise should be estimated and documented in the medical record according to the scale in Table 3–2. Estimation of the age of bruising is inexact. Factors that affect the appearance or healing of a bruise include body location, depth, amount of tissue bleeding, skin color, and circulatory status of the bruised area.

Warning signs. Child maltreatment should be suspected and reported when bruises are extensive or centrally located. Physical abuse is more likely if the history given does not match the estimated age of the bruise or the mechanism of injury required to explain observed findings. The health care professional must consider the developmental age and motor skills of the victim, or the reported abusive sibling, in assessing the veracity of the history given.

Abrasions and Lacerations

Self-inflicted scratches and nicks on the face are common during the first 3 months of life, when the infant lacks motor control. Thereafter, such minor

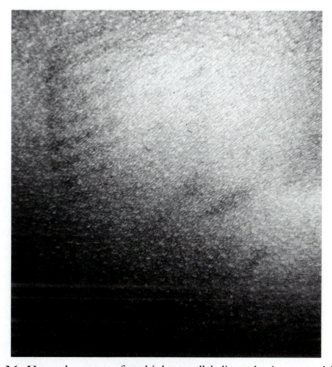

Figure 3–16. Unusual pattern of multiple, parallel, linear bruises caused by kitchen spatula. (Courtesy Dr. Carole Jenny.)

Table 3–2. Determination of Age of Bruise or Contusion

Day	1	2	3	4	5	6	7	8	9	10	13	21	28
	Red-blue		Blue-purple			Green		Yellow-brown			Resolved		

Modified from Wilson EF: *Pediatrics* 60:750–752, 1977. Reproduced with permission of *Pediatrics*.

self-inflicted skin injuries are typically limited to irritated skin areas. Nicks or lacerations produced by the fingers of adults are usually larger and may occur in sites the infant or child cannot easily reach.[3] In the older infant or child, accidental scratches and lacerations are located primarily on hands, elbows, and knees. Following bruises, abrasions and scratches are the next most common form of injury from abuse.[1]

Burns

Scope. It has been estimated that 1% to 16% of children with burns had them deliberately inflicted.[49] The two major mechanisms by which children are intentionally burned are the scalding burn and the dry contact burn.[50]

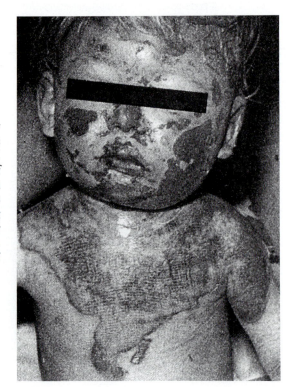

Figure 3–17. Burn caused by small child pulling hot kettle from work surface onto himself. Accidental burns are typically of greatest depth near head, with severity of burn tapering off as hot liquid loses heat running down skin. Inverted triangle or arrowhead appearance results. (From Hobbs CJ: *Br Med J* 298:1302–1305, 1989.)

Examination. The medical provider should note and document the specific burn characteristics, including configuration, depth, extent, and uniformity. The burn configuration may be described as circumferential, splash, or patterned. The depth of burn must be determined as superficial, partial thickness, or full thickness. The estimation of the body surface area involved must also be recorded. Finally, the uniformity of the burn pattern should be noted.[4]

Accidental scalding burns. Most accidental scalding burns occur when a child reaches up and pulls down a container of hot liquid. The resulting burn typically involves anterior surfaces of the body, including areas under the chin and the axillae, chest, hands, and feet. Accidental scalding burns have decreasing, nonuniform depth of burn, often in an arrowhead configuration (Fig. 3–17).

Inflicted scalding and immersion burns. Following a urine or stooling accident, a stressed parent or caretaker may fill the bathtub with hot water with the dual intentions of cleansing and punishment. While the child is held in jackknife fashion against the adult's chest, the child's buttocks and perineum are lowered into the hot water. A uniform, partial- or full-thickness dunking burn involving the buttocks, and possibly the heels or feet, may result (Fig. 3–18).

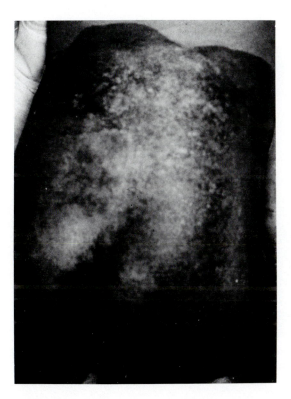

Figure 3–18. Child held tightly against adult's chest and lowered into hot bathtub water sustains "dunking" burn, limited to buttocks, perineum, and heels. (Courtesy Dr. Carole Jenny.)

If the struggling child is held forcibly against the cooler, porcelain bottom of the bathtub during this cleaning or punishment procedure, the buttocks may be spared centrally because of inadequate duration of contact with the hot water. This gives rise to the doughnut burn pattern (Fig. 3–19).

If the child's hands or feet are dipped or held under scalding water, a stocking-glove distribution of partial- or full-thickness burn with uniform depth results (Fig. 3–20).

Dry contact burns. Accidental dry contact burns commonly involve the palms or ventral fingers when a child touches or grabs a hot object in curiosity. A child who accidentally contacts a hot object usually immediately drops the object or moves away, resulting in minimal, nonuniform depth of burn and a partial, incomplete pattern of the offending object.

With intentional dry contact burns the depth of burn is more often uniform and the shape of the burn more closely resembles the offending object (Figs. 3–21 and 3–22), which was placed and held in an abusive manner. Cigarettes leave a characteristic circular burn pattern with typical greater depth of burn centrally, where the cigarette core burns hottest (Fig. 3–23).

Warning signs. Nonaccidental injury should be suspected and reported

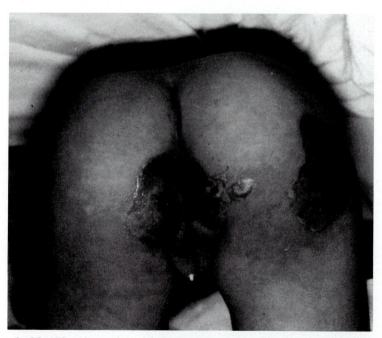

Figure 3–19. When buttocks are held forcibly against bottom of bathtub filled with scalding water, partial- or full-thickness "doughnut" burn may result. (Courtesy Dr. Carole Jenny.)

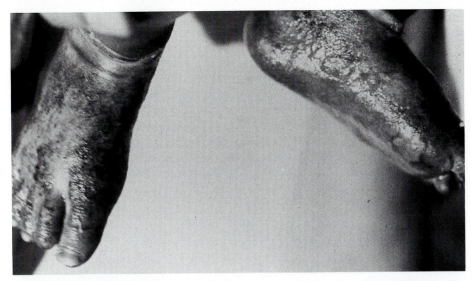

Figure 3–20. Typical "stocking" burn distribution with clear line of demarcation, uniform depth of burn, and no splash marks. Infant is developmentally incapable of accidentally self-inflicting this injury. Infant's feet were forcibly held under hot water. (Courtesy Dr. E. Thomas Sproles III.)

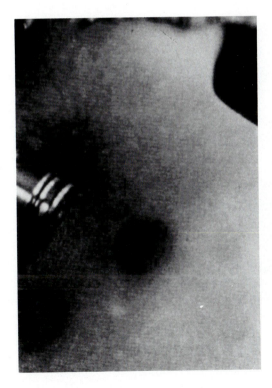

Figure 3–21. Automobile cigarette lighters give characteristic burn pattern. (From Jenny C, Hay TC: *The visual diagnosis of child physical abuse,* Elk Grove Village, IL, 1993, American Academy of Pediatrics and C Henry Kempe Center. Used with permission of the American Academy of Pediatrics.)

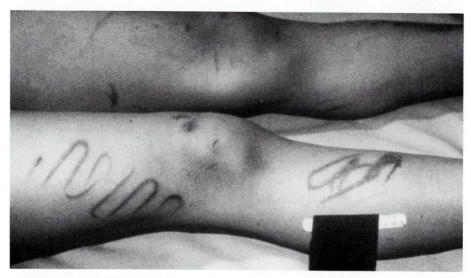

Figure 3–22. Distinctive burn patterns created by hot potato masher. If accidentally acquired, burns would not have been multiple, uniform in depth, and complete in pattern. (Courtesy Dr. Carole Jenny.)

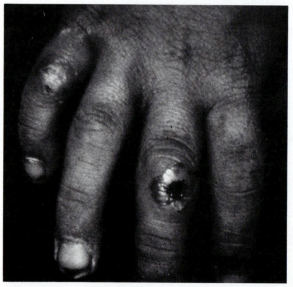

Figure 3–23. Cigarettes are commonly used to inflict dry contact burn. Cigarette burns appear as round, symmetric burns, usually 8 mm in diameter. They are commonly found in clusters. (From Jenny CA, Hay TC: *The visual diagnosis of child physical abuse,* Elk Grove Village, IL, 1993, American Academy of Pediatrics and C Henry Kempe Center. Used with permission of the American Academy of Pediatrics.)

when a scalding burn lacks splash marks, the configuration is circumferential, or the burn depth is uniform. When dry contact burns occur in unlikely areas, such as the dorsum of the hand, the back, the perineum, or the soles of the feet, inflicted injury should also be more strongly considered. Finally, an intentional burn from child maltreatment is more probable when the history of the burn is incompatible with the gross or fine motor capability of the victim or alleged perpetrator.

Fractures

Most common fractures. Diaphyseal fractures, either spiral or transverse, statistically are much more common (4 to 1) in abused children than are epiphyseal-metaphyseal fractures. A transverse fracture (Fig. 3–24) of the midshaft of a long bone results from a direct blow or a bending type of force, whereas the spiral fracture is the result of rotational or torsional forces applied to the

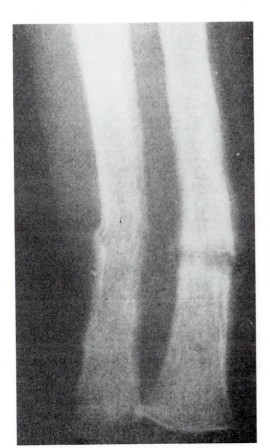

Figure 3–24. A 4-month-old with left spiral fracture of humerus was discovered on skeletal survey to have additional healing transverse fractures of left radius and ulna. (From Merten DF, Carpenter BLM: *Pediatr Clin North Am* 37:815–837, 1990.)

limb.[51,52] Since a diaphyseal fracture is also the most common accidental fracture in children, it is nonspecific for inflicted injury.

Fractures virtually diagnostic of abuse. Metaphyseal "chip" or "bucket handle" fractures in children (Fig. 3–25) probably represent an inflicted injury resulting from shearing forces generated by violent shaking or extremity torsion. Histopathologic study reveals that such injuries are actually a transplanar fracture through primary spongiosa of the metaphysis.[53]

Rib fractures from child abuse are often multiple and bilateral. Rib fractures from abuse may be caused by direct blows, in which case liver or splenic rupture may coexist. Thoracic compression during violent shaking may result in posterior rib fractures (Fig. 3–26) near the attachment to the vertebral bodies, where maximal stress occurs. Such injuries might coexist with trunk encirclement bruising, vertebral compression fractures, or the shaken infant syndrome (see later discussion).

A fracture of the acromion process of the scapula (Fig. 3–27) most often results from a forceful direct blow to the shoulder or violent arm traction. The most common clavicular fracture from accidental or abusive trauma is a fracture of the midshaft, which is therefore not diagnostic of child maltreatment. However, an avulsion fracture of the distal clavicle, although uncommon, is virtually diagnostic of child abuse.[52]

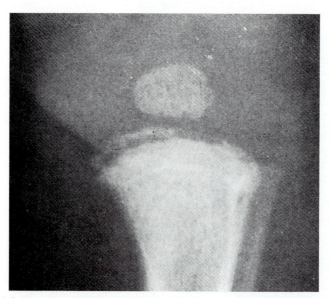

Figure 3–25. Metaphyseal "bucket handle" fracture of tibia of 3-month-old. (From Merten DF, Carpenter BLM: *Pediatr Clin North Am* 37:815–837, 1990.)

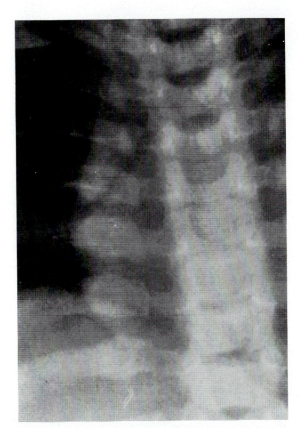

Figure 3–26. This 7-month-old infant with "accidental" skull fracture was discovered to have multiple healing fractures of right sixth through ninth ribs adjacent to costovertebral junctions. In absence of major trauma or preexisting bone disease, rib fractures virtually establish diagnosis of child abuse. (From Merten DF, Carpenter BLM: *Pediatr Clin North Am* 37:815–837, 1990.)

Fractures highly suspect for child abuse. A diaphyseal spiral fracture before 9 months of age (Fig. 3–28) should prompt great concern for nonaccidental injury. When diapering an infant, an angry, abusing caretaker could cause a spiral fracture by violently externally rotating the infant's legs.

However, a spiral fracture below 9 months of age is not absolutely diagnostic of child abuse. I have heard the accidental spiral fracturing of a nonambulatory infant's midhumerus (recorded on video/audio tape), which occurred when an older sibling rolled the prone infant over onto his back with the arm trapped beneath the infant's body.

Anterior compression fracture of the vertebral body (Fig. 3–29) may result

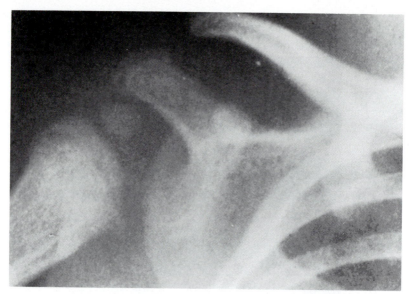

Figure 3–27. Initial skeletal survey on 5-month-old infant with swollen, tender elbow revealed avulsion fracture of tip of acromion process and distal clavicle, as well as metaphyseal fracture of humerus. (From Merten DF, Carpenter BLM: *Pediatr Clin North Am* 37:815–837, 1990.)

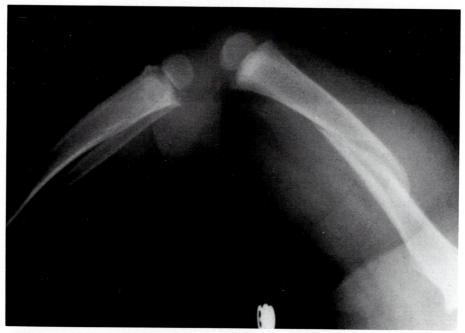

Figure 3–28. Femur radiograph reveals spiral fracture of midshaft femur. Infant was not yet crawling or pulling to standing. Although significant force is required to cause spiral fracture of femur, no history of trauma was given. (From Jenny C, Hay TC: *The visual diagnosis of child physical abuse,* Elk Grove Village, IL, 1993, American Academy of Pediatrics and C Henry Kempe Center. Used with permission of the American Academy of Pediatrics.)

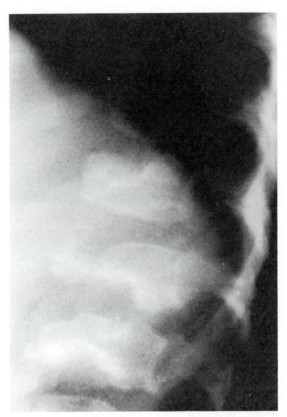

Figure 3–29. Severe fracture deformities of vertebral bodies in 5-year-old boy with history of subdural hematomas at 6 months of age. (From Merten DF, Carpenter BLM: *Pediatr Clin North Am* 37:815–837, 1990.)

from hyperflexion caused by violent shaking of an infant or child. Sternal fractures, indicating direct trauma to a central and protected area of the body, are highly suspect for child abuse. Periosteal elevation, which may be subtle and difficult to detect on plain films (Fig. 3–30), can result from twisting or wrenching of an extremity by an abuser. However, symmetric periosteal elevation of long bones can be normal during the first 6 months of life. Although supracondylar humeral fractures are usually the result of accidental injury, fractures of the middle or proximal humerus are more likely to be inflicted.[54]

    Dating of fractures. The age of a fracture can be roughly estimated from radiographs as detailed in Table 3–3, providing useful information for assessing the reliability of the given history. Skull fractures may be visible for up to 16 weeks and are essentially impossible to date. Metaphyseal fractures are likewise difficult to date radiographically, often heal without callus formation, and may be asymptomatic.

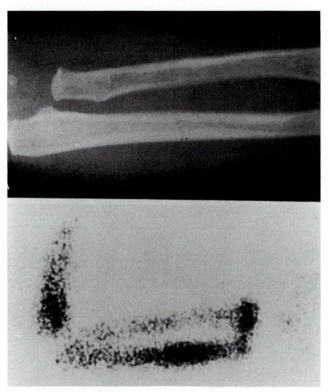

Figure 3–30. Radiograph of left forearm of 6-month-old with subdural hematoma revealed subtle periosteal new bone along medial ulnar midshaft. This was confirmed on skeletal scintigraphy by extensive increased tracer activity in ulnar shaft. (From Merten DF, Carpenter BLM: *Pediatr Clin North Am* 37:815–837, 1990.)

Table 3–3. Estimating the Radiographic Age of Fractures

Category	Early	Peak	Late
Resolution of soft tissue injury	2–5 days	4–10 days	10–21 days
Periosteal new bone formation	4–10 days	10–14 days	14–21 days
Loss of fracture line definition	10–14 days	14–21 days	
Soft callus	10–14 days	14–21 days	
Hard callus	14–21 days	21–42 days	42–90 days
Remodeling	3 months	1 year	2 years to epiphyseal closure

Modified from O'Conner JF, Cohen J: Dating fractures. In Kleinman PK, ed: *Diagnostic imaging of child abuse,* Baltimore, 1987, Williams & Wilkins.

Warning signs. The discovery of multiple fractures in different stages of healing (Fig. 3–31) or fractures inconsistent with the developmental age of the child or the history raises concerns of nonaccidental trauma.

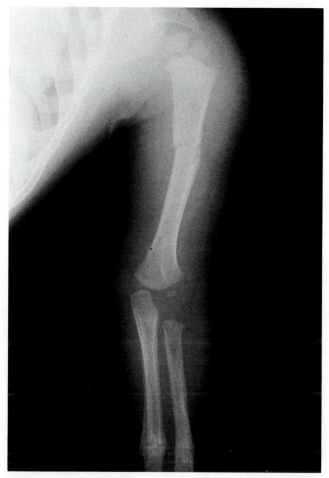

Figure 3–31. Multiple fractures of different ages, including transverse fracture of middiaphysis of humerus with adjacent soft tissue swelling, healing transverse fracture of distal radius with periosteal reaction, and older fracture (nearly completely healed) of distal ulna without periosteal reaction, but with sclerosis at fracture line. These three fractures at different ages strongly suggest child abuse. Child did not receive medical care following first two fractures. (From Jenny C, Hay TC: *The visual diagnosis of child physical abuse,* Elk Grove Village, IL, 1993, American Academy of Pediatrics and C Henry Kempe Center. Used with permission of the American Academy of Pediatrics.)

Abdominal Injuries

Overview. Abdominal injuries, although uncommon, are a leading cause of death from child physical abuse.[55] Children punched or kicked in the abdomen or thrown against a stationary object have sustained serious internal injuries at the hands of adult caregivers. Clinical presentations for life-threatening abdominal injury from child abuse include unexplained shock, anemia, peritonitis, and bilious emesis.[56]

Injuries. Bruises on the anterior abdominal wall, when present, should raise suspicion that serious abdominal injuries may have been inflicted. Internal injuries most likely to result from inflicted blunt abdominal trauma are discussed here in descending order of frequency.[4]

A ruptured liver or spleen (Fig. 3–32) is typically manifest as hypovolemic shock and may be associated with ipsilateral rib fractures from a direct blow. In subtle cases elevations of serum liver transaminase levels may indicate an occult liver laceration caused by child abuse.[57,58] An intestinal perforation may be manifested initially as an acute abdomen with free intraperitoneal air or later as signs of peritonitis.

A child who has sustained epigastric blunt force trauma may have vomiting,

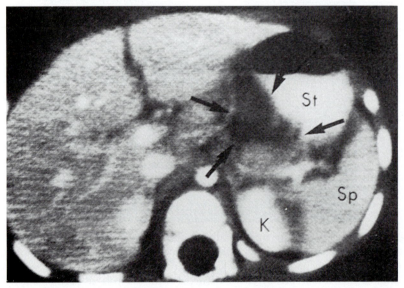

Figure 3–32. Computed tomography scan reveals oblique fracture of liver along falciform ligament. In addition, fluid collection *(arrows)* medial and posterior to stomach eventually evolved into pancreatic pseudocyst. *K,* Kidney; *Sp,* spleen; *St,* stomach. (From Kuhn JP. In Silverman FN, Kuhn JP, eds: *Essentials of Caffey's pediatric x-ray diagnosis,* Chicago, 1990, Year Book.)

pain, and signs of intestinal obstruction. The proximal duodenum, fixed to the spinal column at the ligament of Treitz, may be compressed between the offending object and the spinal column. A duodenal hematoma develops with progressive obstructive effects (Fig. 3–33), eventually causing significant abdominal pain, recurrent vomiting, and dehydration.

When mesenteric vessels are disrupted by abdominal blunt force trauma, hypovolemic shock is usually present. The clinical picture may unfold rapidly

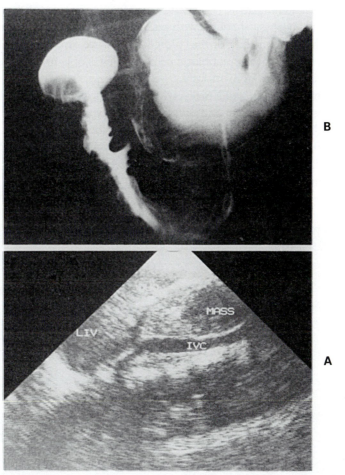

Figure 3–33. A 5-year-old boy with persistent vomiting. **A,** Upper gastrointestinal series reveals intramural hematoma with abrupt narrowing of duodenal lumen just beyond superior flexure. **B,** Longitudinal abdominal ultrasonography demonstrates duodenal hematoma as relatively anechoic mass distal to normal duodenum, containing echogenic gas. (From Merten DF, Carpenter BLM: *Pediatr Clin North Am* 37:815–837, 1990.)

or gradually. The pancreas is frequently injured (Fig. 3–34), even transected, by direct epigastric trauma. Such patients typically have delayed onset of abdominal tenderness, vomiting, and fever. Occasionally, later development of a pancreatic pseudocyst is the only sign of prior abdominal injury from child maltreatment.

Hematuria may be the sign of kidney trauma sustained from a blow to the back. Renal injuries from direct trauma may include parenchymal contusion, laceration, fragmentation, capsular hematoma, pelvocalyceal disruption, or injury to the renal vessels.

Life-threatening acute renal failure may follow massive soft tissue and muscle injury from physical abuse, with resultant rhabdomyolysis and myoglobinuria.[59] Urine appears dark or tea colored. A positive dipstick test for hemoglobinuria in the absence of red blood cells on microscopic urinalysis should raise the suspicion of rhabdomyolysis.

Warning signs. Child maltreatment should be suspected whenever the history presented is incompatible with the force required to produce the internal abdominal injuries. The abdominal injuries described previously are uncommon except in motor vehicle accidents and inflicted trauma. Parents who have abused their child in this manner commonly delay seeking medical attention until significant clinical deterioration occurs.

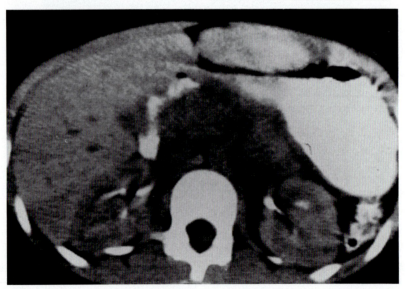

Figure 3–34. A 5-year-old boy with persistent vomiting. Contrast-enhanced abdominal computed tomography image reveals pancreatic contusion. (Same child as in Figure 3–33.) (From Merten DF, Carpenter BLM: *Pediatr Clin North Am* 37:815–837, 1990.)

Head Injuries

Head injuries are the most frequent cause of morbidity and death from child abuse.[60] No central nervous system injury is absolutely specific for and diagnostic of child abuse.[52]

Facial soft tissue injuries. Abrasions, lacerations, contusions, and hematomas of the face are commonly observed in abused infants and children, although underlying facial fractures are rare. Periorbital ecchymoses, if unilateral and nontender, may result from an accidental injury to the forehead. Bilateral, nontender periorbital ecchymoses could occur accidentally only if caused by a midforehead injury. In the case of direct orbital blows the discolored eyelids are tender and swollen (Fig. 3–35). In this setting, careful eye examination is necessary to exclude orbital fracture, hyphema, or retinal hemorrhage.

Lesions of the mouth. A torn frenulum in an infant is almost always inflicted, usually the result of force feeding. The tongue may be bruised or lacerated by teeth when a young child is struck on the jaw. The palate may be injured when an eating utensil is jammed in the mouth of a crying, unconsolable infant or toddler by a stressed parent. Teeth may be traumatized, avulsed,

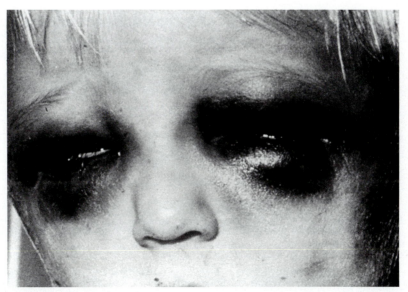

Figure 3–35. Child who has been repeatedly hit about face and eyes with open hand. Swelling and lid tenderness indicate direct eye trauma. If bruising of eyelids is unassociated with swelling and tenderness, basilar skull fracture must also be considered. (From Schmitt BD: *The visual diagnosis of non-accidental trauma and failure to thrive,* Elk Grove Village, IL, 1978, American Academy of Pediatrics and National Center for the Prevention and Treatment of Child Abuse and Neglect. Used with permission of the American Academy of Pediatrics.)

discolored, or dentally neglected. The presence of oral or perioral gonorrhea or syphilis in a prepubertal child is pathognomonic for sexual abuse.[47]

Scalp injuries. Traumatic alopecia may occur as a result of hair pulling. Close scalp inspection reveals petechial hemorrhages and hair shafts broken off at varying lengths. A tender, spongy scalp may indicate a subgaleal hematoma from violent hair pulling or be associated with an underlying skull fracture in the case of a direct blow or impact to the head.

Skull fractures. A simple linear skull fracture is the most common skull fracture resulting from child abuse.[61] Falls from heights less than 4 feet only rarely cause a skull fracture or serious intracranial injury.[61-64] In this accidental setting the fracture is also typically a simple, linear, parietal skull fracture.[61]

Except in the accidental setting of a motor vehicle accident or fall from a significant height, a comminuted, depressed, diastatic, growing, or stellate skull fracture suggests inflicted head injury (Fig. 3–36). Multiple, bilateral, and non-parietal skull fractures also raise suspicion of child abuse.[61]

Although an uncommon result of physical abuse, a fracture of the temporal bone may be associated with an epidural hematoma, a neurosurgical emergency.

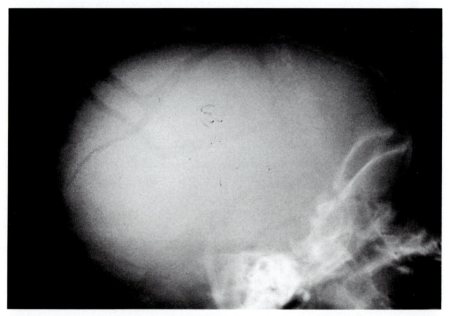

Figure 3–36. Two parietal and occipital skull fractures. Fractures are diastatic (widened), implying increased intracranial pressure. Fractures are complex because they involve more than one fracture line or component. (From Jenny C, Hay TC: *The visual diagnosis of child physical abuse,* Elk Grove Village, IL, 1993, American Academy of Pediatrics and C Henry Kempe Center. Used with permission of the American Academy of Pediatrics.)

Basilar skull fracture should be suspected with findings of postauricular ecchymosis, bilateral nontender periorbital ecchymosis, or hemotympanum.

Clinical presentation of intracranial injury. The acute presentation of more serious intracranial injury from child abuse may include respiratory distress, irritability, lethargy, hypotonia, seizures, coma, vomiting, and poor feeding. Infectious, toxic, or metabolic causes must be excluded. Signs of a direct, inflicted injury may not be readily apparent on initial scalp or cranial inspection. Pupillary dilation to look for retinal hemorrhage may be diagnostically useful.

Intracranial hemorrhage. Subdural (Figs. 3–37 and 3–38), subarachnoid, and especially retinal hemorrhages (Fig. 3–39) are uncommon in accidental injury and common in inflicted injuries.[52,60–65] The presence of a subdural hematoma or retinal hemorrhage requires or implies significant force comparable

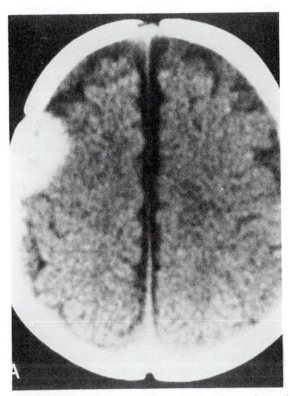

Figure 3–37. A 6-month-old infant with seizures. Axial unenhanced computed tomography reveals focal acute high-density hematoma over right cerebral convexity. Generalized enlargement of extracerebral spaces suggests either chronic subdural hematoma or brain atrophy. (From Merten DF, Carpenter BLM: *Pediatr Clin North Am* 37:815–837, 1990.)

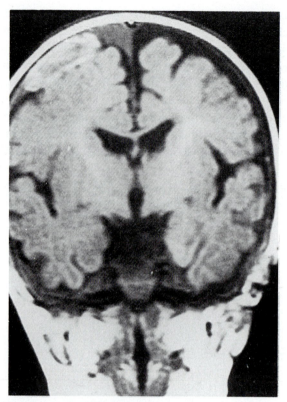

Figure 3–38. Same 6-month-old infant with seizures as in Figure 3–37. Coronal T1-weighted magnetic resonance imaging shows acute right convexity subdural hematoma as high-signal-intensity mass. Lower signal intensity subacute subdural hematoma surrounds acute lesion. (From Merten DF, Carpenter BLM: *Pediatr Clin North Am* 37:815–837, 1990.)

to a motor vehicle accident or a fall from a height of 10 feet or more (usually occurring outdoors).[4,60,62,63]

Subdural hematomas are created by rotational or translational forces, or both, that tear bridging cerebral veins between the brain surface and the dura mater. Such hemorrhage may be caused by a direct blow, violent shaking, or head impact. Severe facial, scalp, and ear contusions, complex skull fracture, and brain contusion may coexist when a subdural hematoma is caused by a direct cranial blow. The shaken infant syndrome and the tin ear syndrome exemplify creation of a subdural hematoma by severe rotational and translational forces (see later discussion).

Shaken infant syndrome. Caffey[66] first postulated a link between severely

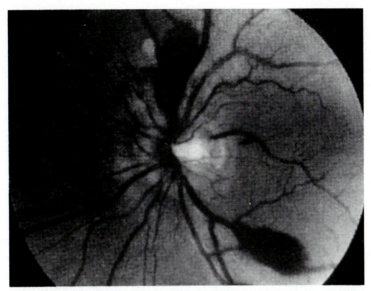

Figure 3–39. Retinal and preretinal hemorrhages are seen in 80% of children with abusive head trauma. (From Jenny C, Hay TC: *The visual diagnosis of child physical abuse*, Elk Grove Village, IL, 1993, American Academy of Pediatrics and C Henry Kempe Center. Used with permission of the American Academy of Pediatrics.)

shaken infants and intracranial and intraocular bleeding, permanent brain damage, and mental retardation. The shaken infant syndrome refers to the constellation of retinal and subdural or subarachnoid hemorrhage in an infant under 2 years of age who lacks external signs of injury.

Although subdural and retinal hemorrhage was originally suspected to result from whiplash caused by manual shaking of an infant held by the extremities or trunk,[67] actual impact of an infant's head may be required to produce such hemorrhage.[68] In light of this postulation, medical providers should look for associated trunk encirclement bruises, vertebral compression fractures, posterior rib fractures, upper extremity metaphyseal fractures, scalp and pinna contusion, subgaleal hemorrhage, and occult skull fracture when making the diagnosis of shaken infant syndrome.

Tin ear syndrome. Tin ear syndrome is the clinical triad of unilateral ear bruising, computed tomography (CT) evidence of ipsilateral cerebral edema and subdural hematoma with obliteration of the basilar cisterns, and hemorrhagic retinopathy. Death occurred in all cases described by Hanigan and associates.[69] They postulate that the children sustained severe unilateral blow to the head and blunt injury to the ear, resulting in significant rotational acceleration of the head, stretching and tearing of cortical veins, production of the subdural hematoma, intracranial hypertension, and tentorial herniation.

Cerebral injuries. Diffuse cerebral edema is the most common cerebral complication of abuse.[70] A relatively common CT finding from inflicted anoxic-ischemic cerebral injury is decreased density of the cerebral cortex with preservation of density of the thalami, brainstem, and cerebellum, a reversal of normal brain densities.[71] Long-term cerebral effects of inflicted cerebral trauma include chronic subdural collections, progressive ventriculomegaly, cerebral atrophy, encephalomalacia, and porencephaly.[70]

EVALUATION
History

Objectives. The objectives of a family interview when child abuse is suspected include the following: (1) to understand the history and mechanism of the child's injury, (2) to assess the veracity of the history, (3) to determine the degree of ongoing risk to the child in the home environment, (4) to take a past medical history of the child and the family members, (5) to form a supportive relationship with the family, and (6) to explain the child protective service process.

Interviews[72]. Separate interviews with the child and parents are ideal. In cases of true child maltreatment, these may reveal historical discrepancies between parents, between child and parents, and over time.

The parental interviews should begin with a discussion of the child's medical condition, the treatment plan, and the prognosis. The practitioner should convey to the parents or caretakers his or her sincere concern for the child's well-being. The child's past medical history is obtained. Once rapport is established, inquiries about family constellation, stresses, dynamics, and crises are made in a supportive manner. Finally, the child's caretakers are asked to describe in detail the events leading up to the injury.

In an interview with a child (suspected victim, child sibling reported to have accidentally caused the injury, or witness), the child's developmental and language capabilities are assessed first. The medical provider should sit at the child's eye level, ask age-appropriate questions, speak quietly, and be willing to listen patiently. The interview should begin with open-ended, general questions such as "Can you tell me what happened?" and "What happened next?" Only when the child provides no additional information to general questions should more specific inquiries be made. Leading questions should be avoided.

Medical records. The entire family's medical records should be reviewed for suspicious trends of "accidental" injuries, failure-to-thrive, missed immunizations and appointments, parental alcoholism or substance abuse, or past concerns of child maltreatment.

Warning signs. Inflicted child maltreatment should be more strongly considered if the history from family and patient reveals (1) delays in seeking medical care, (2) spontaneous or unexplained injury, (3) repetitive patterns of injury, (4) conflicting stories, (5) absent, unavailable, or disinterested parent(s), (6) history incompatible with the child's developmental capability, (7) history incompatible with the developmental capability of the sibling reported to have caused the injury, or (8) history incompatible with the force or means necessary to produce the observed injury.

Physical Examination

In cases of severe or life-threatening injury, immediate intervention by individuals experienced in pediatric trauma life support assumes the highest priority. Serial examination and recording of vital signs, capillary refill, and pulses are needed when serious injury is suspected. Serial neurologic or abdominal examinations may be necessary to diagnose evolving intracranial or intraabdominal injury.

Once the infant's or child's condition is stabilized, a head-to-toe examination should be conducted. General hygiene, adequacy of clothing, and nutritional status are noted and recorded. The entire head, neck, extremities, and trunk are carefully palpated. The entire integument is examined, with the size, location, and estimated age of all injuries entered in the medical record.

Warning signs. Suspicion of child maltreatment is heightened if (1) the child has multiple injuries; (2) injuries noted do not match the history provided with respect to mechanism, developmental capability, or force required; (3) injuries pathognomonic of child abuse are present; (4) the child has multiple injuries at various stages of healing; or (5) different forms of injury are present concurrently.

Laboratory Evaluation

Bleeding disorders. Laboratory evaluation for bleeding diathesis in a child with extensive bruising should include prothrombin time, partial thromboplastin time, thrombin time, fibrinogen level, complete blood cell count (CBC) with platelet count, and bleeding time. If disseminated intravascular coagulation is clinically suspected, measurement of fibrin split products and examination of the peripheral blood smear may also be required. If the "bleeding history" (Table 3–4) and screening laboratory findings are negative, the medical provider can effectively exclude from the diagnosis von Willebrand's disease or more rare bleeding disorders such as factor XIII deficiency, a platelet function defect, or antiplasmin deficiency. Consultation with a pediatric hematologist is recommended when the bleeding history or screening laboratory results are abnormal.

Blood loss or nutritional anemia. Baseline and serial CBCs may aid in

Table 3—4. Evaluation of Bleeding Diathesis

Bleeding History

Frequent or prolonged nasal and oral bleeding
Easy bruising, especially in unusual areas
Gastrointestinal or genitourinary bleeding
Petechiae
Prolonged postoperative bleeding
Positive history of menorrhagia

Screening Laboratory

Prothrombin time (PT)
Partial thromboplastin time (PTT)
Thrombin time (TT)
Fibrinogen
Complete blood cell (CBC) with platelet count
Bleeding time
If disseminated intravascular coagulation is suspected, fibrin split products (FSP) and
  examination of the peripheral blood smear

---

the estimation of gradual blood loss from blunt abdominal trauma. A CBC with indices, examination of the peripheral blood smear, and iron studies should be obtained to aid in the evaluation of nutritional anemia.

Dehydration or water deprivation. Children with hypernatremic dehydration from water restriction or other causes require measurement of serum electrolytes, blood urea nitrogen (BUN), urine specific gravity, and serum and urine osmolarity.

Severe muscle injury. When rhabdomyolysis, myoglobinuria, and possible acute renal failure are clinical concerns because of muscle injury from a severe spanking or beating, assessment of creatinine phosphokinase, renal function (BUN, creatinine, urinalysis, ongoing urine output), and serum myoglobin levels is indicated.

Bone disease. Serum calcium, phosphorus, and alkaline phosphatase should be measured as a baseline evaluation for metabolic or nutritional bone disease when radiographs reveal compatible findings.

Poisoning. Serum and urine toxicology screening is appropriate whenever intentional or accidental poisoning is considered.

Abdominal injury. A CBC, examination of stool for occult blood, and measurement of serum and urine amylase, liver transaminases (aspartate aminotransferase and alanine aminotransferase), and lactate dehydrogenase are appropriate for children who have sustained blunt abdominal injury.

Renal or genital injury. Urinalysis to look for occult hematuria is indicated when children sustain significant flank, perineal, or genital trauma.

Intracranial hemorrhage. Once increased intracranial pressure is excluded, examination of the cerebrospinal fluid (CSF) may be diagnostically important in a child with altered mental status. Bloody CSF should be centrifuged. Xanthochromia is an indicator of trauma in most circumstances.

Radiographic Evaluation[52,73]

Massive trauma. In massively traumatized infants or children, protocols similar to those used for accidental trauma are operative. An initial chest x-ray examination evaluates for pneumothorax, flail chest, pleural effusion, and pulmonary parenchymal injury. An abdominal roentgenogram evaluates for gross pelvic fractures but is inadequate for evaluation of solid visceral injury. An x-ray study of the lateral cervical spine should be obtained before further diagnostic studies are performed in the case of severe trauma.

Fractures or bone injury. The principal imaging study for evaluation of a specific skeletal injury is plain radiography of the injured site.

A precisely written protocol for skeletal survey evaluation of abused children is required. This skeletal survey is mandatory (1) in all cases of suspected physical abuse of children under 2 years of age; (2) for infants under the age of 1 year with significant nutritional neglect or deprivation; (3) for children with severe or multiple fractures; and (4) for children with fractures suspected or known to be caused by physical abuse. The skeletal survey may be clinically indicated for children from 2 to 5 years of age in the presence of specific clinical indicators of abuse. Routine skeletal surveys for all physically abused children over 5 years of age have little value.

Radionuclide bone scans (see Fig. 3–30) provide increased sensitivity for rib fractures, subtle shaft fractures, and areas of early periosteal elevation. Follow-up plain radiographs in 1 to 2 weeks may be useful in some cases.

Abdominal injuries. Abdominal CT (see Figs. 3–32 and 3–34) is effective and sensitive for identifying injuries inflicted on solid and hollow abdominal organs, pneumoperitoneum, or intraabdominal bleeding. In children less than 1 year of age, ultrasonography may be a reasonable initial study when abdominal injury is suspected. On occasion an upper gastrointestinal series is necessary to delineate an obstructive injury such as duodenal hematoma (see Fig. 3–33).

Skull fractures. Skull series radiographs are indicated when impact is suspected or evident. A cranial CT scan using "bone windows" improves definition of depressed or other complex skull fractures.

Intracranial injury. All infants and children with suspected intracranial injury must undergo cranial CT or magnetic resonance imaging (MRI) (see

Figs. 3–37 and 3–38). CT is generally sufficient if the patient has acute injury to the central nervous system. MRI is significantly more sensitive than CT in identifying most intracranial sequelae of abusive assaults, particularly when CT does not adequately explain the clinical findings. Cranial CT or MRI may be indicated to exclude subdural hematoma in an infant or young child with unexplained fractures of the long bones.[74]

Differential Diagnosis

The medical examiner bears the responsibility for thoroughly considering alternate medical diagnoses in the differential diagnosis of child maltreatment. This is necessary to avoid false accusations of child abuse against nonabusive parents and to avoid delaying treatment of alternate diagnoses. Medical conditions have been confused with child sexual abuse, bruising, burns, inflicted fractures, intracranial bleeding, failure-to-thrive, and eye hemorrhage. Table 3–5 represents a child abuse differential diagnostic list compiled from several excellent reviews.[46,75–81]

SPECIFIC MANAGEMENT OF CHILD ABUSE
Reporting to Proper Authorities

Ultimately the primary medical caretaker of an injured child must decide whether the findings exceed a reasonable threshold of suspicion for child abuse. A thorough history and review of medical records, a detailed physical examination, and appropriate laboratory and radiographic evaluations are the prerequisites for this important assessment. Table 3–6 summarizes the warning signs for child abuse.

Medical providers are not required to prove child abuse. If a reasonable suspicion of child abuse exists, the medical provider is mandated by law in every state to report this suspicion to proper authorities. Child protection team professionals in the social work, legal, and law enforcement arenas can assist in this evaluative process. These professionals should be consulted in all clear or equivocal cases of suspected child maltreatment or neglect.

Informing Parents

Medical providers have a duty to inform parents when a report of suspected child maltreatment has been filed, although this responsibility is commonly overlooked or avoided. Parents frequently react with angry denial, but occasionally they show relief. Personal confrontation or accusation should be avoided. The practitioner should stress his or her concern for the child's overall well-being, describe his or her duty by law to report any suspicion of child abuse or neglect, and explain the anticipated upcoming steps in the social service evaluative process. The parents should be told that they will be informed of all

Table 3–5. Differential Diagnosis of Child Abuse

Sexual Abuse

Dermatologic conditions: lichen sclerosus; diaper dermatitis; pinworms; poor hygiene; bubble bath; *Candida;* nonabusive bruising; seborrheic, atopic, or contact dermatitis; lichen simplex chronicus; lichen planus; psoriasis

Congenital conditions: labial fusion, hemangioma, midline defects, prominent medial raphe, linea vestibularis, perianal hyperpigmentation, midline anal skin tags

Injuries: straddle injury, splitting injury, female circumcision, hair tourniquet, seat belt or motor vehicle accident injury to genitalia, excessive masturbation, tampon injury (rare)

Anal conditions: Crohn's disease, postmortem anal dilation, chronic constipation, rectal prolapse, hemolytic uremic syndrome, rectal tumor

Infections: streptococcal vaginitis, perianal cellulitis, perinatally acquired warts, varicella

Urethral conditions: prolapse, caruncle, hemangioma, sarcoma, papilloma, polyps, sarcoma botryoides, ureterocele

Bruising and Integumentary Injuries

Folk medicine practices: coining, spooning, cupping

Mongolian spots

Bleeding disorders: hemophilia, disseminated intravascular coagulation, hemolytic uremic syndrome, vitamin K deficiency (e.g., liver disease), idiopathic thrombocytopenic prupura, von Willebrand's disease

Henoch-Schonlein purpura, erythema multiforme, erythema nodosum, hypersensitivity vasculitis

Dye or ink

Hemangioma or veins

Phytodermatitis from lemons, limes, celery, or parsnips

Aspirin or warfarin toxicity

Type 1 Ehlers-Danlos disease

Meningococcemia

Normal accidental bruising

Eczema, tinea corporis or capitis, granuloma annulare, pityriasis rosea

Allergic periorbital swelling

Alopecia areata

Self-inflicted injuries: childhood depression, mental retardation, Cornelia De Lange syndrome, Lesch-Nyhan syndrome, temper tantrums, rhythmic behaviors, seizures

Burns

Car seat or seat belt burn

Epidermolysis bullosa, staphylococcal scalded skin syndrome

Folk medicine practices: cupping, moxibustion

Impetigo

Chemical burns

Congenital indifference to pain

Chilblains

Herpes

Fixed drug eruption

Mechanical abrasion

Accidental burn

Table continued on following page

Table 3–5. Differential Diagnosis of Child Abuse *Continued*

Intracranial Bleeding

Aneurysm
Brain tumor
Hemorrhagic disease of the newborn
Folk medicine: treatment for "fallen fontanelle"
Meningitis

Eye Hemorrhage

Motor vehicle accident
Subconjunctival hemorrhages: Valsalva effect, hypertension, bleeding disorder, birth
    trauma
Periorbital ecchymosis: bleeding disorder, metastatic neuroblastoma, basilar skull frac-
    ture, forehead trauma
Anterior chamber hyphema: accidental trauma, forceps delivery, juvenile xanthogranu-
    lomatosis
Retinal hemorrhage: meningitis, hypertension, endocarditis, sepsis, vasculitis, bleeding
    disorder, thoracic compression and hypoxia, birth trauma, aneurysm

Fractures

Skeletal dysplasia: osteogenesis imperfecta, infantile cortical hyperostosis (Caffey's dis-
    ease), skeletal anomalies associated with chromosomal disorders
Infections: congenital syphilis, osteomyelitis
Nutritional and metabolic bone disease: rickets, scurvy, secondary hyperparathyroid-
    ism, mucolipidosis II, Menkes' kinky hair syndrome (copper deficiency)
Newborn: obstetric trauma (cephalohematoma, clavicular fracture), prematurity
Drug-induced skeletal reactions: methotrexate osteopathy, prostaglandin therapy, hy-
    pervitaminosis A
Neuromuscular disease: congenital insensitivity to pain, congenital spinal defects (sco-
    liosis, meningomyelocele), cerebral palsy
Innocent accidental trauma (toddler's fracture)
Neoplasm (leukemia)
Cardiopulmonary resuscitation (rare rib fractures), "passive exercise," stress fracture,
    physical therapy
Suboptimal radiographic study

---

medical developments. The clinician's role should remain that of a concerned
medical caretaker.

Disposition

If a case requires further assessment and diagnostic testing that cannot be
easily accomplished in the clinic or emergency room, the child should be admitted to the hospital. This is especially indicated if initial assessment suggests
that the child is at ongoing risk for maltreatment at home. Once inpatient medical

Table 3–6. Warning Signs for Child Abuse

Bruises

Extensive
Centrally located
Specific bruises suspicious for child maltreatment (pinch, slapped cheek, belt or strap, pinna or gluteal cleft, electric cord, rope burn or gag, bizarre shape)

Abrasions and Lacerations

Abrasions and lacerations in sites the infant or child cannot easily reach

Burns

Circumferential configuration
Uniform depth
Scalding second- or third-degree burn lacking splash marks
Dry contact burn in unusual area (soles, dorsum of hand, back, perineum)
Specific burns suspicious for child maltreatment (dunking, doughnut, stocking-glove, cigarette, microwave oven, stun gun)

Fractures

Multiple fractures in different stages of healing
Specific fractures virtually diagnostic of or suspicious for child maltreatment (metaphyseal, rib, acromion, vertebral body, sternal, proximal humerus, or spiral fractures before 9 months)

Abdominal Injuries

Clinical presentation of unexplained shock, peritonitis, anemia, recurrent bloody or bilious emesis
Abdominal wall bruises
Significant delay in seeking medical care
Specific intraabdominal injuries suspicious for child maltreatment in absence of severe accidental injury (ruptured liver or spleen, intestinal perforation, duodenal hematoma, intraperitoneal hemorrhage, rhabdomyolysis)

Head Injuries

Clinical presentation of unexplained respiratory distress, irritability, lethargy, hypotonia, seizures, coma, vomiting, or poor feeding when infectious, metabolic, or toxic causes are excluded
Tender, swollen periorbital ecchymoses
Specific skull fracture(s) suspicious for child maltreatment (multiple, bilateral, nonparietal, comminuted, depressed, stellate, growing, or diastatic)
Retinal, subdural, or subarachnoid hemorrhage in absence of history of motor vehicle accident or severe fall

Table continued on following page

Table 3–6. Warning Signs for Child Abuse *Continued*

History

Conflicting history between parents, between parent and child, or over time
Significant delay in seeking medical care
Repetitive patterns of injury
Absent, unavailable, or disinterested parent(s)
History inconsistent with estimated age of bruising
History inconsistent with estimated age of fracture
History inconsistent with force or mechanism required to produce observed injury
History inconsistent with developmental age and capability of victim (or reported abusive sibling)

Physical Examination

Multiple injuries
Multiple forms of injury
Multiple injuries at various stages of healing
Specific injuries highly suspicious for child maltreatment
Signs of concurrent medical or nutritional neglect

evaluation and therapy are complete, social service professionals evaluate the safety of returning to the family, begin appropriate family therapy, and arrange foster placement if necessary.

Documentation

Medical records must be thorough, accurate, and legible. The detailed medical history should include direct quotations from the child, parents, and siblings. In the physical examination each injury should be carefully described, and sketches and measurements may be included. Professional medical photography of injuries is highly recommended. The results of all laboratory and radiographic evaluations should be recorded, and pending results should be noted.

Because of the likelihood of having to give court testimony[82] in cases of severe or equivocal child abuse, the medical provider should treat the medical record as a legal document. The provider should not enter personal psychosocial and legal conclusions in the medical record.

SUMMARY

The spectrum of child abuse includes physical abuse, sexual abuse, psychologic abuse, and neglect. An estimated 10% of children less than 5 years of age who are brought to the emergency room with traumatic injuries have been maltreated. Any practitioner who is taking care of pediatric trauma patients is also caring for child abuse victims.

National surveys in the United States reveal escalating reports of child abuse, which now affects 45 of every 1000 children yearly. More than three children die each day in the United States from child abuse, half of these before their first birthday. In light of current family economic stresses, the problem is likely to escalate.

Medical professionals must have the courage to intervene in the private lives of families disrupted by child maltreatment. Reporting of suspected child maltreatment to the proper authorities will lead to psychosocial intervention that will begin family healing. First, however, medical providers must learn to recognize traumatic inflicted injuries masquerading as accidental trauma, in the emergency room, in the clinic, or in the neighborhood.

This chapter summarizes the recent explosion of available medical information about child maltreatment. Specific patterns of bruising, burns, abdominal injury, fractures, and head injury should raise concern of inflicted pediatric trauma. More than ever before, physicians caring for pediatric trauma patients have the medical information available to determine if a reasonable clinical suspicion of child abuse exists.

REFERENCES

1. Johnson CF: Inflicted injury versus accidental injury, *Pediatr Clin North Am* 34(4):791–814, 1990.
2. Reece RM, Grodin MA: Recognition of non-accidental trauma, *Pediatr Clin North Am* 32(1):41–60, 1985.
3. Chadwick DL: The diagnosis of inflicted injury in infants and young children, *Pediatr Ann* 21(8):477–483, 1992.
4. Hyden PW, Gallagher TA: Child abuse intervention in the emergency room, *Pediatr Clin North Am* 39(5):1053–1081, 1990.
5. Daro D, McCurdy K: *The National Center on Child Abuse Prevention Research: current trends in child abuse reporting and fatalities; the results of the 1992 annual fifty state survey,* Chicago, April 1993, National Committee for Prevention of Child Abuse (NCPCA).
6. Schlosser P, Pierpont J, Poertner J: Active surveillance of child abuse fatalities, *Child Abuse Neglect* 16(1):3–10, 1992.
7. Kaplan SR, Granik LA, eds: *Child fatality investigative procedures manual,* Child Maltreatment Fatalities Project, Chicago, 1991, American Bar Association and American Academy of Pediatrics.
8. Helfer RM: The etiology of child abuse, *Pediatrics* 51(4):777–779, 1973.
9. Helfer RE: The neglect of our children, *Pediatr Clin North Am* 37(4):923–942, 1990.
10. Jones ED, McCurdy K: The links between types of maltreatment and demographic characteristics of children, *Child Abuse Neglect* 16:201–215, 1992.
11. Frank DA, Zeisel SH: Failure-to-thrive, *Pediatr Clin North Am* 35(6):1187–1206, 1988.
12. Vissing YM, Straus MA, Gelles RT, Harrop JW: Verbal aggression by parents and psychosocial problems in children, *Child Abuse Neglect* 15(3):223–238, 1991.
13. Rosenberg DA: Web of deceit: a literature review of Munchausen syndrome by proxy, *Child Abuse Neglect* 11:547–563, 1987.

14. Alexander RC, Surrell JA, Cohle SD: Microwave oven burns to children: an unusual manifestation of child abuse, *Pediatrics* 79(2):255–260, 1987.

15. Bays J: Substance abuse and child abuse . . . impact of addiction on the child, *Pediatr Clin North Am* 37(4):881–904, 1990.

16. Pickel S, Anderson C, Holliday MA: Thirsting and hypernatremic dehydration—a form of child abuse, *Pediatrics* 45(1):54–59, 1970.

17. Baugh JR, Krieg EF, Weir MR: Punishment by salt poisoning, *South Med J* 76(4):540–541, 1983.

18. Cohle SD, Trestrail JD III, Graham MA, et al: Fatal pepper aspiration, *Am J Dis Child* 142(6):633–636, 1988.

19. Eichelberger SP, Beal DW, May RB: Hypovolemic shock in a child as a consequence of corporal punishment, *Pediatrics* 87(4):570–571, 1991.

20. Frechette A, Rimsza E: Stun gun injury: a new presentation of the battered child syndrome, *Pediatrics* 89(5):898–901, 1992.

21. Press S, Grant P, Thompson VT, Milles KL: Small bowel evisceration: unusual manifestation of child abuse, *Pediatrics* 88(4):807–809, 1991.

22. Reece RM: Unusual manifestations of child abuse, *Pediatr Clin North Am* 37(4):905–921, 1990.

23. Finkelhor D, Hotaling G, Lewis IA, Smith C: Sexual abuse in a national survey of adult men and women, *Child Abuse Neglect* 14(1):19–28, 1990.

24. Feldman W, Feldman E, Goodman JT, et al: Is childhood sexual abuse really increasing in prevalence? An analysis of the evidence. *Pediatrics* 88(1):29–33, 1991.

25. Woodling BA, Kossoris PD: Sexual misuse: rape, molestation, and incest, *Pediatr Clin North Am* 28(2):481–499, 1981.

26. Berliner L, Conte JR: The process of victimization: the victim's perspective, *Child Abuse Neglect* 14(1):29–40, 1990.

27. Singer MI, Hussey D, Strom KJ: Grooming the victim: analysis of a perpetrator's seduction letter, *Child Abuse Neglect* 16(6):877–886, 1992.

28. Beitchman JH, Zucker KJ, Hood JE, et al: A review of the long-term effects of child sexual abuse, *Child Abuse Neglect* 16(1):108–118, 1992.

29. Kinzl J, Bieble W: Long-term effects of incest: life events triggering mental disorders in female patients with sexual abuse in childhood, *Child Abuse Neglect* 16(4):567–573, 1992.

30. Greenwald E, Leitenberg H, Cado S, Tarran MJ: Childhood sexual abuse: long-term effects on psychological and sexual functioning in a nonclinical and nonstudent sample of adult women, *Child Abuse Neglect* 14(4):503–513, 1990.

31. Wozencraft T, Wagner W, Pellegrin A: Depression and suicidal ideation in sexually abused children, *Child Abuse Neglect* 15(4):505–511, 1991.

32. Dejong AR, Rose M: Frequency and significance of physical evidence in legally proven cases of child sexual abuse, *Pediatrics* 84(6):1022–1026, 1989.

33. Berkowitz CD: Sexual abuse of children and adolescents, *Adv Pediatr* 34:275–312, 1987.

34. Paradise JE: The medical evaluation of the sexually abused child, *Pediatr Clin North Am* 37(4):839–862, 1990.

35. Heger A (Sales TB, ed): Response—child sexual abuse: a medical view. New York, 1985, Guilford.

36. Levitt CJ: Sexual abuse in children: a compassionate yet thorough approach to evaluation, *Postgrad Med* 80(2):201–204, 213–215, 1986.

37. Chadwick DL, Berkowitz CD, Kerns D, et al: *Color atlas of child sexual abuse,* Chicago, 1989, Year Book.

38. Heger A, Emans SJ, eds: *Evaluation of the sexually abused child,* New York, 1992, Oxford University Press.

39. Bays J, Chadwick D: Medical diagnosis of the sexually abused child, *Child Abuse Neglect* 17(1):91–110, 1993.

40. Dejong AR, Finkel MA: Sexual abuse of children, *Curr Probl Pediatr* 20(9):489–567, 1990.

41. Committee on Child Abuse and Neglect, American Academy of Pediatrics: Guidelines for the evaluation of sexually abused children, *Pediatrics* 87(2):254–260, 1991.

42. Enos WF: Forensic evaluation of the sexually abused child, *Pediatrics* 78(3):385–398, 1986.

43. McCann J: Use of the colposcope in child sexual abuse examinations, *Pediatr Clin North Am* 37(4):863–880, 1990.

44. Pokorny SF, Pokorny WJ, Kramer W: Acute genital injury in the prepubertal child, *Am J Obstet Gynecol* 166(5):1461–1466, 1992.

45. Feldman KW: Patterned abusive bruises of buttocks and pinnae, *Pediatrics* 90(4):633–636, 1992.

46. Showers J: Scarring for life: abuse with electric cords, *Child Abuse Neglect* 10:25–31, 1989.

47. Gold MH, Roenigk HH, Smith S, Pierce LJ: Human bite marks: differential diagnosis, *Clin Pediatr* 28(7):329–331, 1989.

48. Sterne GG, Chadwick DL, Krugman RD, et al: Oral and dental aspects of child abuse and neglect, *Pediatrics* 78(3):537–539, 1986.

49. Hobbs CJ: Burns and scalds: ABCs of child abuse, *Br Med J* 298:1302–1305, 1989.

50. Feldman KW: Child abuse by burning. In Helfer RE, Kempe RS, eds: *The battered child,* ed 4, Chicago, 1987, University of Chicago Press, pp 197–213.

51. Leonidas JC: Skeletal trauma in the child abuse syndrome, *Pediatr Ann* 12:875–881, 1983.

52. Merten DF, Carpenter LM: Radiographic imaging of inflicted injury in the child abuse syndrome, *Pediatr Clin North Am* 37(4):815–837, 1990.

53. Kleinman PK, Marks SC, Blackbourne B: The metaphyseal lesion in abused infants: a radiologic-histopathologic study, *Am J Roentgenol* 146:895–905, 1986.

54. Leventhal JM, Thomas SA, Rosenfield NS, Markowitz RI: Fractures in young children, *Am J Dis Child* 147(1):87–92, 1993.

55. McCort J, Vaudagna J: Visceral injuries in battered children, *Radiology* 82:424–428, 1964.

56. Cooper A, Floyd T, Barlow B, et al: Major blunt abdominal trauma due to child abuse, *J Trauma* 28:1483–1486, 1988.

57. Coant PN, Kornberg AE, Brody AS, Edwards-Holmes K: Markers for occult liver injury in cases of physical abuse, *Pediatrics* 89(2):274–278, 1992.

58. Hennes HM, Smith DS, Schneider K, et al: Elevated liver transaminase levels in children with blunt abdominal trauma: a predictor of liver injury, *Pediatrics* 86:87–90, 1990.

59. Mukherji SK, Siegel MJ: Rhabdomyolysis and renal failure in child abuse, *Am J Roentgenol* 148:1203–1204, 1987.

60. Billmire ME, Myers PA: Serious head injury in infants: accident or abuse? *Pediatrics* 75(2):340–342, 1985.

61. Hobbs CJ: Skull fracture and the diagnosis of abuse, *Arch Dis Child* 59:246–252, 1984.

62. Duhaime AC, Alario AJ, Lewander WJ, et al: Head injury in very young children: mechanisms, injury types, and ophthalmologic findings in 100 hospitalized patients younger than 2 years of age, *Pediatrics* 90(2):179–185, 1992.

63. Chadwick DL, Chin S, Salerno C, et al: Deaths from falls in children: how far is fatal? *J Trauma* 31(10):1353–1355, 1991.

64. Williams RA: Injuries in infants and small children resulting from witnessed and corroborated free falls, *J Trauma* 31(10):1350–1352, 1991.

65. Eisenbrey AB: Retinal hemorrhage in the battered child, *Childs Brain* 5:40–44, 1979.

66. Caffey J: On the theory and practice of shaking infants, its potential residual effects of permanent brain damage and mental retardation, *Am J Dis Child* 124:161–169, 1972.

67. Caffey J: The whiplash shaken infant syndrome: manual shaking by the extremities with whiplash-induced intracranial and intraocular bleedings, linked with residual permanent brain damage and mental retardation, *Pediatrics* 54(4):396–403, 1974.

68. Duhaime AC, Gennarelli TA, Thibault LE, et al: The shaken baby syndrome: a clinical, pathological, and biomechanical study, *J Neurosurg* 66:409–415, 1987.

69. Hanigen WC, Peterson RA, Njus G: Tin ear syndrome: rotational acceleration in pediatric head injuries, *Pediatrics* 80(5):618–622, 1987.

70. Merten DF, Osborne DRS: Craniocerebral trauma in the child abuse syndrome, *Pediatr Ann* 12(12):882–887, 1983.

71. Han BK, Towbin RB, De Courten-Myers G, et al: Reversal sign on CT: effect on anoxic/ ischemic injury in children, *Am J Roentgenol* 154:361–368, 1990.

72. Newberger EH: Pediatric interview assessment of child abuse, *Pediatr Clin North Am* 37(4):943–954, 1990.

73. Section on Radiology, American Academy of Pediatrics: Diagnostic imaging of child abuse, *Pediatrics* 87(2):262–264, 1991.

74. Caffey J: Multiple fractures of long bones in children suffering from subdural hematoma, *Am J Roentgenol* 56:163–173, 1946.

75. Bays J: Conditions mistaken for child abuse. In Reece R, ed: *Child abuse: medical diagnosis and management,* Malvern, Pa, 1993, Lea & Febiger.

76. Bays J, Jenny C: Genital and anal conditions confused with child sexual abuse trauma, *Am J Dis Child* 144:1319–1322, 1990.

77. Brill PW, Winchester P: Differential diagnosis of child abuse. In Kleinman PK, ed: *Diagnostic imaging of child abuse,* Baltimore, 1987, Williams & Wilkins, pp 221–241.

78. Wheeler DM, Hobbs CJ: Mistakes in diagnosing non-accidental injury: 10 years experience, *Br Med J* 296:1233–1236, 1988.

79. Radkowski MA: The battered child syndrome: pitfalls in radiologic diagnosis, *Pediatr Ann* 12(12):894–903, 1983.

80. Putnam M, Stein M: Self-inflicted injuries in childhood, *Clin Pediatr* 24(9):514–518, 1985.

81. Levin A: Ophthalmic manifestations. In Ludwig S, Kornberg AE, eds: *Child abuse: a medical reference,* New York, 1992, Churchill Livingstone, pp 191–212.

82. Chadwick DL: Preparation for court testimony in child abuse cases, *Pediatr Clin North Am* 37(4):955–970, 1990.

ACUTE CARE OF THE INJURED CHILD

Edward G. Ford

When initially seen by the community emergency department, children with traumatic injuries may have compromise of multiple organ systems. Several authors have designed injury "scores" or tabular evaluations to allow objective evaluation of trauma patients by the community primary health care providers. Such scoring systems categorize the patients' disease severity to allow appropriate and expeditious triage to facilities with the resources necessary to support each patient. Early tabulations were designed to specify mechanism, location, and extent of injury to a given body system. For example, the Glasgow Coma Scale (GCS) is an indicator of severity and projected outcome in head-injured patients (Table 4–1).[1] Such scores have a limited focus and do not convey the overall severity of injury for a patient with multiple organ system trauma.

Scales were next developed to help clinicians classify and study the multiply injured trauma victim. The scales are of two basic types: anatomy based and physiology based.

Anatomic scores focus only on the number of anatomic injuries and the degree of injuries suffered by the patient. Such scores include the Injury Severity Score (ISS; Table 4–2)[2,3] and the Anatomic Index (AI; Table 4–3).[4] These scores provide information only about the type and number of anatomic disruptions. They do not provide information about the physiologic alterations that accompany the anatomic injuries.

The physiologic scores (Trauma Index,[5] Illness/Injury Severity Index,[6] Triage Index,[7] Trauma Score,[8] and APACHE score[9,10]), record alterations in the patient's physiologic status as reflected in changes in blood pressure, heart rate, level of consciousness, and respirations (Tables 4–4 to 4–9). For the most part, these scores and tabulations are large, cumbersome, and not well suited to pediatric patients.

The Modified Injury Severity Scale (MISS) was developed to rectify the apparent shortcomings of the adult scoring systems by considering normal values for children (Table 4–10).[11] The MISS documents multiple prehospital aspects

95

Table 4–1. Glasgow Coma Scale Score

1. Eye opening		
	Spontaneous	4
	To voice	3
	To pain	2
	None	1
2. Verbal response		
	Oriented	5
	Confused	4
	Inappropriate	3
	Incomprehensible words	2
	None	1
3. Motor response		
	Obeys commands	6
	Purposeful movement (pain)	5
	Withdraw (pain)	4
	Flexion (pain)	3
	Extension (pain)	2
	None	1
Total GCS points (1 + 2 + 3) _____		

of care (e.g., mode and mechanism of injury, prehospital medical care, transport) and describes injured body systems at length. MISS anatomic descriptions are primarily subjective, so evaluations by several different investigators may lead to varying scores for the same patient.

Tepas and colleagues[12] designed the Pediatric Trauma Score (PTS) to be a short, concise, objective triage tool that takes into consideration the differences between children and adults (Table 4–11). It provides a scoring system that can be easily used and understood by all members of the health care team, from the first-on-scene emergency medical technicians to the emergency department physician to the accepting physician at a tertiary referral center.[13] This chapter focuses on the PTS. Occasionally, tertiary care providers are unfamiliar with the PTS, so for reference all the standard scoring systems are presented in tabular form.

PEDIATRIC TRAUMA SCORE

For each of the six categories of the PTS the patient is assigned a grade: −1 for the most severely injured children, +1 for moderately injured, or +2 for minor or no injury. The sum of the scores from the six categories represents the pediatric trauma score (see Table 4–11). The six components of the PTS

Text continued on page 101

Table 4–2. Sample Section of the Injury Severity Score

Injury Description	Code
Head (Face, Including Ear and Eye)	
Whole area	
Skin (including eyelid, lip and external ear) [see EXTERNAL]	
Penetrating injury	
NFS	30101.1
No tissue loss	30102.1
Superficial tissue loss	30103.2
Major tissue loss	30104.3
Nerves (see CRANIAL NERVES, HEAD)	
Vessels (see NECK)	
Internal organs	
Ear injury NFS	30201.1
Ear canal injury	30301.1
Inner or middle ear injury	30401.1
Ossicular chain (ear bone) dislocation	30501.2
Tympanic membrane (ear drum) rupture	30601.2
Eye injury NFS	30701.1
Canaliculus (tear duct) laceration	30801.1
Choroid rupture	30901.1
Conjunctive injury	31001.1
Cornea	
NFS	31101.1
Abrasion	31102.1
Contusion	31103.1
Laceration	31104.2

From American Association for Automative Medicine: Abbreviated Injury Scale, 1985
The Injury Severity Score was developed in an attempt to render the Abbreviated Injury Scale (AIS) more usable. The AIS is a booklet of 68 pages that assigns injury severity via a complex system of scoring based on International Classification of Diseases (ICD) codes. Each injury is characterized by body area—(1) head or neck, (2) face, (3) chest, (4) abdominal or pelvic contents, (5) extremities, (6) pelvic girdle, (7) general—and by severity—1 minor; 2 moderate: 3 severe, not life threatening; 4 severe, life threatening, survival probable; 5 critical, survival uncertain. The Injury Severity Score (ISS) is the sum of the squares of the highest AIS grade in each of the three most severely injured areas. Use of the ISS has dramatically increased correlation between severity of injury and mortality, but the scoring system is extremely cumbersome to use.

Table 4–3. Anatomic Index

HICDA-8 Code	Diagnosis		Conditional Probability (p)	Effective Probability (p)
800.0	Fractured vault of skull (closed)		0.28	0.13
800.1	Fractured vault of skull (open)		0.38	0.18
801.0	Fractured base of skull (closed)		0.32	0.19
801.1	Fractured base of skull (open)		0.38	0.22
802.0	Fractured nasal bones (closed)		0.13	0
802.1	Fractured nasal bones (open)		0.12	0
802.2	Fractured mandible (closed)		0.18	0
802.3	Fractured mandible (open)		0.08	0
802.4	Other facial features (closed)		0.17	0
802.5	Other facial features (open)		0.18	0
805.0	Fractured cervical spine (closed)		0.24	0.10
805.1	Fractured cervical spine (open)	*Without*	1.00	1.00
805.2	Fractured thoracic spine (closed)	*cord*	0.04	0
805.3	Fractured thoracic spine (open)	*lesion*	0	0
805.4	Fractured lumbar spine (closed)		0.04	0
806.0	Fractured cervical spine (closed)		0.23	0.21
806.2	Fractured thoracic spine (closed)	*With*	0	0
806.4	Fractured lumbar spine (closed)	*cord*	0.11	0
806.6	Fractured sacrum and coccyx (closed)	*lesion*	0	0
807.0	Fractured ribs (closed)		0.23	.02
807.2	Fractured sternum (closed)		0.20	0
807.6	Flail chest		0.33	.30
808.0	Fractured pelvis (closed)		0.18	.07
808.1	Fractured pelvis (open)		0.33	.33
810.0	Fractured clavicle (closed)		0.17	0
811.0	Fractured scapula (closed)		0.12	0
812.0	Fractured upper end of humerus (closed)		0.04	0
812.2	Fractured shaft humerus (closed)		0.43	0
812.3	Fractured shaft humerus (open)		0.31	0
812.4	Fractured lower humerus (closed)		0.15	0
813.0	Fractured upper radius and ulna (closed)		0.21	0

The Anatomic Index (AI) was developed to circumvent the cumbersome nature of the Abbreviated Severity Injury scale and the Injury Severity Score (ISS). The ISS is determined by data abstracted from hospital records by trained personnel, and its rankings of severity are based on subjective impression. The AI is based on expected mortality from HICDA codes. This information is readily extracted from hospital records by computer-based systems and personnel with little or no medical training.

Table 4–3. Anatomic Index *Continued*

HICDA-8 Code	Diagnosis	Conditional Probability (p)	Effective Probability (p)
813.1	Fractured upper radius and ulna (open)	0.14	0
813.2	Fractured shaft radius and ulna (closed)	0.15	0
813.3	Fractured shaft radius and ulna (open)	0	0
813.4	Fractured lower radius and ulna (closed)	0.04	0
813.5	Fractured lower radius and ulna (open)	0	0
814.0/1	Fractured carpal bones	0.18	0
815.0	Fractured metacarpal bones	0.10	0
820.0	Fractured neck of femur (closed)	0.32	0
820.1	Fractured neck of femur (open)	0	0
820.2	Fractured trochanteric section (closed)	0.14	0
820.3	Fractured trochanteric section (open)	0	0
820.4	Fractured femur (closed)	0.22	0
820.5	Fractured femur (open)	0	0
821.0	Fractured shaft (closed)	0.31	.02
821.1	Fractured shaft (open)	0.17	0
821.2	Fractured lower end femur (closed)	0.11	N/A
821.3	Fractured lower end femur (open)	0.21	0
822.0	Fractured patella (closed)	0.04	N/A
822.1	Fractured patella (open)	0.21	0
823.0	Fractured upper tibia and fibula (closed)	0.32	0.01
823.1	Fractured upper tibia and fibula (open)	0.18	0.03
823.2	Fractured shaft tibia and fibula (closed)	0.10	0
823.3	Fractured shaft tibia and fibula (open)	0.08	0
824.0	Fractured ankle (closed)	0.15	0
824.1	Fractured ankle (open)	0.08	0
825.0	Fractured tarsal or metatarsal (closed)	0.09	0
825.1	Fractured tarsal or metatarsal (open)	0	0
826.0	Fractured phalanges foot (closed)	0	0
826.1	Fractured phalanges foot (open)	0	0
831.0	Dislocation of shoulder	0.09	0
832.0	Dislocation of elbow	0	0
833.0	Dislocation of wrist	0	0
835.0	Dislocation of hip	0.08	0
836.0	Dislocation of knee	0.33	0.14
837.0	Dislocation of ankle	0	0
838.0	Dislocation of foot	0	0
850.0	Concussion	0.03	0.02
851.0	Cerebral contusion (closed)	0.25	0.05
851.1	Cerebral contusion (open)	0.56	0.67
851.2	Cerebral contusion (mild)	0.73	0.14
851.3	Cerebral contusion (moderate)	0.69	0.67
851.4	Cerebral contusion (severe)	0.82	0.83
851.5	Cerebral laceration	1.00	1.00

Table continued on following page

Table 4–3. Anatomic Index *Continued*

HICDA-8 Code	Diagnosis	Conditional Probability (p)	Effective Probability (p)
851.6	Brain stem contusion	0.52	0.48
851.7	Cerebellar contusion	N/A	N/A
851.8	Brain stem or cerebellar laceration	1.00	1.00
852.0	Intracranial hemorrhage	0.53	0.52
852.2	Extradural hemorrhage	0.33	0.33
852.3	Subdural (acute hemorrhage)	0.44	0.44
852.6	Subarachnoid hemorrhage	0.50	0.50
853.0	Other intracranial hemorrhage	0.56	0.40
853.2	Cerebral hemorrhage	0.33	N/A
854.1	Unspecified head injury	0.70	0.70
860.0	Pneumohemothorax	0.31	0.18
861.0	Myocardial contusion	0.44	0.44
861.2	Lung contusion or laceration	0.23	0.10
862.0	Ruptured aorta, bronchus, esophagus	0.43	0.37
863.0	Injury to GI tract	0.23	0.25
864.0	Closed liver injury	0.35	0.30
865.0	Closed splenic injury	0.31	0.10
866.0	Closed kidney injury	0.38	0.25
867.0	Closed injury to pelvic organs	0.44	0.42
868.0	Other intraabdominal injuries	0.31	0.17
870.0	Eye injury	0.04	0.12
870.1	Complicated eye injury	0.17	0
872.0	Ear injury	0.06	0
873.0	Scalp lacerations	0.12	0.01
873.2	Nasal laceration	0	0
873.7	Facial lacerations	0.10	0.01
874.0	Neck lacerations	0.17	0
874.1	Complicated neck lacerations	0.19	0.06

Table 4–4. Trauma Index

	1	3	4	6
Region	Skin or extremities	Back	Chest or abdomen	Head or neck
Type of injury	Laceration or contusion	Stab wound	Blunt	Missile
Cardiovascular status	External hemorrhage	Blood pressure <100 Pulse >100	Blood pressure <80 Pulse >140	Absent pulses
Central nervous system status	Drowsy	Stupor	Motor or sensory loss	Coma
Respiratory status	Chest pain	Dyspnea or hemoptysis	Evidence of aspiration	Apnea or cyanosis

Table 4–5. Illness/Injury Severity Index

Parameter Scored	Point Score			
	0	1	2	3
Pulse	60–100	<60 (100–140)	>140 or irregular	Absent
BP $\left(\dfrac{\text{systolic}}{\text{diastolic}}\right)$	100–150 / 60–90	80–100, 150–200 / 90–120	<80, >200 / >120	Absent
Skin color	Dry and normal	Reddish coloration	Ashen and/or moist	Cyanotic
Respiratory condition	12–20 resp.	≥20	<12 or labored breathing or chest pain	Absent respirations
Consciousness	Alert and oriented	Incoherent or obtunded	Difficult to awaken	Unconscious
Bleeding	None	Controllable	Hard to control	Uncontrollable
Region of injury	Extremities	Back	Chest	Head, neck, abdomen
Type of injury	Laceration, contusion	Fracture	Stab wound	Blunt trauma, missile

Add 1 point for patients under 2 or over 60 years of age.

Total _____

The Illness/Injury Severity Index is a triage tool developed for emergency medical technicians to indicate those patients who may be released from the hospital, admitted to the hospital, or admitted to critical care areas. A score of 0, 1, 2, or 3 is given for each of six clinical conditions. Predictably, a score of 0–6 results in release of the patient from the emergency department, patients with a score of 6–13 will be admitted to the hospital, those with scores of 14–24 will most likely be admitted to critical care areas of the hospital including surgery, the intensive care unit, or coronary care unit, and a score of 24 or greater predicts patient death in the emergency department.

include body weight, patency of the airway, central nervous system activity, blood pressure, wounds, and skeletal injuries.

Size

The most obvious difference between adults and children is a disparity in size. Differences in mass lead to differences in relative momentum achieved during a traumatic event; that is, equal amounts of force applied during a traumatic episode (e.g., motor vehicle accident, fall) are dissipated less and dispersed more extensively in smaller persons. Relatively high-energy injuries produce multiple-system injury in a child as a rule, rather than as an exception.

Smaller children, with a relatively large body surface area, are at risk for heat transmission by convection and conduction and for direct heat and water transfer to the environment by surface moisture evaporation. As the core temperature drops, the child is placed at risk for coagulopathy and cardiac arrhythmias, either of which may prove fatal to an unstable trauma patient. If severe enough, loss of water to the environment may further complicate the child's hemodynamic status.

Table 4–6. Triage Index

Variable	Definition	Score
Respiratory expansion (visual inspection of chest wall movement)	Normal	0
	Shallow	2
	Retractive	2
	None	3
Capillary refill (nail bed or finger pad pressure)	Immediate (less than 2 seconds)	0
		2
Eye opening (spoken or shouted verbal commands or standard pain stimulus)	Delayed (more than 2 seconds)	0
	Spontaneous	1
	To voice	2
	To pain	3
	None	
Verbal response (conversational ability, e.g., sentences, words only, sounds only)	Oriented	0
	Confused	1
	Inappropriate words	2
	Incomprehensible words	3
	None	4
Motor response (spoken or shouted verbal commands or standard pain stimulus)	Obedience	0
	Withdrawal	1
	Flexion	2
	Extension	3
	None	4

Children larger than 20 kg are considered relatively hearty and assigned a +2 score. Children less than 10 kg are considered fragile and are assigned a −1 score. Children of intermediate size (10 to 20 kg) receive a score of +1.

Airway

Anatomic variations in the younger age groups may make the attainment and maintenance of a secure airway difficult. In smaller children the midface is disproportionately smaller than the cranium. The unconscious child's head may lie on the chest in such a way that the upper airway "buckles" and obstructs the flow of air (see Chapter 1). The neutral or "sniffing" position of the child's head, in relation to the axial spine and chest, is usually sufficient to correct any apparent airway obstruction.

Intubation of the small child is difficult. Laryngeal structures are considerably smaller than in older children, and the larynx is relatively anterior. In the very young the epiglottis is quite large and may obscure the larynx. Orotracheal intubation may be attempted with an assistant maintaining axial cervical traction.

Table 4–7. Trauma Score

Trauma Score		Value	Points	Score
A. Respiratory rate		10–24	4	
Number of respirations in 15 seconds, multiply by 4		25–35	3	
		>35	2	
		<10	1	
		0	0	A. _____
B. Respiratory effort				
Shallow—markedly decreased chest movement or air exchange		Normal	1	
Retractive—use of accessory muscles or intercostal retraction		Shallow or retractive	0	B. _____
C. Systolic blood pressure		>90	4	
Systolic cuff pressure—either arm, auscultate or palpate		70–90	3	
		50–69	2	
		<50	1	
No carotid pulse		0	0	C. _____
D. Capillary refill				
Normal—forehead, lip mucosa, or nail bed color refill in 2 seconds		Normal	2	
Delayed—more than 2 seconds of capillary refill		Delayed	1	
None—no capillary refill		None	0	D. _____
E. Glasgow Coma Scale		Total GCS Points	Score	
1. Eye opening				
Spontaneous	4			
To voice	3			
To pain	2			
None	1			
2. Verbal response				
Oriented	5	14–15	5	
Confused	4	11–13	4	
Inappropriate words	3	8–10	3	
Incomprehensible words	2	5–7	2	
None	1	3–4	1	E. _____
3. Motor response				
Obeys commands	6			
Purposeful movement (pain)	5			
Withdraw (pain)	4			
Flexion (pain)	3			
Extension (pain)	2			
None	1			
Total GCS Points (1 + 2 + 3) _____			Trauma Score _____ (Total points A + B + C + D + E)	

Table 4–8. APACHE Scoring System (Acute Physiology Score*)

Points	+4	+3	+2
Cardiovascular			
Heart rate ventricular response (beats/min)	≥180	141–179	111–140
Mean blood pressure (mm Hg)	≥160	131–159	111–130
Right atrial pressure/central venous pressure (mm Hg)			≥26
CPK-MB or ECG evidence of acute myocardial infarction	Yes		
ECG arryhthmias		Atrial arrhythmias + hemodynamic instability	Atrial arrhythmias alone
Serum lactate (mEq/L)	>8	3.5–8	
Blood pH	≥7.7	7.6–7.69	
Respiratory			
Respiratory rate, total nonventilated (breaths/min)	≥50	35–49	26–34
P(A-a)O₂ (100%) or †	>500	351–499	
Paco₂ (mm Hg)	≥70	61–69	50–60
Renal			
Urine output/day			≥5 L
Serum blood urea nitrogen (mg/dl)	>150	101–150	81–100
Serum creatinine (mg/dl	>7	3.6–7	2.1–3.5
Gastrointestinal			
Serum amylase (IU)	≥2000	500–1999	
Serum albumin (mg/dl)	>8		
Bilirubin (total) (mg/dl)		≥15	5.1–14.9
Serum alkaline phosphatase (IU)			>160

*The Acute Physiology Score establishes physiologic injury severity based on laboratory evaluation.
ECG, Electrocardiographic; *CSF*, cerebrospinal fluid.
†P(A-a)O₂ = (FIO₂[713] − PaO₂).
‡Total anergy is no response to any provocative skin tests, including mumps and fungal. Relative anergy is reduced response to skin tests medicative of compromised cellular immunity.

Lifting the jaw with a laryngoscope usually allows adequate visualization of the laryngeal structures and tracheal cannulation.

In a child the normal angle of passage from the nasopharynx into the larynx is an acute angle, which makes nasotracheal intubation difficult if not impossible. In the child suffering a significant head injury, there is a substantial risk of passing a nasotracheal tube into the sphenoid sinus, or directly through the cribriform plate into the brain. Nasotracheal intubation should be avoided in a child with acute traumatic injury.

Bag-mask ventilation is a reasonable option for airway maintenance when

+1	0	+1	+2	+3	+4
	70–110		56–69	41–55	≤40
	70–110		51–69		≤50
16–25	1–15	<1			
	No				
				>6 periventricular contractions/min	Ventricular tachycardia or fibrillation
0–3.4 7.51–7.59	7.33–7.5		7.25–7.32	7.15–7.24	<7.15
	12–25	10–11	7–9		≤6
200–350	<200				
	30–49		25–29	20–24	<20
3501–4888 ml	700–3500 ml		480–699 ml (20–29 ml/hr)	120–479 ml (5–20 ml/hr)	<120 ml/day
21–80	10–20				
1.6–2	0.6–1.5	<0.6	<10		
	≥500				
	3.5–8	2.5–3.4	<2.5		
0–5					
0–160					

Table continued on following page

direct endotracheal intubation is unlikely. In the event of bag-mask ventilation an orogastric tube should be placed to decompress the stomach. Positive pressure from bag-mask ventilation invariably forces a substantial amount of air down the esophagus and into the stomach. Distention of the stomach may cause a vasovagal reflex response with profound bradycardia and hypotension, which may complicate emergency management. Maintenance of cervical axial traction and close attention to providing a tight fit of the mask over an infant's or child's face are keys to successful ventilatory management.

If the injuried child's airway is completely patent and the child is supporting

Table 4–8. APACHE Scoring System (Acute Physiology Score*) *Continued*

Points	+4	+3	+2
Gastrointestinal *Continued*			
Serum glutamic oxaloacetic transaminase			≥1500
Anergy‡	Total		Relative
Hematologic			
Hematocrit (%)	>60		51–60
White blood cell count (total) (per mm³)	>40,000		20,001–40,000
Platelets (per mm³)			>1,000,000
Prothrombin time (in sec > control), no anticoagulants	>12	5.1–12	3.1–5
Septic			
CSF positive culture	Yes		
Blood positive culture	Yes		
Fungal positive culture	Blood and/or CSF	Two sites other than blood or CSF	
Temperature (degrees celsius, rectal)	>41.0	39.1–40.0	
Metabolic			
Serum calcium (mg/dl)	≥16		14–15.9
Serum glucose (mg/dl)	>800	500–800	
Serum sodium (mEq/L)	>180	161–180	156–160
Serum potassium (mEq/L)	>7	6.1–7	
Serum HCO₃ (mmole/L)		>40	
Serum osmolarity (mOsm)	>350	321–350	
Neurologic			
Glasgow Coma Score	3	4–6	7–9

his or her own respiration, a score of +2 is assigned. If moderate measures, such as nasal oxygen or an oral airway, are necesary to support ventilation, a score of +1 is assigned. If invasive procedures, such as intubation or cricothyroidotomy, are required to maintain the airway, a score of −1 is assigned.

Central Nervous System Status

Seventy percent of children who die of multiple traumatic injuries have head injuries as part of their disease complex. The most important prognostic factor in evaluation of the central nervous system is a *history* of loss of consciousness. Regardless of how awake and alert the patient appears when initially encountered, any child who has lost consciousness should be considered potentially seriously injured. Adverse effects occur not only from a direct and

+1	0	+1	+2	+3	+4
101–1499	None				
47–50	30–46		20–29		<20
15,001–20,000	3,000–15,000		1,000–2,999		<1,000
600,001–1,000,000	80,000–600,000		20,000–79,999		<20,000
	0–3				
	No				
	No				
One site other than blood or CSF	None				
38.6–39.0	36.0–38.5	34.0–35.9	32–33.9	30.0–31.9	≤29.9
11.1–13.9	8–11.0		5.0–7.9		<5
251–499	70–250		50–69	30–49	<30
151–155	130–150		120–129	110–119	<110
5.6–6	3.5–5.5	3–3.4	2.5–2.9		<2.5
31–40	20–30	10–19		5–9	<5
301–320	260–300		240–259	220–239	<220
10–12	13–15				

apparently insignificant blow, but also from a subsequent intracranial hemorrhage or cerebral edema. A child may be lucid and alert immediately after the injury but quickly deteriorate and die as a result of unrecognized intracranial traumatic changes.

The PTS divides children with head injuries into three distinct groups. The patient who is totally awake without signs of head injury and without a *history* of loss of consciousness is assigned a +2. The child who is comatose or decerebrate or who has unmistakeable severe injury to the central nervous system is scored a −1. Most children fall between these extremes. They are unresponsive but manifest some degree of impaired response, or they have a history of central nervous system changes (loss of consciousness). These children are assigned a score of +1.

Table 4–9. APACHE Scoring System (Chronic Health Evaluation*)

Qualifying Questions†	Chronic Health Evaluation	Brief Description
Did the patient have weekly visits to a physician? Was the patient unable to work because of illness? Was the patient bedridden or institutionalized because of illness? Had the patient suffered a relapse after systemic treatment for carcinoma?	D	Severe restriction of activity due to disease; includes persons bedridden or institutionalized due to illness
Was the patinet's usual daily activity limited? Did symptoms occur with mild exertion? Had the patient received treatment for neoplasm with remission or uncomplicated hemodialysis?	C	Chronic disease producing serious but not incapacitating restriction of activity
Did the patient see a physician monthly? Did the patient take medication chronically? Was the patient mildly limited in activity level because of illness? Had the patient had diabetes mellitus, chronic renal failure, a bleeding disorder, or chronic anemia?	B	Mild to moderate limitations of activity because of a chronic medical problem
(Negative response to all of the above questions.)	A	Prior good health; no functional limitations

*The Chronic Health Evaluation provides scores for follow-up of the acute injury.
†All answers are based on health status 3 to 6 months before admission.

Circulation

Exsanguinating hemorrhage may occur through obvious external wounds, by bleeding into the thoracic cavity, by hemorrhage into the abdominal cavity, or by hemorrhage into the retroperitoneal tissues. In a hypotensive patient a simple physical examination usually identifies sources of exsanguinating hemorrhage. Loss of bilateral breath sounds, a distended abdomen, obvious external wounds, or severe orthopedic malformations may be clues to a significant hemorrhage. A simple scalp laceration may appear innocent, but the vascularity of the region may allow exsanguination. The degree of such blood loss may not be realized until the patient is rolled on his or her side to inspect the back and is then found to be lying in a large pool of blood.

Although "normal" vital signs vary widely depending on the child's age, a child with a systolic blood pressure of less than 50 mm Hg or a child whose pulse is palpable only at the neck or groin probably has sustained a severe hemorrhagic injury. This type of patient requires an aggressive approach to volume support. Ringer's lactate solution remains within the vascular space and is an efficient adjunct to blood pressure support. Heta-Starch (Hespan, McGaw, Inc.) can also be used as a short-term volume expander, beginning with a 20 ml/kg bolus.

The PTS assigned to children with a systolic blood pressure of 90 mm Hg or greater is +2 (minimally injured). A +1 is assigned if the pressure is 50 to 90 mm Hg, and −1 if the pressure is 50 mm Hg or less.

Occasionally, proper-size blood pressure cuffs are not available. The blood pressure portion of the PTS may then be assessed by assigning a score of +2 for a pulse palpable at the wrist, +1 for a pulse palpable only at the carotid artery or groin, and −1 for no palpable pulse.

Skeletal Injuries

Orthopedic injuries are the most common pathologic traumatic changes in pediatric trauma patients. Orthopedic injuries may play a significant role in the early phases of the management of acute injury by being the source of inconspicuous but significant hemorrhage. Limb dysfunction also complicates long-term management by necessitating recumbency and eventual rehabilitative support.

Orthopedic injuries occur not only in the extremities, where they are obvious, but also to a significant extent in central areas such as the cranial vault and pelvis. Pelvic fractures with lacerations of the retroperitoneal pelvic veins may quickly lead to a patient's death if the retroperitoneal hemorrhage remains unrecognized.

The PTS assigns a +2 for patients without orthopedic injuries, a +1 for simple closed fractures, and −1 for multiple open or closed fractures.

Cutaneous Wounds

Interruptions of the integument that seem minor in adults may be significant in children because of their smaller body surface area. Multiple abrasions, minor burns, and lacerations that appear trivial may actually have an adverse affect on survival or recovery of the injured child. A major penetrating injury (stab wound, gunshot wound, or shotgun wound) must be considered a significant threat to the life of a child.

A child without cutaneous injury receives a score of +2, a child with minor wounds a +1, and a child with major open wounds, penetrating wounds, or tissue loss a −1.

The PTS has proved to be an effective scoring system in pooled patient populations. When 615 children entered into the National Pediatric Trauma Registry from April 1985 to December 1985 were compared on the basis of ISS and PTS, the comparison showed a statistically significant similarity

Table 4–10. Modified Injury Severity Score

	Score	Minor (1)	Moderate (2)
Neurologic	1	GCS 15	GCS 13–14
	2		
	3		
	4		
	5		
Face and neck	1	Abrasion/contusion of ocular apparatus, lid	Undisplaced facial bone fracture
	2		
	3	Vitreous or conjuctival hemorrhage	Laceration of eye, disfiguring laceration
	4		
	5	Fractured teeth	Retinal detachment
Chest	1	Muscle ache or chest wall stiffness	Simple rib or sternal fracture
	2		Major abdominal wall contusion
	3		
	4		
	5		
Abdomen	1	Muscle ache, seat belt abrasion	
	2		
	3		
	4		
	5		
Extremities	1	Minor sprains	Compound fracture
	2	Simple fractures/dislocations	Undisplaced long-bone or pelvic fractures
	3		
	4		
	5		

Calculation of MISS

	Score	Squared	
Neurologic	_____	_____	0 = No Injury
Facial and neck	_____	_____	1 = Minor
Chest	_____	_____	2 = Moderate
Abdomen	_____	_____	3 = Severe, but not life threatening
Extremities and pelvis	_____	_____	4 = Severe, life threatening, survival probable
			5 = Critical, survival uncertain

MISS score _____
(3 most severe only)

The MISS retains the Abbreviated Injury Scale (AIS) categories of injury, with the exception of deletion of the category "General" and substitution of a Glasgow Coma Scale (GCS) score for the neurologic injury category. The MISS is an improved method of scoring as compared with the AIS and the Injury Severity Scale. However, the scoring system is still quite cumbersome and subjectively based.

Severe, Not Life Threatening (3)	Severe, Life Threatening (4)	Critical, Survival Uncertain (5)
GCS 9–12	GCS 5–8	GCS ≤4
Loss of eye, avulsion optic nerve Displaced facial fractures "Blow-out" fractures of orbit	Bony or soft tissue injury with minor destruction	Injuries with major airway obstruction
Multiple rib fractures Hemothorax or pneumothorax Diaphragmatic rupture Pulmonary contusion	Open chest wounds Pneumomediastinum Myocardial contusion	Laceration of trachea, hemomediastinum Aortic laceration Myocardial laceration or rupture
Contusion of abdominal organ Retroperitoneal hematoma Extraperitoneal bladder rupture Thoracic/lumbar spine fractures	Minor laceration of abdominal organs Intraperitoneal bladder rupture Spine fractures with paraplegia	Rupture or severe laceration of abdominal vessels or organs
Displaced long-bone or multiple hand/foot fractures Single open long-bone fractures Pelvic fracture with displacement Laceration of major nerves/vessels	Multiple closed long bone fractures Amputation of limbs	Multiple open long bone fractures

Table 4–11. Pediatric Trauma Score

Score	+2	+1	−1
Size	≥20 kg	10–20 kg	<10 kg
Airway	Normal	Maintainable	Unmaintainable
Systolic blood pressure	≤90 mm Hg	50–90 mm Hg	<50 mm Hg
Central nervous system	Awake	Obtunded/loss of consciousness	Coma/decerebrate
Open wound	None	Minor	Major/penetrating
Skeletal	None	Closed fracture	Open/multiple fractures

($p < .001$). Tepas compared 170 children in combined retrospective and prospective series and also determined that the PTS accurately reflected the degree of injury and outcome when compared with the ISS, which is a significant similarity ($p < .001$).

UNIVERSITY OF TEXAS HEALTH SCIENCE CENTER AT HOUSTON EXPERIENCE

During one calendar year, 34,607 patients were seen in the emergency center of our institution, the University of Texas Health Science Center at Houston; 4867 (14%) were children up to 15 years of age. The pediatric surgical service evaluated and admitted 333 children (7.3%) for management of polytrauma.

Data presented here represent a retrospective review of 327 patient records. The average monthly number of admissions from January through April is double that for the remainder of the year (41 versus 19). Patients were relatively evenly distributed among age groups.

Seventy-one patients were transported via Life-Flight helicopter ambulance service. Of these, 42 came directly from the scene of the injury and 29 were transferred from local hospital emergency centers. Thirty-nine patients arrived by ground ambulance, 27 directly from the accident scene and 12 from local emergency centers. Thirty-nine patients were brought by private ambulance. The mode of arrival is not specified in 181 records.

Forty-three patients were passengers in motor vehicle accidents (Fig. 4–1). Auto-pedestrian accidents accounted for the injuries of 36 patients, 24 patients were injured in motorcycle accidents, 109 in falls, 16 by firearms (15 by single missiles and 1 by shotgun), and 24 by "other" penetrating wounds (stabbing). Nineteen patients suffered near-drowning, 10 ingested harmful substances, 29 had thermal burns, and 17 were hurt playing sports.

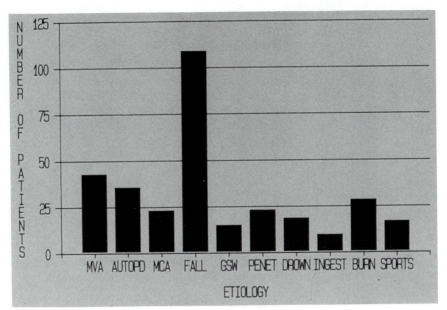

Figure 4–1. Causes of traumatic injuries in the Houston experience. The preponderance of injuries resulted from motor vehicle accidents and falls. *MVA,* motor vehicle accident; *Auto Ped,* auto-pedestrian accident; *MCA,* motorcycle accident; *GSW,* gunshot wound; *Penet,* penetrating injury other than gunshot wounds; *Ingest,* ingestions.

Of the 10 body region categories specified, the most commonly injured was the head region (230) (Fig. 4–2). Of the head-injured patients, 138 (60%) had intracranial damage. Twelve had open skull injuries, 40 had closed skull fractures, seven had subdural hematomas, and two had cervical cord injuries. In addition, 72 of the head-injured patients (31%) had soft tissue injuries, 13 (6%) had facial fractures, and 18 (8%) had eye injuries.

Among the 92 patients with extracranial head injuries, 8 (8.6%) suffered neck injuries (esophagus 1, trachea 2, soft tissue 6). Eight of these patients sustained chest wall injuries, and 13 (14%) had intrathoracic injuries (pulmonary contusion 3, hemothorax 1, pneumothorax 3, tension pneumothorax 3, other 5).

Nine patients underwent exploratory laparotomy. Injured organs included the small bowel 1, liver 2, spleen 2, and other 3. Ten patients had genitourinary injuries, all of which were managed nonoperatively (kidney 4, urethra 1, bladder 1, other 5). Two patients had vascular injuries, one to the subclavian artery and the other to the femoral artery.

Orthopedic injuries in 39 patients included closed pelvic fractures 6, ankle

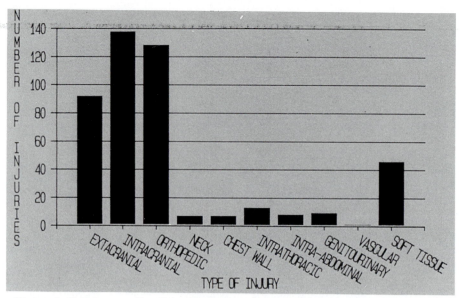

Figure 4–2. Injury profile of the Houston experience. The preponderance of injuries included extracranial and intracranial central nervous system injuries and orthopedic fractures.

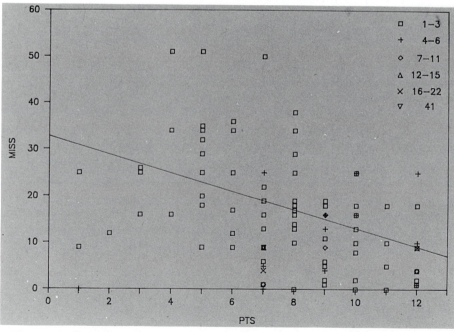

Figure 4–3. Comparison of the Modified Injury Severity Score and the Pediatric Trauma Score. Linear regression slope = −0.63, showing a good correlation between the scoring systems. Numbers and symbols in the right upper corner indicate the number of patients for the given symbol.

114

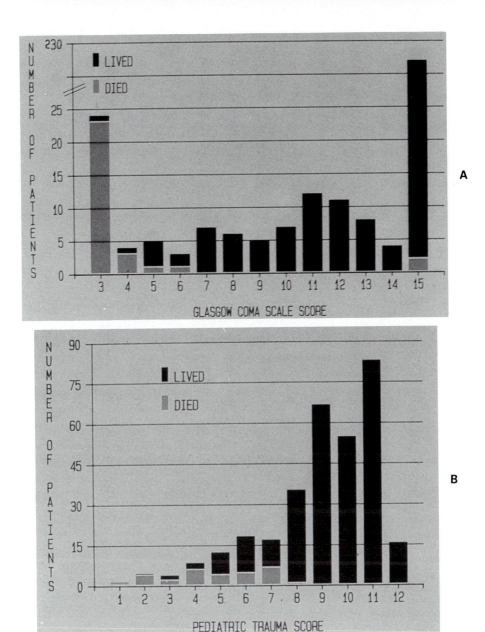

Figure 4–4. Comparisons of mortality as predicted by the Glasgow Coma Scale (GCS) score and Pediatric Trauma Score (PTS). **A,** GCS score and mortality. Predictably, as patients progress from a GCS score of 6 to 3, the rate of mortality increases. However, among patients with a GCS of 15, there is a group of patients who die from injuries other than central nervous system trauma. **B,** In comparison, when the PTS is compared with number of deaths, all deaths occurred at a PTS of 7 or less. As with the GCS, the mortality rate increased as the PTS progressed from 7 to 1. These comparisons clearly show the PTS to be a better predictor of overall mortality than other scoring systems.

fractures 6, foot fractures 3, clavicular fractures 7, femur fractures 12, elbow fractures 5, radius fractures 15, knee fractures 4, and tibia fractures 31.

When the mechanisms of injury were identified, some patients were not assigned a score for either the MISS or the PTS. The MISS is designed to evaluate multiple trauma, so scores for patients classified under burns, substance ingestion, or sexual assault were not indicative of the true level of injury and have been omitted.

The MISS and PTS were calculated for 288 patients and compared (Fig. 4–3). Mean MISS of the group was 10.9 (range 0 to 51). Thirty-seven children (12.8%) were severely injured (MISS greater than 20). Mean MISS was 9.1 for children surviving and 28.9 for those who died ($p < .001$). Of patients classified as severely injured by the MISS, 97.3% had a PTS of 8 or less. Of patients classified as not severely injured, 100% had a PTS greater than 8. Based on a PTS less than or equal to 8, the sensitivity of identifying the severely injured child is 80.4%, linear regression slope $= -0.63$. Twenty-seven patients (9.4%) died. All deaths occured in patients assigned a PTS of 7 or less (Fig. 4–4). The mean GCS of patients surviving was 13.8; the mean GCS was 3.3 in those who died. The GCS correlated well with both the PTS ($+.61$) and the MISS ($-.73$).

In an ongoing study at our institution the PTS is continually put to a stringent prospective clinical evaluation. We have the advantage of a large patient population in a single institution. Our data are compiled and stored in a computer data base by a single observer who is not involved in patient care. Computer data may be used to generate the GCS, the MISS, and the PTS for each patient. We have compared the MISS with the PTS and found an excellent correlation in statistical analysis by linear regression, correlation analysis, sensitivity, and specificity.

We have found that the short, objective, concise nature of the PTS facilitates its use by members of the medical subspecialties and those providing first-responder care.

Children with a PTS of 8 or greater are appropriately cared for at local facilities. Children with a PTS of less than 8 should be considered for immediate triage to a tertiary trauma care center.

REFERENCES

1. Jennet B, Teasdale G, Breakman R, et al: Predicting outcome in individual patients after severe head injury, *Lancet* 1:1031–1034, 1976.
2. Baker SP, O'Neill B, Haddon W, et al: The Injury Severity Score: a method for describing patients with multiple injuries and evaluating emergency care, *J Trauma* 14:187–196, 1974.
3. Baker SP, O'Neill B: The Injury Severity Score: an update, *J Trauma* 18:882–888, 1976.
4. Champion HR, Sacco WJ, Lepper RL, et al: An anatomic index of injury severity, *J Trauma* 20(3):197–202, 1980.

5. Kirkpatrick JR, Youmans RL: Trauma Index: an aid in the evaluation of injury victims, *J Trauma* 11:711–715, 1971.
6. Bever DG, Veenker CH: An illness-injury severity index for non-physician emergency medical personnel, *EMT J* 3:45–49, 1979.
7. Champion HR, Sacco WJ, Hannan DS, et al: Assessment of injury severity: the Triage Index, *Crit Care Med* 8(3):201–208, 1980.
8. Champion HR, Sacco WJ, Carnazzo AJ, et al: Trauma Score, *Crit Care Med* 9:672–676, 1981.
9. Knaus WA, Zimmerman JE, Wagner DP, et al: APACHE—Acute Physiology and Chronic Health Evaluation: a physiologically based classification system, *Crit Care Med* 9(8):591–597, 1981.
10. Knaus WA, Draper EA, Wagner DP, Zimmerman JE: *APACHE II: final form and national validation results of a severity of disease classification system* (abstract), Presented at the Annual Meeting of the Society for Critical Care Medicine, San Francisco, May 1984.
11. Mayer T, Matlak ME, Johnson DG, et al: The Modified Injury Severity Scale in pediatric multiple trauma patients, *J Pediatr Surg* 15:719–726, 1980.
12. Tepas JJ, Bryant M, Mollitt DL, Talbert JL: The Pediatric Trauma Score as a predictor of injury severity in the injured child, *J Pediatr Surg* 22(1):14–18, 1987.
13. Ford EG, Jennings LM, Gibson AE, Andrassy RJ: The Pediatric Trauma Score: accuracy of prediction of injury severity in a single large urban pediatric trauma experience, *Contemp Orthop* 16(1):35–39, 1988.

CHAPTER

5

Emergency Pediatric Imaging

Sue C. Kaste

Emergency radiologic imaging of the traumatized child differs from that of the adult in several ways: (1) the nature of some injuries, (2) imaging techniques, (3) patient management techniques, and (4) equipment.

Although the proper diagnosis frequently is suggested by a careful history and physical examination, diagnostic imaging plays an important role in patient care and management. Such evaluation must be expeditious, accurate, appropriate for the case at hand, and tailored to the individual child. Imaging priorities must be orchestrated with the triage team and surgeons to provide optimal care to the injured child; alleviate unnecessary risks to the child during evaluation; prevent delayed diagnosis, particularly of critical injuries; and provide the clinician with the quickest and most informative assessment possible.

To these ends, this chapter presents an organized approach to emergency imaging of the injured child, emphasizing the optimal imaging modality for a particular anatomic area, encouraging the radiologist to be aware of unsuspected injuries, and addressing present-day controversies.

BASIC PRINCIPLES OF PEDIATRIC IMAGING

It is important to realize that a child is not a miniature adult but has individual needs, thought processes, and pathologic entities. Similarly, a child's corporeal homeostasis is vastly different from an adult's and is extremely fragile. The type and severity of injury may vary in children of different ages with the same mechanism of injury because the characteristic physical makeup varies depending on the child's age. For example, incomplete bony ossification may protect an infant from nasal fracture but predispose the abdominal viscera to injury because of a lack of protection from the unossified costal margins.[1] In addition, a "twisted ankle" predisposes a young child to a Salter I fracture instead

---

Supported in part by the National Cancer Institute, Cancer Center Support (CORE) grant P30CA21765, and by the American Lebanese Syrian Associated Charities.

of a ligamentous tear, which might well have resulted were the physes fused. Toddlers, through their environmental exploration, may injure their lower legs, resulting in toddler's fractures. Infants rarely injure themselves, so child abuse must be considered when an unusual injury occurs in a young patient.

As the child grows and matures, the patterns of accidental injury change. Falls are common during the elementary school years. With maturity the number of injuries from pedestrian-vehicular accidents and motor vehicular accidents increases. Violent crimes and penetrating wounds, similar to those in adults, manifest during middle and late adolescence.[2,3]

As implied in the preceding discussion, the care and management of pediatric patients vary widely with their age, development, injuries, and environment.[4,5] Individualized evaluation and imaging are a must in the pediatric population. The primary care providers for the injured child must be caring, flexible, and inventive personnel who have both patience and interest in working with children.

The ABCs of emergency care must be followed, regardless of the patient's age or injury. The airway must be protected. The smaller and younger the child, the more life threatening any degree of airway compromise. Hemodynamic stabilization is next sought. Imaging is then tailored to the patient, his or her injuries, and available imaging modalities. Imaging, which is limited to diagnosing critical injuries first, must be expedient and purposeful. Nonvital imaging should be temporarily delayed.[6,7] In the critically injured patient only three survey films are required: chest, abdomen and pelvis, and lateral cervical spine. If a chest tube has been placed, a repeat chest radiograph is in order.[9] These most basic of films provide enough information to direct further care—angiographic, surgical, or evaluative.

Children expend tremendous energy in maintaining their body temperature. In the face of trauma or other stress, metabolic requirements are even greater. Therefore the child must be kept warm and comfortable and hypothermia must be prevented.[8] Maintaining homothermia may be difficult in air-conditioned rooms where computer systems support high-technology equipment in the radiology department. Contrast agents used during the emergency evaluation of the patient should be at body temperature to help prevent hypothermia. Overhead lamps are usually ineffective during fluoroscopy.[9]

Children respond favorably to an honest, caring approach. Reassurance that most maneuvers will not be painful and an honest warning of when to expect discomfort or pain will encourage the child to trust the health care providers and to cooperate with their evaluations.

Children 2 years of age and younger are frequently unable to cooperate for physical examination, much less for an imaging study. Sedation may be required. Special immobilizing devices are available when immobility is required.

Simple swaddling provides the child with warmth and security and permits easy movement.[10] Many ambulance crews tape bags of intravenous fluid to the sides of a child's head to maintain alignment of the cervical spine. These bags must be removed before computed tomography (CT) scanning. The uniform density of the fluid in the bags obscures soft tissue densities of the patient. Care must be taken to ensure that respiration or circulation is not compromised by improper application of fixation devices or straps. The immobilized child should never be left unattended.[5]

IMAGING MODALITIES
Plain Radiographs

Plain radiographs are based on attenuation of an electron beam by constituent tissues as the beam passes through the tissues. This provides the basis for the four radiographic densities: air, fat, soft tissue, and bone. Noncontrast radiography is usually the initial imaging modality in the workup of an emergency patient and is the mainstay of orthopedic evaluation.[7] It is readily available, inexpensive, and quickly performed. Plain radiographs are particularly useful in assessing bony architecture because of their high spatial resolution. Soft tissue trauma, however, is not directly evaluated.[6]

The ability to perform portable radiography is essential in evaluating critically injured patients; repeated moving of the patient to and from the radiology department could exacerbate undetected injuries. Although detail is compromised on portable studies because of technical limitations, a fixed radiographic table is inappropriate for use in the trauma room.

Additional information may be gleaned by the administration of various contrast agents such as those administered intravenously for intravenous urography (IVU), orally for esophagography, intravascularly for angiography, and intravesicularly for cystourethrography.[8]

Tomography

Tomography is performed less frequently for children than for adults.[1] This is due both to children's small size and to their usual inability to suspend respiration and motion. The radiographic dose is also considerably higher than that of plain radiography. Tomography has largely been replaced by computed tomography (CT) when additional anatomic detail and information are required. Tomographic evaluation of subtle fractures and skeletal alignment may provide some useful information.

Fluoroscopy

Fluoroscopic examinations require an image intensifier and television viewing system. Videotaping of the examination is a useful adjunct in pediatric radiology, allowing review of the study and selection of appropriate images without increasing the patient's radiation dose.[1]

Fluoroscopic evaluation of joints, fractures, and the spine for assessment of skeletal alignment and stability is a useful adjunct to plain films. Gastrointestinal motility and anatomy may also be assessed fluoroscopically. Useful information about the airway may also be obtained fluoroscopically.

Ultrasound

Diagnostic ultrasound developed as a noninvasive, adaptable, and readily available imaging modality that uses nonionizing sound waves. The images created result from computer-generated reconstruction of sound waves reflected from density interfaces of the examined tissues. Size, shape, and internal architecture of normal and abnormal tissues may be assessed. More recently, the development of duplex and color Doppler imaging has permitted noninvasive assessment of vascular anatomy and its integrity.

Advantages of ultrasound examinations in the pediatric population include the following[1]:

- Lack of ionizing radiation
- Flexibility of scanning
- Lack of contraindications to ultrasound imaging
- Relative painlessness and acceptance of the modality by patients
- Lack of requirement for a contrast agent
- Portability (may be taken to the patient rather than requiring the patient's transport to the ultrasound suite)
- Lack of sedation as a requirement
- Amenability of the child's abdomen to ultrasound evaluation because of its relative lack of fat
- Affordability
- Exquisite lesion characterization

Despite all its advantages, ultrasound evaluation has some drawbacks[1]:

- Imaging is compromised by gas and air (aerophagia is common in injured children) which limits an abdominal study if an "acoustic window" through which the sound beam may be directed cannot be found.
- The examination is operator dependent.
- Only a limited area of interest may be imaged at one time, making the modality inappropriate as a generalized screening tool

As with fluoroscopy, ultrasound examinations may be recorded on tape and reviewed as needed, or images may be selected for filming from the recorded examination.

Computed Tomography

CT is based on computer-generated cross-sectional images of data acquired from multiple passes of tightly collimated electron beams through tissue slices. Scanning is done principally in the axial plane but may be reconstructed in several planes. Direct coronal imaging is frequently performed for facial evaluation but requires both patient cooperation and physical flexibility.

Advantages of CT include the following[1]:

- Rapid imaging of relatively large areas
- Lack of operator dependency
- Superb anatomic detail and tissue characterization
- Assessment of the vascular system, particularly with intravenous administration of contrast medium
- Ability to obtain some physiologic information about organ function even in the presence of organ failure
- Less interference by bowel gas and bone artifact than in ultrasound

CT limitations include these[1]:

- Frequent contrast administration (intravenous or oral or both)
- Moderate expense
- Use of ionizing radiation to obtain the images
- Lack of portability
- Possible limited retroperitoneal and mediastinal evaluation in children because of relative paucity of fat
- Some compromise of the examination by bone and metallic artifacts
- Necessity of immobilizing the patient to avoid degrading the image, so that sedation may be required

CT is a vital tool in emergency radiology and probably ranks second only to plain films in frequency of use.[7] It is the most important modality in assessing head trauma and evaluating blunt abdominal and pelvic trauma.

Nuclear Medicine Imaging

Nuclear scintigraphy provides a physiologic assessment of organs through their selective avidity for various radiotracers. In acute trauma evaluation the usefulness is limited primarily to assessing hepatic and splenic lacerations and renal and cerebrovascular integrity. Nuclear scintigraphy is useful in evaluating occult and stress fractures because of its sensitivity to altered bone metabolism at these sites. Cardiac injury, such as contusion, may be assessed with nuclear scintigraphy, but success has been limited.[7]

Magnetic Resonance Imaging

Magnetic resonance imaging (MRI) has developed rapidly as a less invasive means of body imaging, particularly for evaluation of the musculoskeletal and central nervous systems. Magnetic fields across tissues are used for selectively altering the magnetic fields of the individual protons in the tissues. As these protons "relax," they emit energy, which is detected by radiofrequency coils. Computer manipulation of these tissue-generated signals creates images for interpretation. Assessment in virtually any plane is standard.[10-14]

The multiplanar capability of MRI, as well as its excellent intrinsic soft tissue contrast, makes it ideal for imaging the central nervous system (CNS) and musculoskeletal system. MRI is exquisitely sensitive to motion, which severely degrades the images, especially when MRI is used for imaging the chest and abdomen (because of respiratory and bowel motion). Children virtually always need sedation because they cannot lie still for the time required to complete most MRI examinations.[10,11] Whether or not a trauma victim should be sedated for an examination must be determined on a case by case basis. Technologic improvements that make examinations faster should alleviate this problem. The length of the imaging gantry does not allow adequate visual monitoring of even unsedated patients. An additional difficulty in the use of MRI is the careful attention to safety required because of the tremendous magnetic fields surrounding the imaging unit. In particular, any ferromagnetic substance (e.g., nonaluminum wheelchairs, respirators, monitoring devices, oxygen tanks) may become a projectile missile as it is pulled toward, and sometimes into, the magnet. Such occurrence may severely damage the equipment and any person between the "missile" and its final target—the magnet. For the same reason, special patient support and monitoring equipment that is not made of ferromagnetic materials must be used during an MRI study.[10,11]

In most cases unstable patients and trauma patients should be evaluated by imaging modalities other than MRI. Time and again, CT has proved its usefulness and sensitivity in the evaluation of trauma patients. MRI can exquisitely demonstrate aortic dissection, although because of clinical instability and difficulty in monitoring, these patients are usually best evaluated by CT or angiography.[7,10,11]

Contrast agents have been developed for use with MRI to enhance tissue characteristics. The administration of contrast agents, as with CT, makes MRI a "less invasive" rather than a "noninvasive" modality. MRI is expensive and less readily available than CT or ultrasound.

Angiography and Interventional Procedures

The development of newer imaging modalities and continual improvements in technology have modified the role of angiography and expanded the arena of the interventional radiologist. Angiography is an invasive procedure requiring arterial or venous access, as well as the use of intravascular contrast agents. Sedation or general anesthesia is almost invariably required for performance of these procedures in children. In the setting of trauma, angiography is used primarily to assess vascular integrity. In fact, it is the only modality that directly assesses vessels and should be used liberally when any question exists regarding vascular integrity or a source of bleeding.[7]

More recently the use of interventional radiology and expertise with embolization procedures have decreased the trauma patient's morbidity and mortality from extensive surgical interventions.[7] Inherent in invasive procedures are risks and benefits. The indications for invasive vascular procedures are strictly defined, and the relative risks and benefits beyond the defined indications must be weighed.

An experienced pediatric interventionalist can safely perform angiography and interventional procedures for specific clinical indications. A dedicated angiography suite, appropriate selection of catheters, needles, and wires, and the presence of trained, experienced technologic and nursing personnel are required for efficient, safe completion of these diagnostic examinations.[1,7]

IMAGING OF HEAD TRAUMA

One of the most common reasons for hospital admission after trauma is closed head injury.[6,7,10,11] The vast majority of head injuries may be considered minor. Controversy persists concerning the utility of imaging neurologically intact patients after minor head trauma, whether such patients should be hospitalized for observation, and, which, if any, screening head imaging should be performed.[15–18]

Recent reports based on patients of all ages have addressed these issues with the following findings[15,16,19]:

- CT scanning is a reliable means of screening patients with minimal head injury and determining those who require hospital admission for observation.
- No patient with minor head injury, a Glasgow Coma Scale (GCS) score of 14 or 15, and a normal head CT showed neurologic deterioration.
- As with more serious head trauma, there were no factors (i.e., physical examination, history, GCS score) that predicted which patients would have an abnormal CT scan.[15,16]

The most common acute finding is cerebral contusion (Fig. 5–1), followed by subarachnoid hemorrhage (Fig. 5–2) and subdural hematoma.[19]

Plain radiographs were obtained in only 15% of 2766 patients evaluated in a recent multicenter study. Of patients whose plain films showed a fracture, 39.3% had an associated relevant CT finding, whereas only 13.9% of those without fracture had a relevant positive CT scan.[17]

This study also found the following[17]:

- Twenty percent of patients with minor head injury have an acute lesion seen on CT.

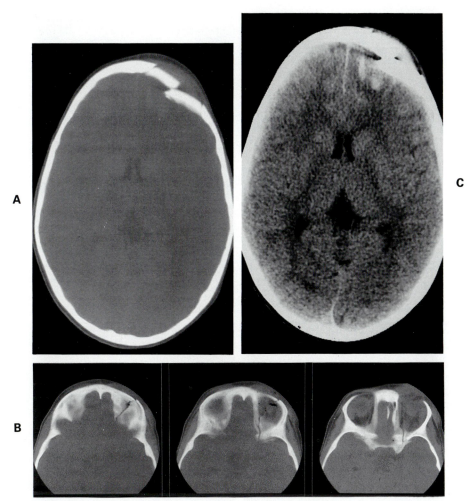

Figure 5–1. A and **B,** Selected computed tomographic images of a 3-year-old girl who fell head first onto a cement curb. The child suffered an orbital-frontal fracture that extended into the left orbital roof, crossed the roof and the optic foramen, and extended into the left temporal bone with 5 mm of depression. **C,** Subjacent hemorrhagic contusions and subarachnoid hemorrhage are present. Soft tissue swelling overlies the fracture site. (Courtesy Dr. Robert Kaufman.)

- One third of patients with a GCS score of 13 and minor head injury have an acute lesion, and 10% of those patients require craniotomy.
- Twenty percent of patients with minor head injury and abnormal neurologic findings require central nervous system–specific treatment.
- Twenty-five percent of patients with minor head injury and positive CT require treatment.

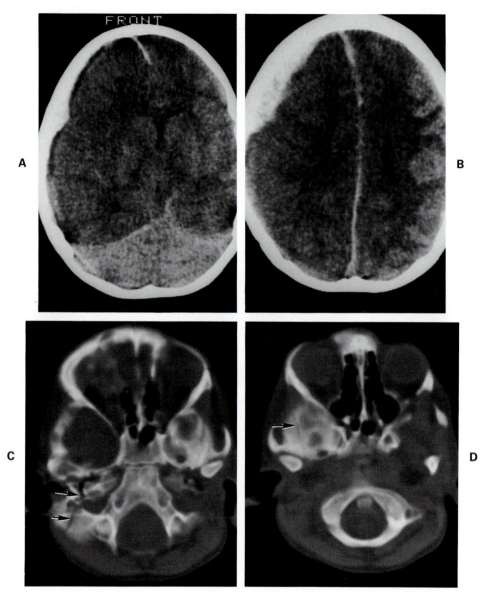

Figure 5–2. A and **B,** Axial unenhanced computed tomographic (CT) scan of the head in a 7-year-old boy, a victim of child abuse. The CT scan exquisitely demonstrates the marked diffuse cerebral edema with decreased attenuation throughout the cerebral parenchyma, more so on the right, and the concurrent marked mass effect across the midline, subfalcine herniation, and near-complete effacement of the right lateral ventricle. Interhemispheric hemorrhage is demonstrated by the abnormal intensity along the falx. Dense extraaxial fluid along the right frontal parietal distribution also represents hemorrhage. **C** and **D,** CT images filmed with bone window of the same child demonstrate right basilar skull fractures coursing through the right petrous bone and middle ear and posteriorly through the right occiput *(arrows).*

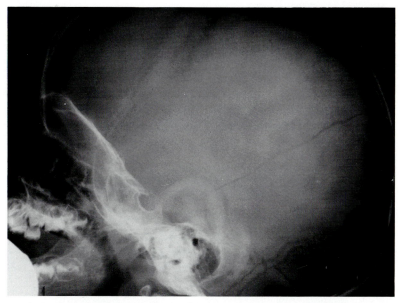

Figure 5–3. Lateral plain radiograph of 1-year-old girl with a linear left parietal skull fracture caused by a fall. Notice the straight configuration of the fracture in contrast to the irregular wavy configuration of the sutures.

- Two of five patients with minor head injury, abnormal neurologic findings, and positive CT require treatment, and 25% need intracranial pressure monitoring or craniotomy.
- Two percent of patients with minor head injury and no abnormalities on neurologic examination or CT require treatment, and none require craniotomy.

Head trauma in children is common, but as discussed previously, information gained from plain radiographs is limited unless obtained for a specific reason (further delineating a depressed fracture configuration or delineating a missile's tract).[7,10,20] At best, only 25% of children with head trauma have an associated skull fracture (Fig. 5–3).[20] The presence or absence of a fracture is an unreliable indicator of intracranial damage.[15–24]

For evaluation of the comatose patient, plain films are readily available, may offer insight into the mechanism of injury, and may be obtained at the same time as the screening cross-table lateral cervical spine films.[7,10,20]

Since CT's advent, it has repeatedly proved its efficacy in the evaluation of cranial trauma and now is the imaging modality of choice.[7,15–17,19] Its sensitivity for detection of intracranial abnormality is well documented.* The position of

---

*References 6, 7, 9, 10, 13-15, 17, 18, 21, 22, 25–47.

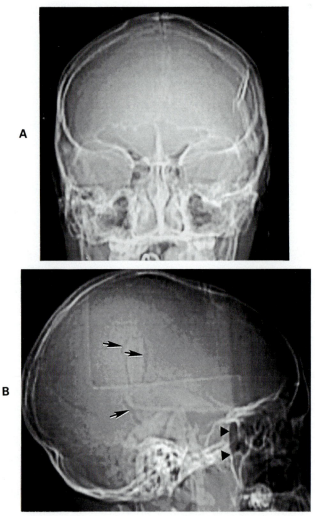

Figure 5–4. Unenhanced computed tomographic scan of a 12-year-old boy who sustained severe left parietal head injury as an unrestrained passenger in a motor vehicle accident. **A,** Anteroposterior digital radiograph demonstrating severely depressed left parietal skull fracture. **B,** Lateral topogram demonstrating the depressed skull fracture *(arrows)* and air-fluid level in the sphenoid sinus *(arrowheads)*.

orbital and intracranial foreign bodies may also be clearly delineated with CT.[32,40,41,43]

While CT's delineation of skull fractures (particularly linear) may be limited, its detection of depressed bone fragments and basilar skull fractures far exceeds that of plain radiographs, particularly in patients who are uncooperative or comatose (Figs. 5–2 and 5–4).[48] CT also demonstrates intracranial manifes-

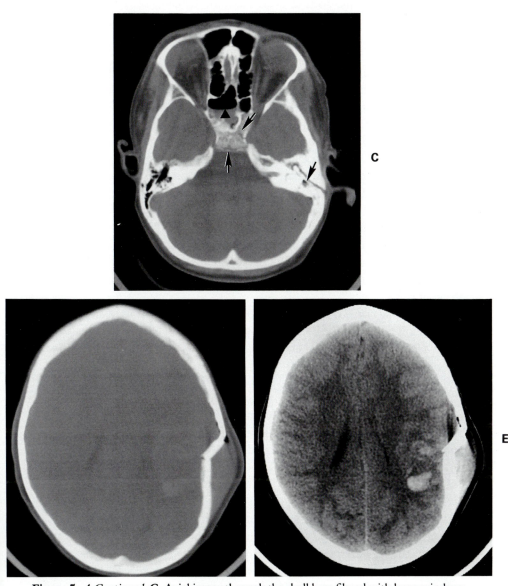

Figure 5–4 *Continued* **C,** Axial image through the skull base filmed with bone windows demonstrates extension of the fracture into the left petrous bone, sphenoid bone, sphenoid sinus, and clivus *(arrows)*. The air-fluid level within the sphenoid sinus *(arrowhead)* is also apparent on the digital radiograph in **A. D** and **E,** Axial soft tissue and bone window images through the level of the fracture demonstrate the degree of depression and associated hemorrhagic contusion of the left parietal lobe. (Courtesy Dr. Robert Kaufman.)

tations of head trauma such as acute subdural hematomas, contusions, acute epidural hematomas, intraparenchymal hematomas, acute traumatic aneurysms, cerebral edema, shear injuries, and traumatic pneumocephalus (Figs. 5–5 and 5–6).[20-22,25–41,48]

Complex facial fractures are exquisitely depicted by CT, which clearly shows positioning of fracture fragments, the complex facial anatomy, and its relationship to the mechanism of injury (see Fig. 5–1).*

Regardless of the imaging modality used, assessment of symmetry of facial structures is critical. The goal in imaging facial trauma is detection of all fractures, which allows classification of injuries, delineation of bone fragment positions and associated soft tissue injuries, and determination of associated intracranial, spinal, and calvarial injuries.[39,49] Above all, airway patency and security must be obtained and maintained before and during imaging. Patients with facial injury are particularly prone to airway compromise.

Recently the use of MRI in patients with acute head and face trauma has attracted widespread interest. MRI's role as currently defined, the significance of MRI findings not detected with CT, and MRI's limitations are beyond the scope of this chapter.†

In summary, CT is the modality of choice for evaluation of head trauma. Plain radiographs play the limited but specific role of delineating depressed skull fractures, missile trajectories, and foreign bodies.

Imaging of Spinal Trauma

Plain radiography is the initial imaging technique of choice following spine trauma (Fig. 5–7). Excellent film technique is imperative in diagnosis but may be difficult when patients are belligerent, frightened, or comatose.[9,58-71] The initial film should be a well-penetrated, brow-up, cross-table lateral view that includes all seven cervical vertebral bodies. If all seven are not adequately delineated, the original views should be augmented with a swimmer's view—all performed without moving the patient.[9,58–60,67,68] Most spinal fractures and subluxations are defined in this manner. Early delineation of fractures is necessary so that additional injuries do not result from moving a patient with unstable spinal fractures.[9] Anteroposterior and open-mouth odontoid views improve the sensitivity of the cross-table lateral view from 82% to 93%.[66] Thirty-degree oblique views complete the cervical spine series.

Delineating upper cervical spine injuries can be difficult. C1 and C2 fractures are best shown by the open-mouth odontoid view. Familiarity with normal spinal anatomy and its relationships, particularly in the pediatric population, is

---

*References 9, 20, 39, 43, 44, 47, 49–51.
†References 7, 12, 30, 33, 44, 52-57.

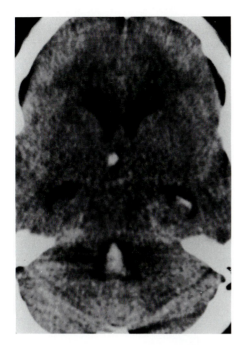

Figure 5–5. Axial unenhanced computed tomographic scan of the head of a young man demonstrates acute intraventricular hemorrhage and associated acute obstructive hydrocephalus.

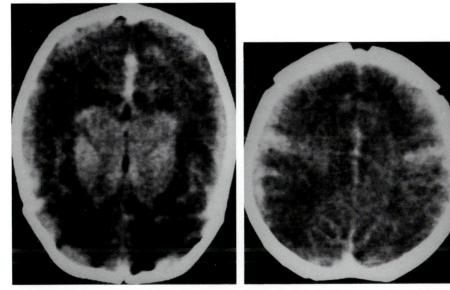

Figure 5–6. Axial unenhanced computed tomographic scan of a neonate who has suffered an anoxic event, such as may be seen with strangulation. Note the marked decrease in attenuation of the cerebral hemispheres and accentuation of the thalami. High cortical sulci are enhanced by subarachnoid hemorrhage.

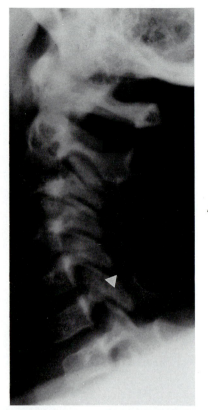

Figure 5–7. Lateral and bilateral oblique views of the cervical spine of a young girl who had fallen from her bicycle and complained of neck pain. **A,** Lateral cervical spine film demonstrates widening of the intervertebral distance between C6 and C7 with a nondisplaced fracture through the facet of C6 *(arrowhead)*. **B** and **C,** Bilateral oblique views demonstrating abnormal relationship between the facets of C6 and C7 with the right facet of C6 subluxed superiorly and anteriorly to that of C7 *(arrowhead)* and the left facet of C6 distracted superiorly *(arrow)*. These findings are consistent with the rupture of the posterior longitudinal ligament at C6-7 and associated joint capsule rupture at this level.

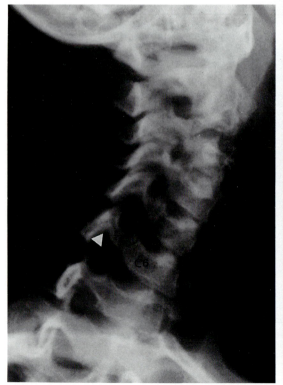

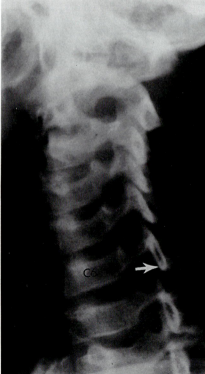

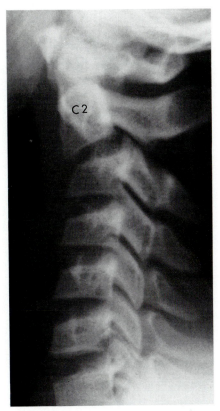

Figure 5–8. Posttraumatic lateral cervical spine radiograph demonstrates anterior sub-luxation of C2 on C3 resulting from ligamentous injury. (Courtesy Dr. Barry Gerald.)

helpful in detecting injuries.[60,66-68] Familiarity with injury mechanisms particular to children provides further insight into detection of lesions,* such as whiplash injuries from child abuse,[52] high cervical spine fractures and subluxations in young children riding in forward-facing car seats,[74] and predilection for upper cervical spine injuries in children in contrast to lower cervical spine injuries in adults (Figs. 5–8 to 5–11).[60-65]

Plain film tomography may be used for further definition of the spinal bony architecture and requires little or no movement of the patient. Soft tissue injuries are diagnosed by secondary signs on plain radiographs; for example, disruption of normal bony alignment without evidence of fracture implies ligamentous

---

*References 52, 58, 60, 65, 66, 72–75.

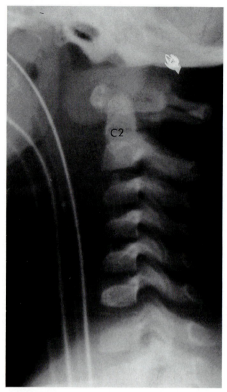

Figure 5–9. Young girl who suffered extensive cervical ligamentous injuries in a motor vehicle accident. Note marked increase in distance between skull base and C1, between C1 and C2, and between C6 and C7. An associated prevertebral hematoma is present. (Courtesy Dr. Barry Gerald.)

strain, tear, or rupture, and prevertebral soft tissue swelling may imply hemorrhage or soft tissue injury (Fig. 5–12).[72]

CT has rapidly become the definitive imaging modality for spinal trauma,* but MRI's role is still being defined.† Bony definition and localization of fragments are exquisitely depicted by CT.‡ CT also provides more information about associated soft tissue abnormalities than plain radiographs,[6,79] although less than MRI (Figs. 5–13 and 5–14).[79]

MRI shows soft tissue structures in exquisite detail. In assessment of spinal

*References 9, 58, 66, 67, 69, 70, 76–81.
†References 61, 64, 71, 72, 76, 82–89.
‡References 6, 58, 66, 67, 69, 70, 78, 81, 82, 89.

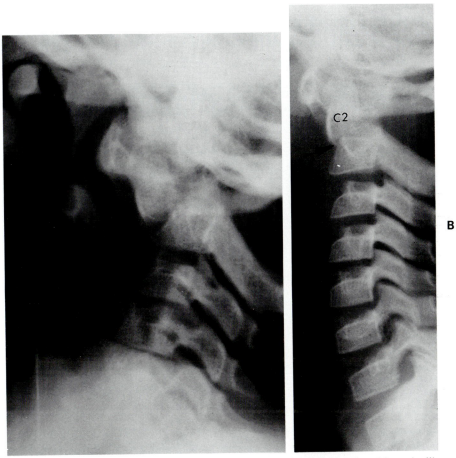

Figure 5–10. Young female victim of a motor vehicle accident who awoke with torticollis and neck pain after 5 days in a coma. **A,** Initial portable cross-table lateral radiograph demonstrating subcutaneous emphysema. The occipitoatlantal and atlantoaxial relationships are difficult to assess. **B,** Follow-up radiograph showing anterior displacement of C1 and the odontoid process with resultant narrowing of the spinal canal. Arrow marks the fracture site. (Courtesy Dr. Barry Gerald.)

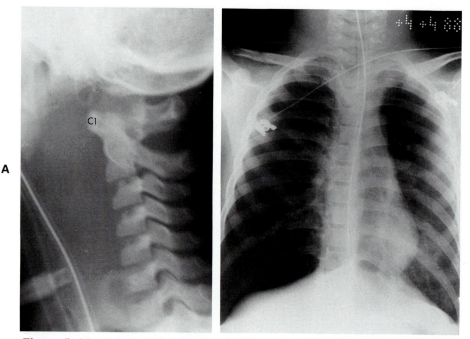

Figure 5–11. A 6-year-old black boy who was struck by a "hit and run" driver. **A,** Portable cross-table lateral radiograph of the cervical spine demonstrating atlantooccipital dislocation. The head is dislocated anteriorly on the neck. The marked prevertebral soft tissue swelling has caused airway occlusion (in this case hematoma) and anteriorly displaced both the nasogastric and the endotracheal tubes. **B,** Portable anteroposterior chest radiograph of the same child in a recumbent position demonstrates a pneumothorax on the right side, most apparent in the base of the right hemithorax, and pulmonary contusion of the left lower lobe. The soft tissues of the neck are swollen. (Courtesy Dr. Tom Boulden.)

injuries it plays an important role in evaluation of cord injury, ligamentous integrity, and cartilaginous and diskal injuries.* This is particulary important in children, who may have extensive cord and soft tissue injury without bony injury or external signs of trauma. This deceptive nature of pediatric injuries is due to the hypermobility of the pediatric spine, the top-heaviness of children, and their underdeveloped supporting musculature.[58,60]

When MRI is not available or spinal MRI cannot be performed, CT myelography (MCT) may provide the needed information regarding injury to the nerve roots, spinal cord, and dura.[58,69,76,79,80] Neither of these modalities, however, is performed on an unstable patient.

---

*References 58, 61, 63, 66, 67, 78–80, 82–87, 89.

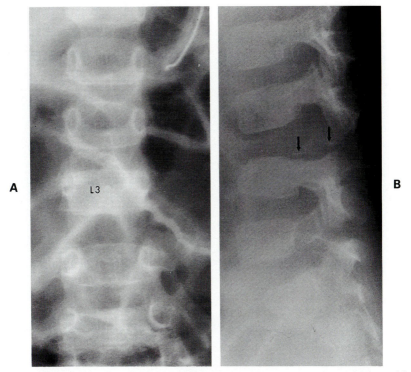

Figure 5–12. A 5-year-old boy who had been involved in a motor vehicle accident. **A,** Anteroposterior abdominal and, **B,** lateral spine radiographs demonstrate fracture-dislocation of L3-4 associated with perched facets. Note compression of L4 body and avulsed fragments *(arrows)*. (Courtesy Dr. Gary Hedlund.)

In summary, plain radiographs remain the initial imaging modality for spinal trauma. Further workup by CT, MCT, and MRI depends on the plain film findings and clinical evaluation.

IMAGING OF CHEST TRAUMA

As with other injuries, the mechanism of injury and the sequelae of thoracic trauma in the pediatric population vary significantly from those in the adult population.[4,90–93] Blunt chest trauma, usually from motor vehicle accidents, is a major cause of death in children.[91,94–96] The chest of a child is considerably more pliable and tolerates greater deformity than an adult's chest. The manifestations of injury therefore vary from those in adults. Because of the pliability of the thoracic cage in children, its usefulness as a barrier to external trauma is somewhat limited. The majority of force to the thoracic cage is transmitted through the chest wall to the lung where it is absorbed, resulting in pulmonary

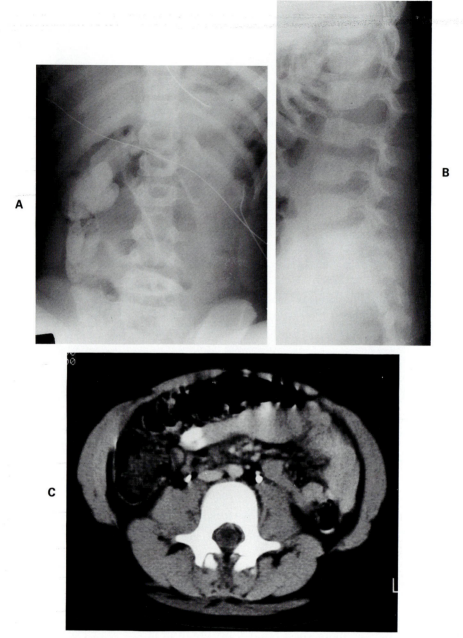

Figure 5–13. A 4-year-old girl who was wearing a lap belt when involved in a motor vehicle accident. **A,** Anteroposterior portable abdominal radiograph with the child recumbent demonstrates marked widening of the intraspinous distance between L2 and L3. **B,** Portable lateral spine radiograph confirms the finding and shows marked cephalad displacement of articulating facets of L2 relative to L3, the result of ligamentous injury. Also note soft tissue edema over the back. **C,** Axial computed tomographic scan through the abdomen shows posterior soft tissue edema. (Courtesy Dr. Gary Hedlund.)

contusions and less commonly pulmonary laceration.[91,97–100] In addition, the mediastinal structures are more loosely fixed in children and therefore may shift considerably within the chest, causing significant compromise of the great vessels, airway, heart, and lungs in the form of acute angulation, compression, and displacement.[91,101]

Certain injuries are uncommon in the pediatric population: flail chest, open pneumothorax, ruptured diaphragm, and aortic rupture.[91,92,94] Whereas fractured ribs may readily be appreciated in teenagers, such fractures are rare in younger children. When they occur, they may be difficult to detect because they tend to be "greenstick" or "bowing" fractures. In the pediatric population, thoracic injury is commonly complicated by aspiration of gastric contents.[91]

Isolated blunt thoracic injuries are uncommon in children. Blunt chest injury is usually seen in concert with cranial or abdominal trauma and often results from pedestrian-vehicle accidents, child abuse, and falls.[90,92,94,101] Blunt chest injuries are more common in children less than 7 years of age.[90,92] Penetrating injuries are uncommon in children but occur with increasing frequency in adolescence.[2,3,5,92,102]

In evaluating pediatric chest trauma the physician should remember that in children the thoracic cage terminates more cephalad in the abdomen than in adults, which places the child at increased risk of upper abdominal trauma.[91] As with many other forms of injury, the severity cannot be accurately assessed on the basis of external manifestations.

Once a patient's airway is secured, hemodynamic resuscitation begun, and clinical assessment performed, initial imaging evaluation consisting of an anteroposterior chest radiograph is indicated.[7,93,96,103–108] Although portable radiography is often suboptimal, a great deal of needed information regarding the chest and thorax may be obtained from such a study. Careful evaluation of the radiograph must include assessment of pleural, pulmonary parenchymal, and bony thoracic structures (Fig. 5–15). The approach to the chest radiograph must be systematic and all encompassing. The distribution of any detectable rib fractures may provide insight into associated injuries.[93,99,103,109,110] Brachial plexus or vascular pedicle trauma should be considered if upper rib fractures are present. Lower rib fractures should raise concern about hepatic and splenic injuries. Even the slightest widening of the mediastinal contour implies significant trauma and necessitates evaluation of the integrity of the mediastinal vasculature and thoracic spine.* Rupture of the esophagus from blunt trauma is exceedingly rare, but when present it frequently has no abnormal radiographic findings.[111] Pleural effusions, also indicative of significant injury, often "cap" the lung apices on the

---

*References 7, 93, 103, 105, 106, 110.

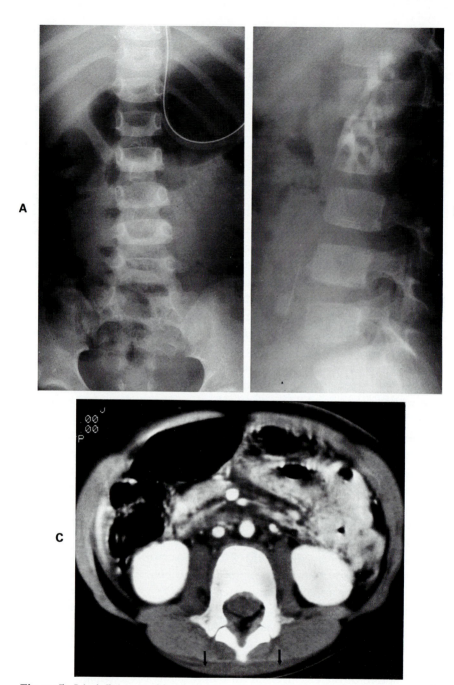

Figure 5–14. A 5½-year-old girl who was wearing a lap belt at time of a motor vehicle accident. **A,** Anteroposterior abdominal radiograph of recumbent patient shows a very subtle increased interspinous distance between L2 and L3. **B,** Lateral lumbar radiograph shows a widened L2-3 interspinous distance without fracture, indicative of ligamentous injury. **C,** Axial enhanced computed tomography through the abdomen demonstrating soft tissue edema at the L2-3 level *(arrows).*

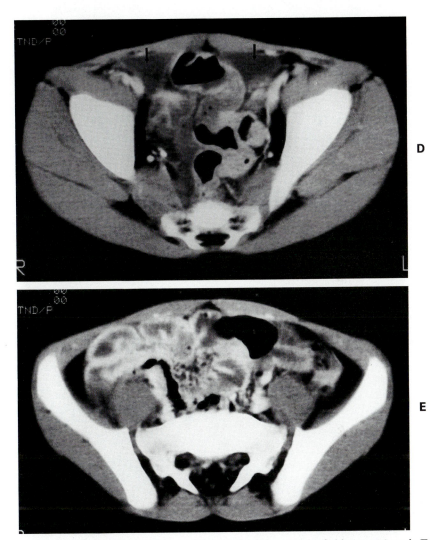

Figure 5–14 *Continued* **D,** This patient also had free pelvic fluid *(arrows)* and, **E,** marked, intense, abnormal bowel wall enhancement. (Courtesy Dr. Gary Hedlund.)

anteroposterior recumbent film as fluid layers dependently. Similarly, pneumothoraces collect anteriorly and may be missed by the "vertical beam" (anteroposterior portable) technique.[112,113] Careful assessment of the chest radiograph for symmetry of the hemithoraces, secondary signs of unilateral volume loss, and symmetry of hemithoracic density improves detection of subtle abnormalities (see Fig. 5–11B).

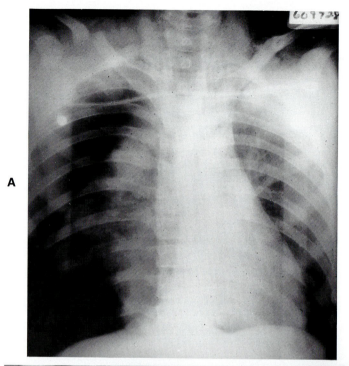

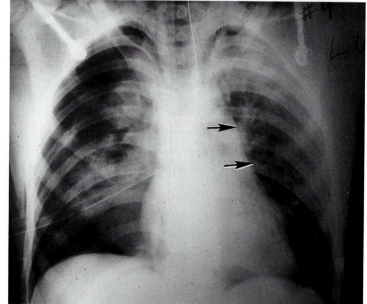

Figure 5–15. A 14-year-old boy whose dirt bike overturned, throwing him chest down onto the ground. Clinical examination revealed ecchymosis on his right shoulder and anterior midchest just to the right of the midline. **A,** The initial portable anteroposterior chest radiograph demonstrates a collapsed right lung, fractured right clavicle, subcutaneous emphysema in the neck, and left upper lobe pulmonary contusion. **B,** Even with placement of a right thoracostomy tube, the lung did not reexpand. Bronchial rupture was diagnosed and surgically repaired. Also note pneumomediastinum *(arrow)* and progression of the left upper lobe contusion. (Courtesy Dr. Thom Lobe.)

When possible, upright posteroanterior and lateral views of the chest should also be obtained.[93,103] In selected cases decubitus views of the chest, with the side in question nondependent or "up," or a cross-table lateral view may demonstrate pneumothorax, pulmonary parenchymal disease, or pleural effusion.

Direct assessment of vascular integrity can be determined only by angiography, which may be quickly and safely performed by a radiologist experienced in pediatric interventional procedures.* The thoracic aorta is at particular risk because of its fixations in the mediastinum at the level of the proximal descending aorta, just distal to the fixed aortic root, and less commonly at the aortic hiatus.[93,105,116] No reliable correlation exists between external signs of chest trauma and the presence or absence of aortic rupture. The most important clinical information is that of a rapid deceleration injury.[93,96,106,110]

Controversy exists over the utility of CT and more recently MRI or transesophageal color Doppler echocardiography (TEE) in the assessment of vascular integrity.[114,117] In a hemodynamically stable trauma patient, CT or MRI may be used to evaluate the chest, usually in concert with imaging for abdominal trauma. As mentioned previously, MRI has limited use in an emergency situation because the patient cannot be adequately observed while being imaged, nonferromagnetic equipment is necessary, and the examination takes a long time to complete. For follow-up assessment or for clarification of a mediastinal abnormality, MRI's demonstration of mediastinal structures, particularly the heart and great vessels, is exquisite (see Fig. 5–16).

CT is a sensitive imaging modality that frequently demonstrates abnormalities not readily appreciated on plain radiographs (Fig. 5–17).[90,107,112,118] Although CT is more sensitive, the additional findings it demonstrates may be of clinically limited significance.[107] CT does contribute, however, to evaluation of the mediastinum, extent of pulmonary parenchymal disease, and diagnosis of pneumothoraces. In this respect it may be used to clarify findings on the plain chest radiograph or clinical findings.† Detection of unsuspected or previously undetected pneumothoraces may be particularly important when mechanical ventilation is being considered.[97]

Cardiac injury is rare in the pediatric population where blunt trauma predominates.[101] Imaging assessment of myocardial injury is mainly by nuclear scintigraphy in the form of thallium imaging[120] and more recently MRI or echocardiography.[93,121,122] Plain film findings of cardiac injury are extremely limited,[101,121,123] and when present they are usually referable to secondary signs of cardiac decompensation in the form of pulmonary vascular congestion and

---

*References 7, 96, 106, 110, 112–114.
†References 96, 108, 110, 113, 119, 121.

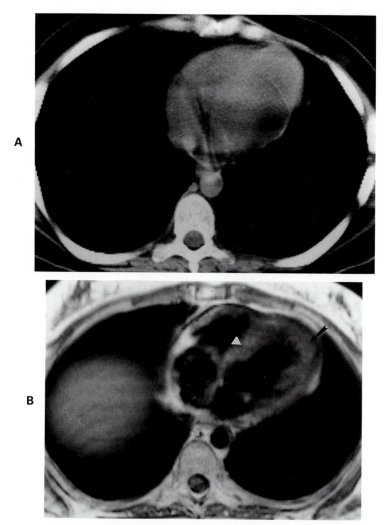

Figure 5–16. A, Axial enhanced computed tomographic scan through the level of the heart, descending aorta, and azygous vein, demonstrating poor delineation of intracardiac and mediastinal anatomic detail. **B** and **C,** Axial and coronal T1-weighted magnetic resonance images of the chest through the heart, descending aorta, and azygous vein. The cardiac chambers and atrioventricular valves are exquisitely delineated. The left ventricular muscular thickness *(arrow)* and intraventricular septal wall thickness *(arrowhead)* may be readily assessed.

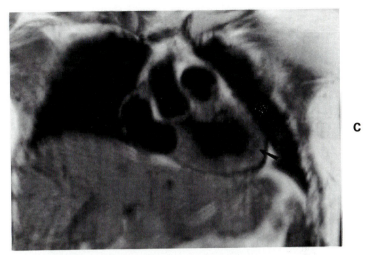

C

Figure 5–16, *Continued.*

interstitial edema. Seldom does the transverse diameter of the heart increase even in cases of acute pericardial effusion.[121,123]

Thus, although modern-day imaging has refined the sensitivity and specificity of injury detection, the standard portable anteroposterior (preferably upright) plain radiograph remains the baseline examination for thoracic trauma.

Once the patient has been stabilized, additional imaging may be performed. Although invasive, angiography remains the only direct means of assessing vascular integrity. The roles of CT, MRI, and TEE as alternative, less invasive means of evaluating the vasculature are to be determined.

IMAGING OF ABDOMINAL TRAUMA

A high index of suspicion must be maintained in the evaluation of a child with blunt abdominal trauma. Multiorgan injury is the norm. Associated head injury is common, often making the abdominal examination unreliable.[124–127] It is imperative that the mechanism of injury be determined and that characteristically associated injuries be sought to minimize morbidity and mortality.[7,128–137] Delay in diagnosis of vascular perforation, hollow viscous rupture, or pancreatic injury may be catastrophic.[119,138–145]

Abdominal trauma in children is usually of the nonpenetrating or "blunt" type, resulting from motor vehicle accidents, pedestrian-vehicle accidents, being kicked or punched as in sports-related injuries, or child abuse.[135,136] Initial clinical evaluation of the patient in the field or in the emergency room directs subsequent evaluation and treatment. Since the development of the emergency medical

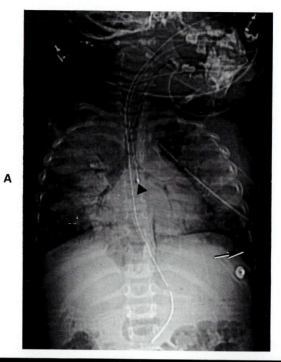

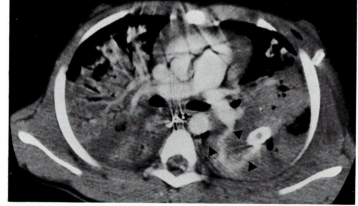

Figure 15–17. A 4-year-old girl whose 7-year-old brother shot her in the chest while playing with a gun. **A,** Anteroposterior digital chest radiograph after intubation and placement of a nasogastric tube and left thoracostomy tube. Note extensive bilateral pulmonary parenchymal injury and small residual pneumothorax on the left side *(arrow)*. The bullet fragments overlie the midthoracic spine *(arrowhead)*. **B,** Axial enhanced computed tomographic scan of the midchest, performed for bullet localization once the patient was hemodynamically stable. Note extensive bilateral pulmonary consolidations. An unexpected finding was contrast extravasation from the left pulmonary artery *(arrowheads)*.

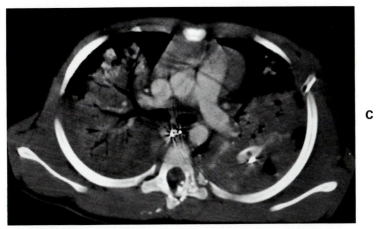

Figure 15–17 *Continued* **C,** Bone window image one level cephalad shows bullet fragments anterior to the vertebral bodies, within the spinal canal, and posteriorly in the paraspinal muscles. Fractures of the posterior elements and adjacent rib can be seen. The course of the bullet may be followed from the subcutaneous emphysema in the left anterolateral chest wall through to the spinal and paraspinal fragments. (Courtesy Dr. Chris Rickman.)

system with its rapid triage of patients in the field, early resuscitation, and rapid transport to established trauma centers, more critically injured children are brought to the emergency room than ever before.[146]

Children who are clinically and hemodynamically stable and have minor injuries may need relatively few tests and may be treated primarily by close observation. If the child has life-threatening head or abdominal injuries or is hemodynamically unstable, emergency surgery for definitive therapy may be indicated. Imaging should not delay treatment.

For children who have severe abdominal injuries but are or have become clinically stable, additional imaging may be warranted to delineate injury or clarify clinical findings.[7,138,147–151]

Treatment of blunt abdominal trauma in children is more conservative (i.e., nonoperative) than in adults. Expectant observation of solid organ injuries has repeatedly demonstrated the healing capability of abdominal solid viscera.[136,137,146,152–155] For this reason, means of noninvasively evaluating the pediatric abdomen have been developed.

Plain Films

Plain radiographs of the abdomen offer the least information of all radiologic modalities. In the trauma setting, however, they are useful for identifying intraabdominal free air, retroperitoneal air, and associated fractures and for

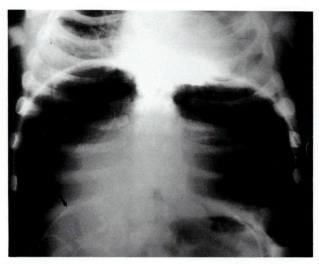

Figure 5–18. Portable anteroposterior abdominal film in a recumbant infant demonstrating massive pneumoperitoneum as demonstrated by large subdiaphragmatic air collections. The borders of the diaphragms on both the thoracic and abdominal sides are well defined and both sides of the bowel wall are exquisitely delineated *(arrow).* (Courtesy Dr. William Kauffman.)

localizing radiopaque foreign bodies (Fig. 5–18). Additional imaging may then be performed as indicated.[131,152,156]

Nuclear Studies

Nuclear scintigraphy is infrequently used in emergency situations but may be helpful after the patient is stabilized for noninvasive assessment of cerebral and solid organ perfusion.[157–163] Scintigraphic identification and follow-up of hepatic and splenic lacerations are also well documented.[154,158,164,165] In the absence of CT or angiography capability, nuclear scintigraphy may be used as an emergency imaging modality.

Ultrasound

Ultrasound use in the trauma setting has not gained the popularity in the United States that it has in Europe. Free peritoneal fluid, solid organ lacerations and contusions, and subcapsular hematomas have all been diagnosed with ultrasound.* Solid organ contusions may be missed depending on their size, age,

---

*References 125, 136, 149, 150, 166–168.

and location.[136] Technologic advances now allow assessment of vascular integrity by use of pulsed and color Doppler ultrasound, although its place in the evaluation of acute pediatric trauma has not yet been fully defined.

The noninvasiveness, portability, and adaptability of ultrasound make it an ideal imaging modality for pediatric patients. Adequacy and diagnostic sensitivity are operator dependent. In patients with abdominal pain and tenderness, or those with rib fractures, the pressure of the transducer on the skin may be intolerable.

Computed Tomography

Over the past decade, CT has emerged as the diagnostic testing modality of choice for pediatric abdominal injury, virtually replacing diagnostic peritoneal lavage (DPL), urography, and nuclear scintigraphy in clinically stable children. This is due partly to its relative noninvasiveness (which parallels the trend toward conservative therapy in the pediatric trauma population), the ease with which the retroperitoneum (an area inaccessible to DPL) may be evaluated, organ injury specificity (but arguably less sensitivity than DPL), and overall assessment of organ function and perfusion.* CT quickly provides anatomic and functional evaluation of all intraabdominal, pelvic, and retroperitoneal structures. Abdominal examinations are seldom isolated studies but rather are combined with head or pelvic examinations.[131,138,173] The two examinations (CT and DPL) are not mutually exclusive.†

In critically injured and unstable patients DPL predominates because of its ready accessibility, its high diagnostic sensitivity, and the speed with which it may be performed.[125,131,138,175–177]

The indications for abdominal CT include any patient who has sustained blunt abdominal trauma[125] and has suspected intraabdominal injury, but whose abdominal examination findings are equivocal or cannot be assessed. Patients with head trauma frequently fit into this category because of an altered sensorium. Abdominal CT should not be used as a screening modality in patients who lack clinical or laboratory evidence of abdominal injury,[151,178,179] regardless of the level of sensorium. In these patients evidence of intraabdominal injury may be evident as hypovolemia, ecchymosis (as in "lap belt injuries"), hematuria, hyperamylasemia, or abdominal tenderness. Although abdominal CT of patients lacking these signs and symptoms occasionally demonstrates unsuspected abnormalities, in the series reported none altered patient outcome or therapy.[178]

---

*References 7, 127, 136, 138, 146–149, 152, 153, 169–172.
†References 125, 133, 138, 149, 153, 174–176.

Conversely, in children in whom there is the slightest suggestion of intraabdominal injury, whether in the form of nonspecific pain, vomiting, or hematuria, underlying injury should be aggressively sought, particularly in light of the poor correlation between physical findings and underlying damage.

Solid Organ Injury

In children, as in adults, the most frequently injured abdominal organ is the spleen, followed by the liver and the kidneys.[125,132,139,166,179] Injury to these organs occurs frequently without associated rib fractures. Splenic fracture (the most common manifestation), fragmentation, contusion, and hematoma formation may all be seen (Figs. 5−19 to 5−21). Experience has taught that even apparently severe injuries may heal without laparotomy.[137,138,146,153−155] CT optimally demonstrates solid organ injuries even when they are subtle. Demonstration of periportal tracking by CT may be the only indication of liver or internal trauma.[180,181]

In the absence of CT availability, or for follow-up examinations, liver-spleen scintigraphy or ultrasound may be used with good results. In the presence of congenital variations, especially accessory spleens, false-positive diagnoses may occur with liver-spleen scans.[136,158,159,164] False-negative studies may result with either CT or ultrasound, depending on the location of injury, its extent, its age, and the technique used for examination.*

Hemobilia is rare and usually results from fracture of the liver center. The source of hemobilia is difficult to diagnose; angiography remains the procedure of choice for diagnosis.[184]

Pancreatic Injury

Pancreatic injury is often difficult to diagnose and occurs relatively frequently in children.[167] Hyperamylasemia may not be present initially, and abdominal pain, if present, may be nonspecific.[131,136,138,168] CT or ultrasound is the preferred imaging modality. Because of the lack of retroperitoneal fat in most children, early CT may not adequately demonstrate abnormality.[182,185] Ultrasound usually delineates the pancreas, but in the presence of bowel distention, the study may be nondiagnostic. In the presence of abdominal pain, pressure from the ultrasound transducer may be intolerable for the young patient. Plain abdominal radiography may demonstrate a "sentinel loop" of dilated transverse colon, ileus, and pleural effusion.[149,167] Delay in diagnosis of pancreatic injury significantly increases patient morbidity and mortality because of peritonitis and the formation of abscess, pseudocyst, and fistula. Clinical symptoms may be

---

*References 136, 153, 155, 167, 182, 183.

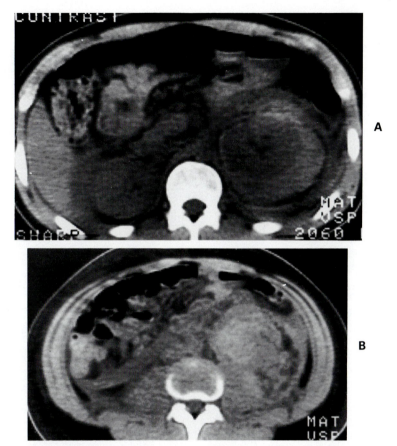

Figure 5–19. A 16-year-old boy fell from his horse, landing on a rock with his left flank. **A,** The fractured left kidney is seen in these non-contrast-enhanced abdominal computed tomographic images as having an irregular outline, isodense with the normal contralateral kidney. It is surrounded and anteriorly displaced by subcapsular hematoma of increased density. **B,** Retroperitonal hematoma abuts the left psoas muscle and extends laterally along the left paracolic gutter. Free fluid can also be seen in the subhepatic space.

subtle before the development of peritonitis from spilled pancreatic enzymes.[129,138,139,146,149] Injury occurs when blunt trauma to the upper abdomen compresses the pancreas against the spine.

Gastrointestinal Injury

Gastric or bowel perforations, which are uncommon, may also be difficult to diagnose. Intestinal injuries occur in 4% to 5% of patients with major injury from blunt abdominal trauma and may be present in up to 15% of pediatric

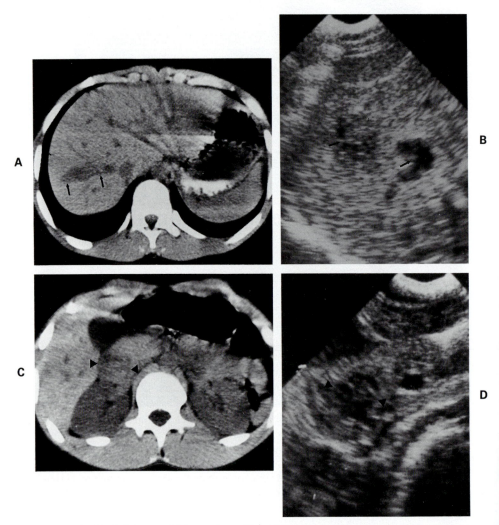

Figure 5–20. A 14-year-old boy who suffered blunt abdominal trauma with resultant hepatic laceration and obstructing duodenal hematoma. **A,** Axial contrast-enhanced computed tomographic scan through the upper abdomen showing a linear hepatic laceration *(arrows)*. **B,** Concurrent ultrasound demonstrating the hepatic lacerations and surrounding hematoma. **C,** Axial computed tomographic scan through the midabdomen and, **D,** concurrent ultrasound showing duodenal hematoma *(arrowheads)*, which over the course of several days increased in size, obstructing the common bile duct. Subsequently the patient did well with conservative therapy.

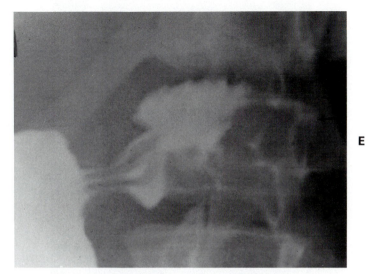

Figure 5–20 *Continued.* **E,** Image from initial upper gastrointestinal series showing complete proximal duodenal obstruction (arrow points to proximal level of obstruction).

patients who are hospitalized because of blunt abdominal trauma.[131,139] The presence of pneumoperitoneum, diagnosed by abdominal radiography or CT, quickly raises the suspicion of bowel perforation. However, perforation may occur without pneumoperitoneum.[138,140,144,182,186] The most common site of rupture is the retroperitoneal duodenum.[138,182,187] In these children retroperitoneal air may be seen outlining the kidney or psoas muscle, but pneumoperitoneum is unusual. Small sites of bowel perforation may quickly seal and prevent pneumoperitoneum. Small bowel hematoma is more common in children, whereas perforation occurs more frequently in adults.[136,138,167,186,188]

Plain abdominal radiographs may be useful for detection of pneumoperitoneum, hydropneumoperitoneum, ileus, scoliosis, and associated injuries.[173,186–189] Although plain films lack both sensitivity and specificity, the demonstration of retroperitoneal free air establishes the diagnosis of duodenal rupture and the demonstration of a large volume of intraabdominal free air warrants emergency laparotomy.

The incidence of bowel injury may be increasing with the use of seat belts. Knowledge of injuries associated with seat belts (bowel rupture, vascular tear, bladder rupture, lumbar spine injury) significantly improves the physician's ability to detect these injuries and decrease subsequent morbidity and mortality.[139,190] Close attention should be paid to the presence and distribution of skin ecchymoses, which may be the only sign of an associated injury.

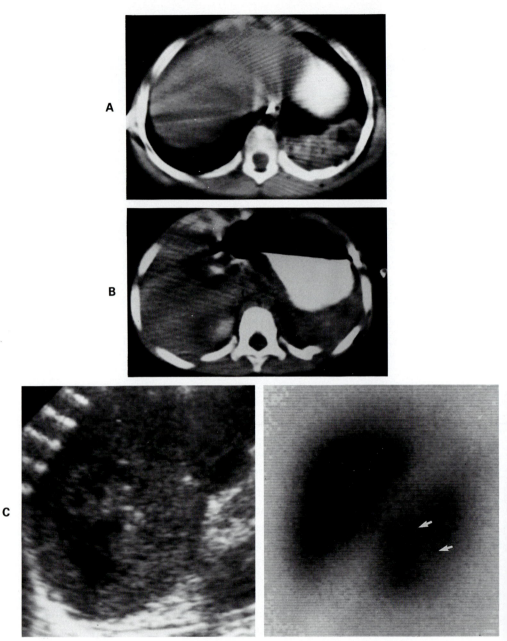

Figure 5–21. A 7-year-old boy hit by a car while bike riding. **A** and **B,** Axial enhanced computed tomographic images through the lower chest and upper abdomen showing left posterior rib fractures, pulmonary contusion of the left lower lobe, and subcutaneous emphysema along left posterolateral chest wall. Note poor definition of the splenic contour with inhomogeneous enhancement of the splenic parenchyma, indicative of splenic hematoma. **C,** Ultrasound shows inhomogeneous echotexture of the splenic pulp with hypoechoic areas of liquefying hematoma. **D,** Left lateral view of the abdomen from a liver-spleen scan demonstrating a linear band of photopenia and an irregular contour posteroinferiorly *(arrows)*.

Gastric rupture from blunt abdominal trauma is rare. Reported cases in children have usually occurred immediately after a meal when the stomach was full, resulting in a "balloon-bursting" type of injury, or from child abuse. This injury is associated with high rates of mortality and morbidity. The clinical presentation is usually shock, with or without subcutaneous emphysema. Abdominal radiography or CT usually shows a large amount of free intraperitoneal air and fluid. Extensive peritoneal contamination by gastric contents ensues, and rapid diagnosis and treatment are necessary to decrease associated morbidity and mortality.[141-143]

CT and ultrasound are exquisitely sensitive in detecting hemoperitoneum, which may be the only clue to the diagnosis of bowel perforation. Although hemoperitoneum is frequently present with hepatic and splenic trauma, the unexplained presence of large amounts of fluid in the abdomen or pelvis should immediately suggest bowel injury.[186,191-193] The exact location of the injury may be difficult to discern preoperatively, but localized bowel edema (bowel wall more than 3 mm thick) and focal hematoma or clot may give indication of the point of injury.[187,188,191] Additional imaging by CT or plain radiography with oral contrast medium may be helpful in delineating the point of injury.[138,140,186]

Specific to children has been the hypoperfusion complex, described initially on CT by Taylor and associates.[194] The complex may be seen in young children whose initial hemodynamic stability is followed by decompensation. The CT findings of the complex include the following:

- Small abdominal aorta, inferior vena cava, superior mesenteric artery, and superior mesenteric vein
- Dilated fluid-filled bowel
- Abnormally exaggerated enhancement of bowel wall, mesentery, kidneys, and pancreas
- Moderate to large volume of peritoneal fluid
- Hypoperfusion of pancreas and spleen

Patients with these CT findings have a poor prognosis[153,170,194-196] (Fig. 5–22).

Genitourinary Injury

Renal injury is the third most common injury in blunt abdominal trauma. Injury may be so minor as to be undetectable by imaging or so major as to be life threatening.

In the past, asymptomatic microscopic hematuria was an indication for performing intravenous urography (IVU) or abdominal CT. More recently quantitation of hematuria and correlation with imaging and surgical findings have modified imaging guidelines in children.[131,182,197,198] Taylor and co-workers[197] reported the low yield of abdominal CT in children with blunt abdominal trauma in whom microscopic hematuria was the only indication for

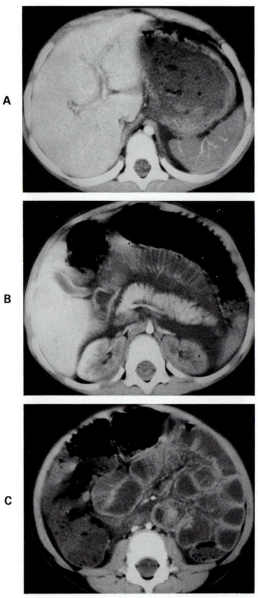

Figure 5–22. A 9-year-old victim of a motor vehicle accident who was hemodynamically stable at the outset of computed tomographic (CT) examination of the abdomen. On computed tomography, acute deterioration was evidenced by signs of shock bowel syndrome: **A,** periportal low density from blood or lymph, small-caliber aorta, poor splenic perfusion, and hemoperitoneum; **B,** inhomogeneous and poor renal perfusion, abnormally intense pancreatic and gallbladder wall enhancement, and abundant hemoperitoneum; and **C,** diffusely distended bowel with abnormally intense bowel wall enhancement and very small-caliber inferior vena cava and aorta. (Courtesy Dr. Robert Kaufman.)

CT. Subsequently, Burbridge and associates[198] reported the same findings concerning emergency excretory urography.

Although IVU (with or without tomography) may be appropriate for evaluation when isolated renal trauma is suspected or when the patient's condition is too unstable to permit CT examination, CT provides more information about intraabdominal and retroperitoneal structures, is more sensitive and specific, and uses a lower total radiation dose than IVU with tomograms.[138,148,149,153,170] CT's ability to define the presence, size, and rate of growth of retroperitoneal hematoma has recently been evaluated as an indicator for emergency surgery versus observation.[131,199,200] Even in the presence of major injuries such as a shattered kidney or renal vascular pedicle injuries, treatment approaches vary as summarized in Chapter 8.[153]

Ultrasound provides excellent anatomic information about the kidneys but lacks the additional functional assessment offered by CT. Pulsed and color Doppler imaging can be used to assess renal vascular integrity. Either CT or ultrasound is excellent for follow-up of renal injury and monitoring of healing.

When intravenous contrast material is to be administered for either IVU or CT, the presence of bladder or urethral injury should first be ruled out. These structures are best initially studied via retrograde urethrography and, if indicated, retrograde cystography. This order of events allows CT assessment of upper genitourinary tract integrity without obscuration by a full bladder.[151]

Bladder and urethral injuries are relatively common, particularly in association with pelvic fractures. When blunt trauma to a distended bladder results in perforation, it is usually an intraperitoneal rupture of the dome.[151,168] Extraperitoneal rupture is the more common form and is usually associated with pelvic fracture.[138] The most common form of bladder injury, however, is contusion.[151] Associated bladder wall thickening may be easily demonstrated by CT but less commonly by cystography. Urethral injuries are usually seen in males and occur at the junction of the posterior urethra and bladder neck.[151,168] They are best assessed by retrograde urethrography.

Plain pelvic radiographs are the initial imaging choice for multiple trauma victims. They are an excellent method of assessing bony integrity of the pelvis and hips.[151]

As with abdominal trauma, CT is the preferred imaging modality for the assessment of pelvic trauma because it evaluates not only the bony pelvis, but also the soft tissue structures (Fig. 5–23). Pelvic fractures vary from simple avulsion fractures of the iliac spines to complex life-threatening fractures. Associated vascular injury is common and may be massive.[151,201,202] Retroperitoneal hematoma is usually the result of bleeding from the rich venous plexuses in which lacerations are frequently associated with posterior pelvic fractures. Such bleeding and fractures are readily demonstrated with CT.[151] Arterial injury from

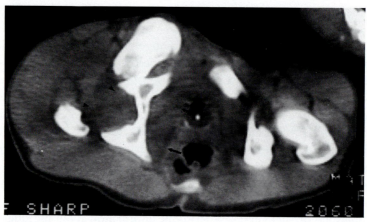

Figure 5–23. An 18-year-old man who was involved in a motor vehicle accident. Axial computed tomographic scan through the pelvis demonstrates fracture dislocation of the right hip. Note large pelvic hematoma *(arrows)* and hemorrhage at the fracture site *(arrowheads)*. The patient had concurrent hematoma of the anterior abdominal wall.

pelvic fracture is uncommon and may be life threatening, but it can be diagnosed and treated angiographically.[151,202–204]

Summary

Blunt trauma to the abdomen results in a wide spectrum of injuries. Knowledge of the mechanism of injury greatly enhances lesion detection. Plain radiographs are the initial imaging modality, followed by CT in hemodynamically stable patients and DPL or surgery or both in unstable patients.

When CT is not available or the patient's condition is too unstable for it, IVU may be used as a screening tool to assess renal integrity. Ultrasound is gaining popularity for evaluating pediatric trauma patients in emergency situations.

Angiography and, if indicated, embolization are excellent means of diagnosing and treating arterial injuries and may be lifesaving.

IMAGING OF VASCULAR AND PENETRATING WOUNDS

Angiography remains the only direct means by which the vascular tree may be assessed.[7] Modifications of this procedure include digital subtraction angiography and occasionally dynamic CT. Although MRI has been demonstrated to evaluate the great vessels, its use in the emergency trauma situation is not justified and it is not readily accessible or safe for patient monitoring.[7,10,11]

During the past 10 to 15 years angiographic and interventional radiologic procedures in the pediatric population have gained acceptance.[205–212] This in part is due to technologic improvements in and subspecialization of pediatric angiographic interventional procedures. Staff experienced in pediatric angiography can perform these procedures safely, quickly, and judiciously. As in the adult population, they offer an alternative to surgical exploration. In some instances, such as with pelvic fracture, surgical exploration to determine the point of bleeding may be difficult at best, and angiographic assessment with embolization of the bleeding vessel may be the preferred approach.[7,212,213–216]

Whenever the question of vascular injury arises, angiographic evaluation should be performed without delay. Angiography may be performed preoperatively, intraoperatively, or in certain cases postoperatively. Concurrent interventional or therapeutic angiographic procedures may be indicated as well.

Injury to the extremity arteries in children presents a challenge to the trauma team, particularly the surgeon. Missing the diagnosis of an arterial injury, or even delaying it for several hours, subjects the child to significant morbidity, including limb length discrepancy, loss of function of the extremity, blood pressure differentials, bone age retardation, and even the necessity for amputation. Surgical exploration of extremity injuries carries a risk (see Chapter 13), particularly in children. Arterial integrity must therefore be aggressively evaluated.[7,211,216–221] The rationale for and sequence of evaluation are fully discussed in Chapter 13.

THE ABUSED CHILD

Caffey initially described the radiographic manifestations of the "abused child" in 1946, when he described long bone fractures in association with infantile subdural hematoma.[222] Silverman in 1953 expounded upon this topic, further defining the prognostic implications of these injuries and refining the radiographic manifestations.[223]

Since that time the literature has become replete with entries about child abuse and its multifactorial presentation.[4,9,224–230] In essence, nonaccidental trauma should be suspected anytime radiographic findings are discrepant with the clinical history. Typically described epiphyseal-metaphyseal injuries of the long bones in children are present in only approximately 50% of abused children. Spiral and transverse diaphyseal fractures are reported to be four times as common as epiphyseal-metaphyseal injuries (Fig. 5–24).[227] The skull was the second most common skeletal injury in 34% of a series of 563 cases reported. Frequency of additional injuries varied and in part were contingent upon the age of the child and the mechanism of abuse.

Approximately two thirds of abused children have radiographic manifestations, and over half have detectable fractures. The abused child may have a single acute fracture resulting from a single occurrence of abuse, but a multiplicity of fractures in varying stages of healing is more commonly seen (Fig. 5–25). Abundant and exaggerated callus formation is not uncommon and is usually due to repeated trauma. Such injury usually occurs when an adult holds the

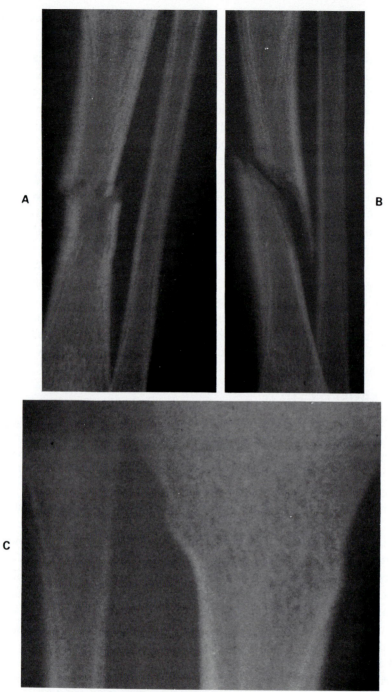

Figure 5–24. Infant victim of child abuse. Plain radiographs of the extremities revealed multiple fractures. **A,** Anteroposterior and, **B,** lateral radiographs of the left lower extremity showing an oblique midtibial diaphyseal fracture. **C,** The child also had torus fracture of the proximal right tibial metaphysis.

160

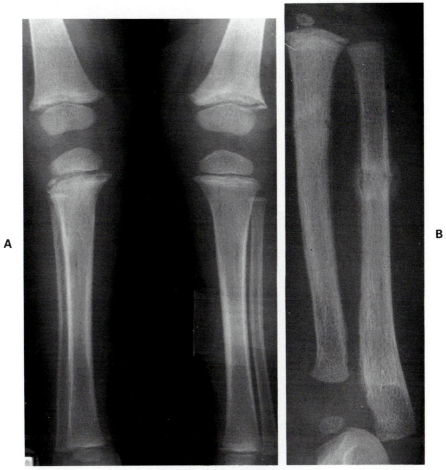

Figure 5–25. A 10-month-old male victim of child abuse. Plain radiographs of the extremities demonstrate multiple fractures of various ages. **A,** Anteroposterior views of the legs reveal bilateral distal femoral and proximal right tibial metaphyseal bucket-handle fractures typical of abuse. Soft tissue around the left knee is swollen. **B,** The same patient with a healing fracture of the mid–left ulnar diaphysis, a more acute distal left radial diaphyseal fracture, and periosteal reaction along the shafts of both the radius and the ulna.

child by the extremities and severely shakes him or her. Injuries occur not from direct blunt trauma, but rather from acceleration-deceleration forces, stretching, and pulling.[224,227]

Whenever child abuse is suspected, a skeletal survey should be performed. The utility of nuclear medicine scintigraphy remains controversial.[4,229,230] A radiographic survey including anteroposterior and lateral views of the skull, anteroposterior views of the thorax and of the abdomen, and views of the pelvis and extremities usually suffices. Any suspicion of intracranial injury with or without external signs of abuse warrants CT or MRI.

Among the conditions that may be diagnostically confused with child abuse are the following, although clinical, sociologic, and radiographic findings can usually differentiate abuse from one of these diagnoses: congenital syphilis, multifocal osteomyelitis, rickets, scurvy, infantile cortical hyperostosis (Caffey's disease), osteogenesis imperfecta, leukemia, metastatic neuroblastoma, normal periosteal reaction of infancy, congenital insensitivity to pain, hypophosphatasia, meningococcemia, frostbite, and electrical burns.[232,233]

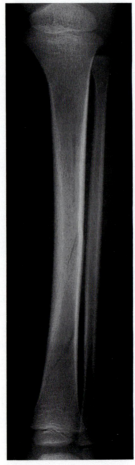

Figure 5–26. Typical toddler's fracture showing torque fracture of the tibia.

TODDLER'S FRACTURES

Fractures during toddlerhood most frequently result from a spiral torque on the child's tibia (Fig. 5–26). The child refuses to walk. Clinical and radiographic signs are usually sparse, although there may be focal warmth and tenderness at the point of the fracture. Early radiographic signs may be nothing more than subtle soft tissue swelling.[1,229,230,231]

When visible, the fracture may not be seen on all views. Characteristically it is an oblique or spiral hairline fracture of the tibial diaphysis. During the subacute phase, subperiosteal new bone formation may be visualized on the radiograph. From its appearance, new bone formation may be difficult to differentiate from a bone tumor.

SPORTS INJURIES

Sports-related injuries, particularly ligamentous injuries, are much more common in midadolescence than in childhood. Children in parentally supervised and organized athletics have a greater incidence of injuries than those who play unsupervised games. This seems to be related to adult pressures forcing children to extend themselves beyond their physical limits.[232]

Muscular development may exceed the strength of the apophysis, leading to avulsion fractures (Figs. 5–27 and 5–28).[232] Knowing the locations of the more common avulsion fractures can expedite diagnosis and prevent these be-

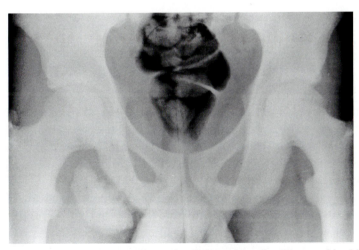

Figure 5–27. Anteroposterior radiograph of the pelvis of a 15-year-old athletic boy complaining of right leg pain. He has a large avulsion fracture of the ischial tuberosity, the origin of the hamstring muscles. (Courtesy Dr. Tom Boulden.)

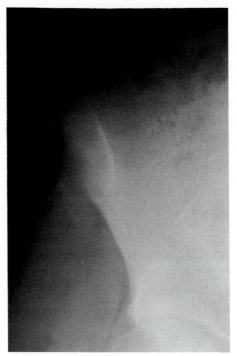

Figure 5–28. A 15-year-old boy felt pain and heard a "pop" in his right hip while running track. An anteroposterior view of the pelvis shows avulsion fracture of his right superior iliac spine at the insertion of the sartorius muscle.

nign traumatic conditions from being misdiagnosed as infectious or neoplastic processes on the basis of radiography.[230]

PHYSEAL INJURIES

Injuries to the physis occur only in children. Approximately 15% of childhood fractures involve specifically the physis. Ligamentous injuries around a joint seldom occur in childhood because the cartilaginous and ligamentous structures surrounding a joint are considerably stronger than the cartilaginous growth plate in a child.[229,233]

The type I injury (Fig. 5–29), accounting for approximately 6% of physeal injuries,[234] involves only the growth plate[229,233,234] and usually results from a shearing or avulsion stress.[233] Type I injuries may be difficult to visualize radiographically. Subtle widening of the growth plate or surrounding soft tissue edema may be all that is apparent. Comparison views of the anatomically contralateral side may provide insight into the abnormality. Follow-up radiographic examinations in 7 to 10 days can improve the detection rate of these fractures.

The most common physeal injury is the type II fractures (Fig. 5–30),

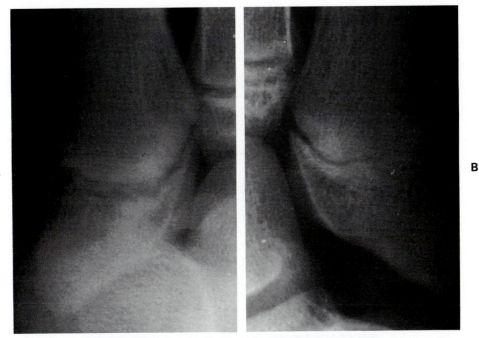

Figure 5–29. Salter-Harris type I injury with fracture across the growth plate in a 16-year-old boy who twisted his ankle. **A,** Plain radiograph of the injured ankle shows widening of the right fibular physis. **B,** Comparison view of the normal left ankle confirms the presence of a Salter I fracture of the right distal fibula.

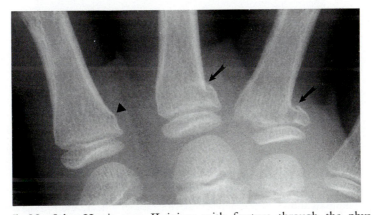

Figure 5–30. Salter-Harris type II injury with fracture through the physis and adjacent metaphysis. Anteroposterior radiograph of a child who had suffered hand trauma. Note Salter II fractures of the proximal metaphyses of the third and fourth proximal phalanges *(arrow)*. The fracture of the fourth proximal phalange is also displaced. There is an associated buckle fracture of the second proximal phalanx *(arrowhead)*.

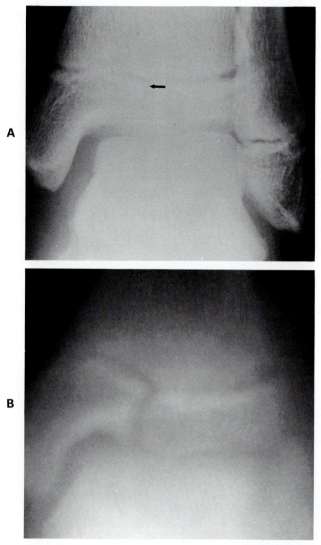

Figure 5–31. Salter-Harris type III injury with fracture through the physis and extending into the epiphysis shown in this anteroposterior radiograph, **A,** and tomogram **B.**

which accounts for 75% of physeal injuries.[234] The type II fracture extends through the physis and the adjacent metaphysis and is most commonly seen in children older than 10 years of age.[233,234] This type of fracture most frequently results from an avulsion or shearing injury.[233]

Eight percent of physeal injuries are type III (Fig. 5−31), which is a fracture through the physis and extending through the epiphysis.[229,233,234] These fractures are intraarticular.[229,233] There may be displacement of the epiphyseal fragment, which may also undergo abnormal rotation. Type III injuries commonly occur at the knee or ankle. When the distal tibial epiphysis is involved as the physis is closing, it is termed a Tillaux fracture.[229]

The type IV injury (Fig. 5−32), accounting for 10% of physeal injuries, is a vertical fracture through the metaphysis, physis, and epiphysis.[229,233,234] Open reduction is frequently required.[229,233,234] Traumatic epiphysiodesis with limb shortening may result.[229,233]

The most uncommon of the physeal fractures is the type V injury, which accounts for only 1% of physeal injuries and results from a crushing injury to the physis, commonly at the ankle or knee.[229,233,234] Radiographic diagnosis of this injury at its acute stage is difficult, if not impossible.[229,230,233,234] The morbidity related to this fracture is due to premature traumatic epiphysiodesis, which may not be manifest until years after the initial injury.[229,234]

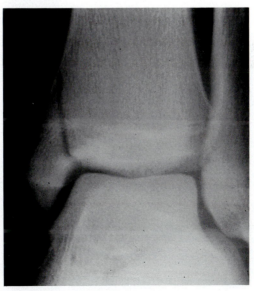

Figure 5−32. Salter-Harris type IV injury with fracture through the physis and extending into both the metaphysis and the epiphysis.

The morbidity related to Salter-Harris type fractures depends on diagnosis, classification type, location, and developmental age of the child at the time of the injury.

NAVICULAR FRACTURE

Carpal fractures are uncommon in children, but when they occur, fracture of the carpal navicular (scaphoid) bone is the most common.[230,235,236] The fracture is characterized clinically by "snuff box" tenderness. When nondisplaced, it may be difficult to identify radiographically with a routine wrist series (usually consisting of posteroanterior, lateral, and external oblique views) (Fig. 5–33, *A*). A navicular view (posteroanterior view with ulnar deviation) often aids in radiographic diagnosis (Fig. 5–33, *B*).[235] Further evaluation with CT, MRI, or nuclear scintigraphy may delineate the fracture earlier.[236,237]

If the diagnosis is missed at the time of initial examination, the fracture may be recognized when nonunion and avascular necrosis develop, although these sequelae are more common in adults than in children. They result from disruption of the blood supply to the proximal fragment.[237,238] Because of the

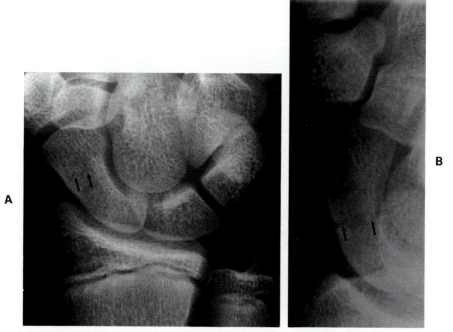

Figure 5–33. Wrist pain after trauma was clinically localizable to the "snuffbox." **A,** Nondisplaced horizontal navicular fracture (*arrows*) is difficult to detect. **B,** The fracture is readily appreciated on the navicular view (*arrows*).

possibility of these sequelae, every attempt should be made to delineate the suspected fracture. If it cannot be identified radiographically, the patient should be treated for presumed fracture and follow-up studies performed.[236]

CONCLUSION

Trauma remains the leading cause of death in children, and its sequelae are seen all too frequently in emergency rooms. The physician's knowledge of the patterns and mechanisms of injury in the pediatric population and particular expertise in dealing with children expedite diagnosis and treatment. Only when physicians are knowledgeable about traumatic injury will they recognize it in patients. Improved technology and teamwork contribute to the goal of reducing morbidity and mortality from pediatric trauma.

REFERENCES

1. Kirks DR: *Practical pediatric imaging: diagnostic radiology of infants and children,* Boston, 1984, Little, Brown.
2. Dove DB, Stahl WM, Del Guerico LRM: A five-year review of deaths following urban trauma, *J Trauma* 20(9):760–766, 1980.
3. Baker CC, Oppenheimer L, Stephens B, et al: Epidemiology of trauma deaths, *Am J Surg* 140(1):144–150, 1980.
4. Holmes MJ, Reyes HM: A critical review of urban pediatric trauma, *J Trauma* 24(3):253–255, 1984.
5. Valentine J, Blocker S, Chang JHT: Gunshot injuries in children, *J Trauma* 24(11):952–956, 1984.
6. Bates D, Raggieri P: Imaging modalities for evaluation of the spine, *Radiol Clin North Am* 29(4):675–690, 1991.
7. Ben-Menacham Y, Fisher RG: Diagnostic and interventional radiology in trauma. In Maddox KL, Moore EE, Feliciano DV, eds: *Trauma,* Norwalk, Conn, 1988, Appleton & Lange.
8. Hey EN, Katz G: The optimum thermal environment for naked babies, *Arch Dis Child* 45(241):328–334, 1970.
9. Poznanski AK: Practical considerations in examining infants in the radiology department. In *Pediatric radiology,* Proceedings of the 75th Scientific Assembly and Annual Meeting, Radiological Society of North America, November 26–December 1, 1989.
10. Shalen PR: Diagnostic challenges in closed head trauma, *Radiol Clin North Am* 19(1):53–68, 1981.
11. Doezema D, King JN, Tandberg D, et al: Magnetic resonance imaging in minor head injury, *Ann Emerg Med* 20(12):1281–1285, 1991.
12. Heiken JP, Brown JJ, eds: *Manual of clinical magnetic resonance imaging,* ed 2, New York, 1991, Raven Press.
13. Lufkin RB: *The MRI manual,* Chicago, 1990, Mosby.
14. Barnes PD: Magnetic resonance in pediatric and adolescent neuroimaging, *Neurol Clin* 8(3):741–757, 1990.
15. Stein SC, O'Malley KF, Ross SE: Is routine computed tomography scanning too expensive for mild head injury? *Ann Emerg Med* 20(12):1286–1289, 1991.

16. Livingston DH, Loder PA, Koziol J, Hunt CD: The use of CT scanning to triage patients requiring admission following minimal head injury, *J Trauma* 31(4):483–489, 1991.

17. Shackford SR, Wald SL, Ross SE, et al: The clinical utility of computed tomographic scanning and neurologic examination in the management of patients with minor head injuries, *J Trauma* 33(3):385–394, 1992.

18. Servdei F: Computed tomographic examination in minor head injury (letter), *Lancet* 337:788–789, 1991.

19. Mohanty SK, Thompson W, Rakower S: Are CT scans for head injury patients always necessary? *J Trauma* 31(6):801–804, 1991.

20. The head. In Swischuck LE: *Emergency radiology of the acutely ill or injured child,* ed 2, Baltimore, 1986, Williams & Wilkins, pp 491–547.

21. Zimmerman RA, Bilaniuk LT, Gennarelli T, et al: Cranial computed tomography in diagnosis and management of acute head trauma, *Am J Roentgenol* 131(7):27–34, 1978.

22. Forbes GS, Shudy II PF, Piepgras DG, Houser OW: Computed tomography in the evaluation of subdural hematomas, *Radiology* 126(1):143–148, 1978.

23. Harwood-Nash DC: Head injuries in child abuse. In *Pediatric radiology,* Proceeding of the 75th Scientific Assembly and Annual Meeting, Radiological Society of North America, November 26–December 1, 1989.

24. Harwood-Nash DC, Hendrick EB, Hudson AR: The significance of skull fractures in children, *Radiology* 101(1):151–155, 1971.

25. Reider-Groswasser I, Fishman E, Razon N: Epidural haematoma: computerized tomography (CT) parameters in 19 patients, *Brain Injury* 5(1):17–21, 1991.

26. Zimmerman RD, Russell EJ, Yurberg E, Leeds NE: Falx and interhemispheric fissure on axial CT. II. Recognition and differentiation of interhemispheric subarachnoid and subdural hemorrhage, *AJNR* 3(11–12):635–642, 1982.

27. Lee J-P, Lui T-N, Chang C-N: Acute post-traumatic intraventricular hemorrhage analysis of 25 patients with emphasis on final outcome, *Acta Neurol Scand* 84:85–90, 1991.

28. LeRoux PD, Haglund MM, Newell DW, et al: Intraventricular hemorrhage in blunt head trauma: an analysis of 43 cases, *Neurosurgery* 31(4):678–685, 1992.

29. Osborne AG: Diagnosis of descending transtentorial herniation by cranial computed tomography, *Radiology* 123(10):93–96, 1977.

30. Barkovitch AJ: MR and CT evaluation of profound neonatal and infantile asphyxia, *AJNR* 13:959–972, 1992.

31. Cohen RA, Kaufman RA, Myers PA, Towbin RB: Cranial computed tomography in the abused child with head injury, *AJR* 146(1):97–102, 1986.

32. Bird CR, McMahan JR, Gilles FH, et al: Strangulation in child abuse: CT diagnosis, *Radiology* 163(2):373–375, 1987.

33. Mendelsohn DB, Levin HS, Harward H, Bruce D: Corpus callosum lesions after closed head injury in children: MRI, clinical features and outcome, *Neuroradiology* 34(5):384–388, 1992.

34. Bešenski N, Brzović Z, Pripić-Vučković R, et al: CT detection of minimal brain lesions in closed cerebral trauma, *Neurol Croat* 41(1–2):33–42, 1992.

35. Meyer CA, Mirvis SE, Wolf AL, et al: Acute traumatic midbrain hemorrhage: experimental and clinical observations with CT, *Radiology* 179(3):813–818, 1991.

36. Sasiadek M, Marciniak R, Bem Z: CT appearance of shearing injuries of the brain, *Bildgebung* 58(3):148–149, 1991.

37. Zepp F, Brühl K, Zimmer B, Schumacher R: Battered child syndrome: cerebral ultrasound and CT findings after vigorous shaking, *Neuropediatrics* 23(4):188–191, 1992.
38. Zimmerman RA, Bilaniuk LT, Bruce D, et al: Computed tomography of craniocerebral injury in the abused child, *Radiology* 130(3):687–690, 1979.
39. Johnson DH Jr: CT of maxillofacial trauma, *Radiol Clin North Am* 22(1):131–144, 1984.
40. Merten DF, Osborne DRS, Radkowski MA, Leonidas JC: Craniocerebral trauma in the child abuse syndrome: radiological observations, *Pediatr Radiol* 14:272–277, 1984.
41. Radkowski MA, Merten DF, Leonidas JC: The abused child: criteria for the radiologic diagnosis, *Radiographics* 3(2):262–297, 1983.
42. Pathria MN, Blaser SI: Diagnostic imaging of craniofacial fractures, *Musculoskel Trauma* 27(5):839–853, 1989.
43. Unger JM: Fractures of the nasolacrimal fossa and canal: a CT study of appearance, associated injuries, and significance in 25 patients, *AJR* 158(6):1321–1324, 1992.
44. Betz BW, Wiener MD: Air in the temporomandibular joint fossa: CT sign of temporal bone fracture, *Radiology* 180(2):463–466, 1991.
45. Ilankovan V, Hadley D, Moos K, el Attar A: A comparison of imaging techniques with surgical experiences in orbital injuries, *J Cranio Maxillofac Surg* 19(8):348–352, 1991.
46. Maguire AM, Enger C, Eliott D, Zinreich SJ: Computerized tomography in the evaluation of penetrating ocular injuries, *Retina* 11(4):405–411, 1991.
47. Assael LA: Clinical aspects of imaging in maxillofacial trauma, *Radiol Clin North Am* 31(1):209–220, 1993.
48. Johnson MH, Lee SH: Computed tomography of acute cerebral trauma, *Radiol Clin North Am* 30(2):325–352, 1992.
49. Meservy CJ, Towbin R, McLaurin RL, et al: Radiologic characteristics of skull fractures resulting from child abuse, *AJNR* 8:455–457, 1987.
50. Johnson MH, Lee SH: Computed tomography of acute cerebral trauma, *Radiol Clin North Am* 30(2):325–352, 1992.
51. Gentry LR: Facial trauma and associated brain damage, *Radiol Clin North Am* 27(2):435–446, 1989.
52. Olson EM, Wright DL, Hoffman HT, et al: Frontal sinus fractures: evaluation of CT scans in 132 patients, *AJNR* 13:897–902, 1992.
53. Sklar EML, Quencer RM, Bowen BC, et al: Magnetic resonance applications in cerebral injury, *Radiol Clin North Am* 30(2):353–366, 1992.
54. Yokota H, Kurokawa A, Otsuka T, et al: Significance of magnetic resonance imaging in acute head injury, *J Trauma* 31(3):351–357, 1991.
55. Ogawa T, Sekino H, Uzura M, et al: Comparative study of magnetic resonance and CT scan imaging in cases of severe head injury, *Acta Neurochir* 55:8–10, 1992.
56. Wilson JTL, Hadley DM, Wiedmann KD, Teasdale GM: Intercorrelation of lesions detected by magnetic resonance imaging after closed head injury, *Brain Injury* 6(5):391–399, 1992.
57. Alexander RC, Schor DP, Smith WL Jr: Magnetic resonance imaging of intracranial injuries from child abuse, *J Pediatr* 109:975–979, 1986.
58. Levin AV, Magnusson MR, Rafto SE, Zimmerman RA: Shaken baby syndrome diagnosed by magnetic resonance imaging, *Pediatr Emerg Care* 5(3):181–186, 1989.
59. Gehweiler JA Jr, Osborne RL Jr, Becker RF: *The radiology of vertebral trauma*, Philadelphia, 1980, WB Saunders.

60. The spine and spinal cord. In Swischuck LE: *Emergency radiology of the acutely ill and injured child*, ed 2, Baltimore, 1986, Williams & Wilkins, pp 556–595.
61. Harris JH Jr, Yeakley JS: Radiographically subtle soft tissue injuries of the cervical spine, *Curr Probl Diagn Radiol* 18(4):165–190, 1989.
62. Byrd SE, Wilczynski MA: Imaging modalities for the pediatric spine, *Curr Opin Radiol* 3(6):906–918, 1991.
63. Zimmerman RA, Bilaniuk LT, Bury EA: Magnetic resonance of the pediatric spine, *Magn Reson Imaging* 5(3):169–204, 1989.
64. Bundschuh CV, Alley JB, Ross M, et al: Magnetic resonance imaging of suspected atlanto-occipital dislocation, *Spine* 17(2):245–248, 1992.
65. Berquist TH: Cervical spine trauma (abstract), *Radiology* 178(2):591, 1991.
66. Pathria MN, Petersilge CA: Spinal trauma, *Radiol Clin North Am* 29(4):847–865, 1991.
67. Murphey MD, Batnitzky S, Bramble JM: Diagnostic imaging of spinal trauma, *Radiol Clin North Am* 27(5):855–872, 1989.
68. Riddervold HO: Easily missed fractures, *Radiol Clin North Am* 30(2):475–494, 1992.
69. Handel SF, Lee Y-Y: Computed tomography of spinal fractures, *Radiol Clin North Am* 19(1):69–89, 1981.
70. Post MJD, Green BA: The use of computed tomography in spinal trauma, *Radiol Clin North Am* 21(2):327–375, 1983.
71. Byrd SE, Wilczynski MA: Imaging modalities for the pediatric spine, *Curr Opin Radiol* 3(6):906–918, 1991.
72. Hudgins PA, Hudgins RJ: Radiology of cervical spine trauma, *Neurosurgery* 37:571–595, 1991.
73. Roshkow JE, Haller JO, Hotson GC, et al: Imaging evaluation of children after falls from a height: review of 45 cases, *Radiology* 175(2):359–363, 1990.
74. Fuchs S, Barthel MJ, Flannery AM, et al: Cervical spine fractures (abstract), *Radiology,* January 1990, p 296.
75. Hayes CW, Conway WF, Walsh JW, et al: Seat belt injuries: radiologic findings and clinical correlation, *Radiographics* 11(1):23–36, 1991.
76. Miller JA, Smith TH: Seatbelt induced chance fracture in an infant, *Pediatr Radiol* 21:575–577, 1991.
77. Ballock RT, Mackersie R, Abitbol J-J, et al: (abstract), *Radiology,* 1992, p 294.
78. Banerian KG, Wang A-M, Samberg LC, et al: Association of vertebral end plate fracture with pediatric lumbar intervertebral disk herniation: value of CT and MR imaging, *Radiology* 177(3):763–765, 1990.
79. Volle E, Assheuer J, Hedde JP, Gustorf-Aeckerle R: Radicular avulsion resulting from spinal injury: assessment of diagnostic modalities, *Neuroradiology* 34(3):235–240, 1992.
80. Nussbaum ES, Sebring LA, Wolf AL, et al: Myelographic and enhanced computed tomographic appearance of acute traumatic spinal cord avulsion, *Neurosurgery* 30:43–48, 1992.
81. Montana MA, Richardson ML, Kilcoyne RF, et al: CT of sacral injury, *Radiology* 161(2):499–503, 1986.
82. Morris RE, Hasso AN, Thompson JR, et al: Traumatic dural tears: CT diagnosis using metrizamide, *Radiology* 152(2):443–446, 1984.
83. Kulkarni MV, McArdle CB, Kopanicky D, et al: Acute spinal cord injury: MR imaging at 1.5 T, *Radiology* 164(3):837–843, 1987.
84. Brightman RP, Miller CA, Rea GL, et al: Magnetic resonance imaging of trauma to the thoracic and lumbar spine, *Spine* 17(5):541–550, 1992.

85. Kerslake RW, Jaspan T, Worthington BS: Magnetic resonance imaging of spinal trauma, *Br J Radiol* 64:386–402, 1991.
86. Yamashita Y, Takahashi M, Matsuno Y, et al: Acute spinal cord injury: magnetic resonance imaging correlated with myelopathy, *Br J Radiol* 64(759):201–209, 1991.
87. Goldberg AL, Baron B, Daffner RH: Atlantooccipital dislocation: MR demonstration of cord damage, *J Comput Assist Tomogr* 15(1):174–178, 1991.
88. Hackney DB: Denominators of spinal cord injury, *Radiology* 177(1):18–20, 1990.
89. Silberstein M, Tress BM, Hennessy O: A comparison between M.R.I. and C.T. in acute spinal trauma, *Australas Radiol* 36(3):192–197, 1992.
90. Bentson JR, Spickler E, Lufkin RB: Magnetic resonance imaging of the spine. In Lufkin RB, ed: *The MRI manual,* St Louis, 1990, Mosby, pp 142–154.
91. Haller JA, Pokorny WJ: Pediatric trauma. In Mattox KL, Moore EE, Feliciano DV, eds: *Trauma,* Norwalk, Conn, 1988, Appleton & Lange, pp 629–644.
92. Meller JL, Little AG, Shermeta DW: Thoracic trauma in children, *Pediatrics* 74(5):813–819, 1984.
93. Dee PM: The radiology of chest trauma, *Radiol Clin North Am* 30(2):291–306, 1992.
94. Sivit CJ, Taylor GA, Eichelberger MR: Chest injury in children with blunt abdominal trauma: evaluation with CT, *Radiology* 171(3):815–818, 1989.
95. Hedlund GL, Kirks DR: Emergency radiology of the pediatric chest, *Curr Probl Diagn Radiol* 19:135–164, 1990.
96. Groskin SA: Selected topics in chest trauma, *Radiology* 183(3):605–617, 1992.
97. Smyth BT: Chest trauma in children, *J Pediatr Surg* 14(1):41–47, 1979.
98. Carrico CJ, Ivey TD, Rusch VW: Injury to the lung and pleura. In Mattox KL, Moore EE, Feliciano DV, eds: *Trauma,* Norwalk, Conn, 1988, Appleton & Lange, pp 349–364.
99. The chest. In Swischuk LE: *Emergency radiology of the acutely ill or injured child,* ed 2, Baltimore, 1986, Williams & Wilkins, pp 105–116.
100. The lung parenchyma. In Rosenberger A, Adler OB, Troupin RH: *Trauma imaging in the thorax and abdomen,* Chicago, 1987, Year Book, pp 49–62.
101. Goodman LR, Putman CE: The S.I.C.U. chest radiograph after massive blunt trauma, *Radiol Clin North Am* 19(1):111–123, 1981.
102. Eichelberger MR, Randolph J: Chest trauma in children. In Brooks BF, ed: *The injured child,* Austin, 1985, University of Texas Press, pp 44–52.
103. Valentine J, Blocker S, Change JHT: Gunshot injuries in children, *J Trauma* 24(11):952–956, 1984.
104. Shuck JM, Snow NJ: Injury to the chest wall. In Mattox KL, Moore EE, Feliciano DV, eds: *Trauma,* Norwalk, Conn, 1988, Appleton & Lange, pp 321–334.
105. Heare MM, Heare TC, Gillespy T III: Diagnostic imaging of pelvic and chest wall trauma, *Radiol Clin North Am* 27(5):873–890, 1989.
106. Mattox KL, O'Gorman RB: Injury to the thoracic great vessels. In Mattox KL, Moore EE, Feliciano DV, eds: *Trauma,* Norwalk, Conn, 1988, Appleton & Lange, pp 385–400.
107. Chest wall and diaphragm. In Rosenberger A, Adler OB, Troupin RH: *Trauma imaging in the thorax and abdomen,* Chicago, 1987, Year Book, pp 16–30.
108. Ben-Menachem Y: Logic and logistics of radiography, angiography, and angiographic intervention in massive blunt trauma, *Radiol Clin North Am* 19(1):9–15, 1981.
109. Smejkal R, O'Malley KF, David E, et al: Routine initial computed tomography of the chest in blunt torso trauma, *Chest* 100(3):667–679, 1991.

110. The mediastinum. In Rosenberger A, Adler OB, Troupin RH: *Trauma imaging in the thorax and abdomen,* Chicago, 1987, Year Book, pp 63–84.
111. Mulder DS, Barkun JS: Injury to the trachea, bronchus, and esophagus. In Mattox KL, Moore EE, Feliciano DV, eds: *Trauma,* Norwalk, Conn, 1988, Appleton & Lange, pp 335–348.
112. Mirvis SE, Templeton P: Imaging in acute thoracic trauma, *Semin Roentgenol* 27:184–210, 1992.
113. The pleural space. In Rosenberger A, Adler OB, Troupin RH: *Trauma imaging in the thorax and abdomen,* Chicago, 1987, Year Book, pp 31–48.
114. Toombs BD, Lester RG, Ben-Menachem Y, Sandler CM: Computed tomography in blunt trauma, *Radiol Clin North Am* 19(1):17–35, 1981.
115. Gundry SR, Burney RE, Mackenzie JR, et al: Assessment of mediastinal widening associated with traumatic rupture of the aorta, *J Trauma* 23(4):293–299, 1983.
116. Cigarroa JE, Isselbacher EM, DeSanctis RW, Eagle KA: Diagnostic imaging in the evaluation of suspected aortic dissection, *N Engl J Med* 328(1):35–43, 1993.
117. Pais SO: Diagnostic and therapeutic angiography in the trauma patient, *Semin Roentgenol* 27:211–232, 1992.
118. Nienaber CA, von Kodolitsch Y, Nicolas V, et al: The diagnosis of thoracic aortic dissection by noninvasive imaging procedures, *N Engl J Med* 328(1):1–9, 1993.
119. Manson D, Babyn PS, Palder S, Bergman K: CT of blunt chest trauma in children, *Pediatr Radiol* 23(3):1–5, 1993.
120. Kiev J, Kerstein MD: Role of three hour roentgenogram of the chest in penetrating and nonpenetrating injuries of the chest, *Surg Gynecol Obstet* 175(3):249–253, 1992.
121. Palder SB, Shandling B, Manson D: Rupture of the thoracic trachea following blunt trauma: diagnosis by CAT scan, *J Pediatr Surg* 26(11):1320–1322, 1991.
122. McCarthy MC, Pavlina PM, Evans DK, et al: The value of SPECT-thallium scanning in screening for myocardial contusion, *Cardiovasc Intervent Radiol* 14(4):238–240, 1991.
123. Mazurek B, Jehle D, Martin M: Emergency department echocardiography in the diagnosis and therapy of cardiac tamponade, *J Emerg Med* 9:27–31, 1991.
124. Indrani S, Raji V, Kalyani N, et al: Sonographic diagnosis of blunt trauma causing delayed hemopericardium and cardiac tamponade, *J Ultrasound Med* 10(5):291–293, 1991.
125. Tenzer ML: The spectrum of myocardial contusion: a review, *J Trauma* 25(7):620–627, 1985.
126. Laasonen EM, Penttila A, Sumuvuori H: Acute lethal trauma of the trunk: clinical, radiologic, and pathologic findings, *J Trauma* 20(8):662–665, 1980.
127. Taylor GA, Sivit CJ: Computed tomographic imaging of abdominal trauma in children, *Semin Pediatr Surg* 1(4):253–259, 1992.
128. Thal ER, Meyer DM: The evaluation of blunt abdominal trauma: computed tomography scan, lavage, or sonography? *Adv Surg* 24:201–228, 1991.
129. Cooney DR: Splenic and hepatic trauma in children, *Surg Clin North Am* 61(5):1165–1180, 1981.
130. Foley RW, Harris LS, Pilcher DB: Abdominal injuries in automobile accidents: review of care of fatally injured patients, *J Trauma* 17(8):611–615, 1977.
131. Feliciano DV, Marx JA, Sclafani SJA: Abdominal trauma, *Patient Care* 26(18):44–83, 1992.

132. Sivit CJ, Taylor GA, Eichelberger MR: Visceral injury in battered children: a changing perspective, *Radiology* 173(3):659–661, 1989.
133. Ross P Jr, Perkal MF, Degutis LC, Baker CC: Clarification of the role of CT scan in the acute evaluation of blunt abdominal trauma, *Conn Med* 55(6):330–332, 1991.
134. Sivit CJ, Taylor GA, Newman KD: Safety-belt injuries in children with lap-belt ecchymosis: CT findings in 61 patients, *AJR* 157(1):111–114, 1991.
135. National Safety Council: *Accident facts,* Chicago, 1982, The Council.
136. Kaufman RA, Babcock DS: An approach to imaging the upper abdomen in the injured child, *Semin Roentgenol* 19:308–320, 1984.
137. Touloukian RJ: Abdominal injuries in children: a perspective for the 1980s. In Brooks BF, ed: *The injured child,* Austin, 1985, University of Texas Press, pp 53–60.
138. Ben-Menachem Y, Fisher RG, Ward RE: Are "occult" intra-abdominal and extraperitoneal injuries really occult? *Radiol Clin North Am* 19(1):125–140, 1981.
139. Hayes CW, Conway WF, Walsh JW, et al: Seat belt injuries: radiologic findings and clinical correlation, *Radiographics* 11(1):23–36, 1991.
140. Kakos GS, Grosfeld JL, Morse TS: Small bowel injuries in children after blunt abdominal trauma, *Ann Surg* 174(2):238–241, 1971.
141. Vassy LE, Klecker RL, Koch E, Morse TS: Traumatic gastric perforation in children from blunt trauma, *J Trauma* 15(3):184–186, 1975.
142. Asch MJ, Coran AG, Johnston PW: Gastric perforation secondary to blunt trauma in children, *J Trauma* 15(3):187–189, 1975.
143. Siemens RA, Fulton RL: Gastric rupture as a result of blunt trauma, *Am Surg* 43(4):229–233, 1977.
144. Schenk WG III, Lonchyna V, Moylan JA: Perforation of the jejunum from blunt abdominal trauma, *J Trauma* 23(1):54–56, 1983.
145. Sivit CJ, Peclet MH, Taylor GA: Life-threatening intraperitoneal bleeding: demonstration with CT, *Radiology* 171(2):430, 1989.
146. Cook DE, Walsh JW, Vick CW, Brewer WH: Upper abdominal trauma: pitfalls in CT diagnosis, *Radiology* 159(1):65–69, 1986.
147. Gay SB, Sistrom CL: Computed tomographic evaluation of blunt abdominal trauma, *Radiol Clin North Am* 30(2):367–388, 1992.
148. McCort JJ: Caring for the major trauma victim: the role of radiology, *Radiology* 163(1):1–9, 1987.
149. Kuhn JP, Berger PE: Computed tomography in the evaluation of blunt abdominal trauma in children, *Radiol Clin North Am* 19(3):503–513, 1981.
150. Amparo EG, Hayden CK, Schwartz MZ, Lobe TE: Computerized tomography and ultrasonography in evaluating blunt abdominal trauma in children: preliminary results of a prospective comparison. In Brooks BF, ed: *The injured child,* Austin, 1985, University of Texas Press, pp 61–70.
151. Taylor GA, Eichelberger MR, O'Donnell R, Bowman L: Indications for computed tomography in children with blunt abdominal trauma, *Ann Surg* 213(3):212–233, 1991.
152. Karp MP, Cooney DR, Berger PE, et al: The role of computed tomography in the evaluation of blunt abdominal trauma in children, *J Pediatr Surg* 16(3):316–323, 1981.
153. Kirks DR, Caron KH, Bisset GS III: CT of blunt abdominal trauma in children: an anatomic "snapshot in time," *Radiology* 182:631–632, 1992.
154. Gelfand MJ: Scintigraphy in upper abdominal trauma, *Semin Roentgenol* 19:296–307, 1984.

155. Bulas DI, Eichelberger MR, Sivit CJ, et al: Hepatic injury from blunt trauma in children: follow-up evaluation with CT, *AJR* 160(2):347–351, 1993.

156. Kaufman RA: CT of blunt abdominal trauma in children: progress, pitfalls, and controversies. In Poznanski AK, Kirkpatrick JA, eds: *Syllabus: a categorical course in pediatric radiology*, Chicago, November 27–December 1, 1989, Radiology Society of North America, pp 57–65.

157. Mindelzun RE, McCort JJ: Upper abdominal trauma: conventional radiology, *Semin Roentgenol* 19:259–268, 1984.

158. Shaffer HA: Perforation and obstruction of the gastrointestinal tract: assessment by conventional radiology, *Radiol Clin North Am* 30(2):405–426, 1992.

159. Treves ST, Kirkpatrick JA: Bone. In Treves ST, ed: *Pediatric nuclear medicine*, New York, 1985, Springer-Verlag, pp 1–48.

160. Bone scanning. In Mettler FA Jr, Guiberteau MJ: *Essentials of nuclear medicine imaging*, New York, 1983, Grune & Stratton, pp 214–247.

161. Parekh JS, Teates CD: Emergency nuclear medicine, *Radiol Clin North Am* 30(2):455–474, 1992.

162. Gastrointestinal tract. In Mettler FA Jr, Guiberteau MJ: *Essentials of nuclear medicine imaging*, New York, 1983, Grune & Stratton, pp 181–213.

163. Treves ST, Markisz JA: Liver. In Treves ST, ed: *Pediatric nuclear medicine*, New York, 1985, Springer-Verlag, pp 129–140.

164. Treves ST, Lebowitz RL, Kuruc A, et al: Kidneys. In Treves ST, ed: *Pediatric nuclear medicine*, New York, 1985, Springer-Verlag, pp 63–103.

165. Treves ST, Strand RL, Crone RK, Lipp A: Brain. In Treves ST, ed: *Pediatric nuclear medicine*, New York, 1985, Springer-Verlag, pp 205–222.

166. Cerebrovascular system. In Mettler FA Jr, Guiberteau MJ: *Essentials of nuclear medicine imaging*, New York, 1983, Grune & Stratton, pp 51–78.

167. Treves ST: Spleen. In Treves ST, ed: *Pediatric nuclear medicine*, New York, 1985, Springer-Verlag, pp 141–156.

168. Filiatrault D, Longpré D, Patriquin H, et al: Investigation of childhood blunt abdominal trauma: a practical approach using ultrasound as the initial diagnostic modality, *Pediatr Radiol* 17:373–379, 1987.

169. Kuligowska E, Mueller PR, Simeone JF, Fine C: Ultrasound in upper abdominal trauma, *Semin Roentgenol* 19(4):281–295, 1984.

170. The abdomen. In Swischuck LE: *Emergency radiology of the acutely ill or injured child*, ed 2, Baltimore, 1986, Williams & Wilkins, pp 153–309.

171. Federle MP: CT of abdominal trauma, *Crit Rev Diagn Imaging* 19(4):257–316, 1983.

172. Berger PE, Kuhn JP: CT of blunt abdominal trauma in childhood, *AJR* 136(1):105–110, 1981.

173. Tan WW, Chen C-C, Chiang HJ: The value and role of computed tomography in blunt injury of the abdomen, *Chin Med J* 48(2):116–120, 1991.

174. Federle MP: CT of upper abdominal trauma, *Semin Roentgenol* 19:269–280, 1984.

175. Taylor GA, Eichelberger MR: Abdominal CT in children with neurologic impairment following blunt trauma: abdominal CT in comatose children, *Ann Surg* 210(2):229–233, 1989.

176. Donohue JH, Federle MP, Griffiths BG: Computed tomography in the diagnosis of blunt intestinal and mesenteric injuries, *J Trauma* 27(1):11–17, 1987.

177. Marx JA, Moore EE, Jorden RC, Eule J Jr: Limitations of computed tomography in the evaluation of acute abdominal trauma: a prospective comparison with diagnostic peritoneal lavage, *J Trauma* 25(10):933–937, 1985.

178. Fabian TC, Mangiante EC, White TJ, et al: A prospective study of 91 patients undergoing both computed tomography and peritoneal lavage following blunt abdominal trauma, *J Trauma* 26(7):602–608, 1986.
179. Gomez GA, Alvarez R, Plasencia G, et al: Diagnostic peritoneal lavage in the management of abdominal trauma: a reassessment, *J Trauma* 27(1):105, 1987.
180. Fried AM, Humphries R, Schofield CN: Abdominal CT scans in patients with blunt trauma: low yield in the absence of clinical findings, *J Comput Assist Tomogr* 16(5):717–721, 1992.
181. Hedlund GL, Kirks DR: *The "unevaluable abdomen": efficacy of abdominal computed tomography in patients with serious closed head trauma,* Presented at the Annual Meeting of the Society of Pediatric Radiology, San Antonio, Tex, Apr 6–9, 1989.
182. Siegel MJ, Herman TE: Periportal low attenuation at CT in childhood, *Radiology* 183(3):685–688, 1992.
183. Patrick LE, Ball TI, Atkinson GO, Winn KJ: Pediatric blunt abdominal trauma: periportal tracking at CT, *Radiology* 183(3):689–691, 1992.
184. Mirvis SE, Shanmuganathan K: Abdominal computed tomography in blunt trauma, *Semin Roentgenol* 27(3):150–183, 1992.
185. Croce MA, Fabian TC, Kudsk KA, et al: AAST organ injury scale: correlation of CT-graded liver injuries and operative findings, *J Trauma* 31(6):806–812, 1991.
186. Sax SL, Athey PA, Lamki N, Cadavid GA: Sonographic findings in traumatic hemobilia: report of two cases and review of the literature, *J Clin Ultrasound* 16:29–34, 1988.
187. Sivit CJ, Eichelberger MR, Taylor GA, et al: Blunt pancreatic trauma in children: CT diagnosis, *AJR* 158(5):1097–1100, 1992.
188. Sherck JP, Oakes DD: Intestinal injuries missed by computed tomography, *J Trauma* 30(1):1–7, 1990.
189. Karnaze GC, Sheedy PF II, Stephens DH, McLeod RA: Computed tomography in duodenal rupture due to blunt abdominal trauma, *J Comput Assist Tomogr* 5(2):267–269, 1981.
190. Rizzo MJ, Federle MP, Griffiths BG: Bowel and mesenteric injury following blunt abdominal trauma: evaluation with CT, *Radiology* 173:143–148, 1989.
191. Bulas DI, Taylor GA, Eichelberger MR: The value of CT in detecting bowel perforation in children after blunt abdominal trauma. *AJR* 153(3):561–564, 1989.
192. Mirvis SE, Gens DR, Shanmuganathan K: Rupture of the bowel after blunt abdominal trauma: diagnosis with CT, *AJR* 159(6):1217–1221, 1992.
193. Sivit CJ, Taylor GA, Bulas DI, et al: Blunt trauma in children: significance of peritoneal fluid, *Radiology* 178(1):185–188, 1991.
194. Orwig D, Federle MP: Localized clotted blood as evidence of visceral trauma on CT: the sentinel clot sign, *AJR* 153(4):747–749, 1989.
195. Sivit CJ, Taylor GA, Newman KD, et al: Safety-belt injuries in children with lap-belt ecchymosis: CT findings in 61 patients, *AJR* 157(1):111–114, 1991.
196. Taylor GA, Fallat ME, Eichelberger MR: Hypovolemic shock in children: abdominal CT manifestations, *Radiology* 164(2):479–481, 1987.
197. Sivit CJ, Taylor GA, Bulas DI, et al: Posttraumatic shock in children: CT findings associated with hemodynamic instability, *Radiology* 182(3):723–726, 1992.
198. Hara H, Babyn PS, Bourgeois D: Significance of bowel wall enhancement on CT following blunt abdominal trauma in childhood, *J Comput Assist Tomogr* 16(1):94–98, 1992.
199. Taylor GA, Eichelberger MR, Potter BM: Hematuria: a marker of abdominal injury in children after blunt trauma, *Ann Surg* 208(6):688–693, 1988.

200. Burbridge BE, Groot G, Oleniuk FF et al: Emergency excretory urography in blunt abdominal trauma, *Can Assoc Radiol J* 42:326–328, 1991.
201. Tong Y-C, Chun J-S, Tsai H-M, et al: Use of hematoma size on computerized tomography and calculated average bleeding rate as indications for immediate surgical intervention in blunt renal trauma, *J Urol* 147:984–986, 1992.
202. Grieco JH, Perry JF Jr: Retroperitoneal hematoma following trauma: its clinical importance, *J Trauma* 20(9):733–736, 1980.
203. Rothenberger D, Velasco R, Strate R, et al: Open pelvic fracture: a lethal injury, *J Trauma* 18(3):184–187, 1978.
204. Gilliland MG, Ward RE, Flynn TC, et al: Peritoneal lavage and angiography in the management of patients with pelvic fractures, *Am J Surg* 144(6):744–747, 1982.
205. Mucha P, Farnell MB: Analysis of pelvic fracture management, *J Trauma* 24(5):379–386, 1984.
206. Selby JB: Interventional radiology of trauma, *Radiol Clin North Am* 30(2):427–439, 1992.
207. Fellows KE Jr: The uses and abuses of abdominal and peripheral arteriography in children, *Radiol Clin North Am* 10(2):349–366, 1972.
208. Pais SO: Diagnostic and therapeutic angiography in the trauma patient, *Semin Roentgenol* 27(3):211–232, 1992.
209. Towbin RB: Pediatric intervention. In *Pediatric radiology,* Proceedings of the 75th Scientific Assembly and Annual Meeting, Radiological Society of North America, November 26–December 1, 1989.
210. Towbin RB, Ball WS: Pediatric interventional radiology, *Radiol Clin North Am* 26(2):419–440, 1988.
211. Kirks DR, Fitz CR, Harwood-Nash DC: Pediatric abdominal angiography: practical guide to catheter selection, flow rates, and contrast dosage, *Pediatr Radiol* 5(1):19–23, 1976.
212. Selby JB Jr: Interventional radiology of trauma, *Radiol Clin North Am* 30(2):427–440, 1992.
213. Kirks DR: Pediatric renal angiography, *Appl Radiol* 11:83–98, 1978.
214. Ben-Menachem Y, Handel SF, Ray RD, Childs TL: Embolization procedures in trauma: the pelvis, *Semin Intervent Radiol* 2(2):158–181, 1985.
215. Fisher RG, Ben-Menachem Y: Embolization procedures in trauma: the extremities—acute lesions, *Semin Intervent Radiol* 2(2):118–124, 1985.
216. Fisher RG, Ben-Menachem Y: Embolization procedures in trauma: the abdomen—extraperitoneal, *Semin Intervent Radiol* 2(2):148–157, 1985.
217. Casarella WJ, Martin EC: Angiography in the management of abdominal trauma, *Semin Roentgenol* 19:321–327, 1984.
218. Phillips CD: Emergent radiologic evaluation of the gunshot wound victim, *Radiol Clin North Am* 30:307–324, 1992.
219. Mills RP, Robbs JV: Paediatric arterial injury: management options at the time of injury, *J R Coll Surg Edinb* 36(1):13–17, 1991.
220. Ben-Menachem Y: Vascular injuries of the extremities: hazards of unnecessary delays in diagnosis, *Orthopedics* 9(3):333–338, 1986.
221. King TA, Perse JA, Marmen C, Darvin HI: Utility of arteriography in penetrating extremity injuries, *Am J Surg* 162(2):163–165, 1991.
222. Caffey J: Multiple fractures in the long bones of infants suffering from chronic subdural hematoma. *Am J Roentgenol Radium Ther* 56(2):163–173, 1946.

223. Silverman FN: The roentgen manifestations of unrecognized skeletal trauma in infants *Am J Roentgenol Radium Ther* 69(3):413–427, 1953

224. Caffey J: On the theory and practice of shaking infants: its potential residual effects of permanent brain damage and mental retardation. *Am J Dis Child* 124(2):161–169, 1972.

225. Caffey J: The whiplash shaken infant syndrome: manual shaking by the extremities with whiplash-induced intracranial and intraocular bleedings, linked with residual permanent brain damage and mental retardation. Pediatrics 54(4):396–403, 1974.

226. Kempe CH, Silverman FN, Steele B, et al: The battered-child syndrome. *JAMA* 181(1):17–24, 1962.

227. Merten DF, Radkowski MA, Leonidas JC: The abused child: a radiological reappraisal *Radiology* 146(2):377–381, 1983.

228. Ludwig S, Warman M: Shaken baby syndrome: a review of 20 cases. *Ann Emerg Med* 13:104–107, 1984.

229. Ogden JA: *Skeletal injury in the child*, ed 2, Philadelphia, 1990, WB Saunders.

230. The extremities. In Swischuck LE: *Emergency radiology of the acutely ill or injured child*, ed 2, Baltimore 1986, Williams & Wilkins.

231. Oestreich AE, Crawford AH: *Atlas of pediatric orthopedic radiology*, Chapter 3, New York, 1985, Georg Thieme Verlag.

232. Fractures associated with pediatric diseases. In Ogden JA: *Skeletal injury to the child*. Philadelphia, 1990, WB Saunders, pp 265–312.

233. Kirks DR: Skeletal system. In *Practical pediatric imaging,* Boston, 1984, Little, Brown & Co, pp 198–324.

234. Resnik CS: Diagnostic imaging of pediatric skeletal trauma. *Radiol Clin North Am* 27(5):1013–1022, 1989.

235. Kerr R: Diagnostic imaging of upper extremity trauma. *Radiol Clin North Am* 27(5):891–908, 1989.

236. The wrist and hand. In Ogden JA: *Skeletal injury to the child,* Philadelphia, 1990, WB Saunders, pp 527–570.

237. Jonsson K, Jonsson A, Sloth M, et al: CT of the wrist in suspected scaphoid fracture. *Acta Radiologica* 33:500–501, 1992.

238. Nakamura R, Imaeda T, Horii E, et al: Analysis of scaphoid fracture displacement by three-dimensional computed tomography. *J Hand Surg* 16(3):488–492, 1991.

6

Central Nervous System Injuries

Bruce P. Jaufmann

Despite aggressive and successful treatment of systemic injuries in multiply traumatized children, central nervous system (CNS) injury may still result in a discouraging ultimate outcome. Craniospinal injury is one of the leading causes of mortality and long-term morbidity in the pediatric population and is a major concern for individuals involved in the acute management of pediatric trauma.[1] As many as 35% of pediatric surgical admissions are due to trauma, and 50% of those patients have head injuries. Long-term sequelae of CNS injury result in enormous financial costs to the family and society. The associated psychosocial devastation is frequently immeasurable. Physicians caring for pediatric patients must be strong advocates of accident prevention, as well as experts in the assessment, initial treatment, and subsequent management of the neurologically injured child.

Physiologic and anatomic characteristics of the developing nervous system and adjacent structures produce a response to trauma unique to infants and children.[2] Deformation characteristics of the immature skull result in a response to trauma that cannot be extrapolated to the adult population. The plasticity of the pediatric CNS at both the structural and physiologic levels is a tremendous asset in recovery from severe neurologic injury.[3] With appropriate management a severe CNS injury in a pediatric patient may have an excellent outcome. These characteristics pose unique challenges for diagnosis, management, and rehabilitation of the traumatized pediatric patient.

This chapter explores the pathophysiology of injury to the craniospinal axis and provides a discussion of diagnostic modalities and their advantages and limitations, the understanding of which is essential to the early and effective assessment and management of patients with CNS injuries. Optimal management strategies are reviewed in detail. The chapter makes it apparent that a team approach is essential for the optimal recovery of infants and children with severe neurologic injury.

180

EPIDEMIOLOGY

Accidents are the major cause of death in individuals between the ages of 1 and 19 years.[4] In the United States head trauma is responsible for 3.6% of hospital admissions and 3.3% of total days spent in the hospital.[5] The estimated incidence of head injuries in children under 15 years of age is 200 to 230 per 100,000 population, with a 5% fatality rate.[4,6] Falls are the most common cause of CNS injury in children less than 5 years of age, but recent studies show a rising incidence of motor vehicle accidents and assault in this age group. In children older than 5 years of age, injuries are commonly caused by recreational activities and motor vehicle accidents, with a 2:1 male/female preponderance. The incidence of child abuse is difficult to assess.[7] Pedestrian and bicycle mishaps are also common in this age group. Children who have suffered previous neurotrauma have a greater statistical probability of experiencing a second injury.[4,8] This is most likely the result of social activities and environments that predispose the patient to both accidental and nonaccidental injury. The rising incidence of violent crimes, especially in urban areas, further predisposes children to neurologic injury.[9]

EVALUATION AND DIAGNOSIS
Minor Neurotrauma

The evaluation and decision-making process concerning the conscious child with head trauma is difficult, with potentially serious implications. Assessment of orientation and cognitive function in a frightened child can be extremely difficult and requires a cautious, patient, thorough approach to triage and management. Thought should be given to the mechanism of injury, which may suggest the possibility of significant injury or hemorrhage from an apparently minor wound. A neurologic examination must be carefully performed and documented (Table 6–1). The level of consciousness must be documented and then serially evaluated in the emergency room, with urgent attention directed to any child with a deteriorating neurologic status. Posttraumatic seizure activity or a loss of consciousness indicates that a force has been applied to the cranium that is severe enough to cause at least transient neurologic dysfunction.

Focal neurologic deficits may indicate the presence of severe injuries. Monoparesis or hemiparesis implies structural injury to the motor cortex. Visual dysfunction may be indicative of injury to optic nerves or the occipital cortex. Cranial nerve abnormalities may result from fracture of the skull base. Clinical symptoms of basilar skull fractures may include hemotympanum seen on otoscopic examination, cerebrospinal fluid (CSF) otorrhea, or rhinorrhea. A "double-ring sign" on the patient's pillow or dressing gauze is indicative of a CSF fistula resulting from injury to the petrous bone (Fig. 6–1). Vestibulocochlear nerve dysfunction is also common with skull base fractures. Orbital or mastoid

Table 6–1. Components of Basic Neurologic Examination

Head	Evidence of fracture, laceration, or depression
Mental status	Awake, alert, stuporous, or unresponsive
Eyes	Pupils, extraocular motions, funduscopic examination, corneal reflexes
Ears	Hemotympanum, cerebrospinal fluid, otorrhea
Motor examination	Follows commands with good strength, withdraws, abnormal posturing
Sensory examination	Pinprick, light touch, proprioception
Deep tendon reflexes	Biceps, triceps, ankle and knee
Babinski reflexes	
Cerebellar examination if possible	Finger to nose, heel to shin

ecchymosis is frequently indicative of significant cranial trauma. These are commonly described as the classic "raccoon's eyes" and "Battle's sign," respectively (Fig. 6–2). Patients with such signs require further radiographic evaluation and directed treatment.

In minor head injury a plain skull series may help determine whether the

A 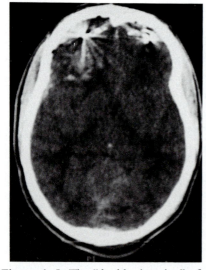 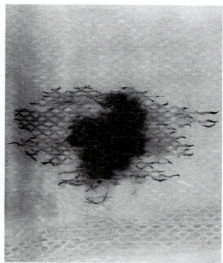 B

Figure 6–1. The "double-ring sign" of cerebrospinal fluid mixed with blood. **A,** This patient suffered a transfrontal gunshot wound with disruption of the cribriform plate and cerebrospinal fluid rhinorrhea. **B,** The bloody discharge forms the "double-ring sign" when allowed to contact filter paper or the patient's dressings. This "double ring" is indicative of cerebrospinal fluid mixed with blood.

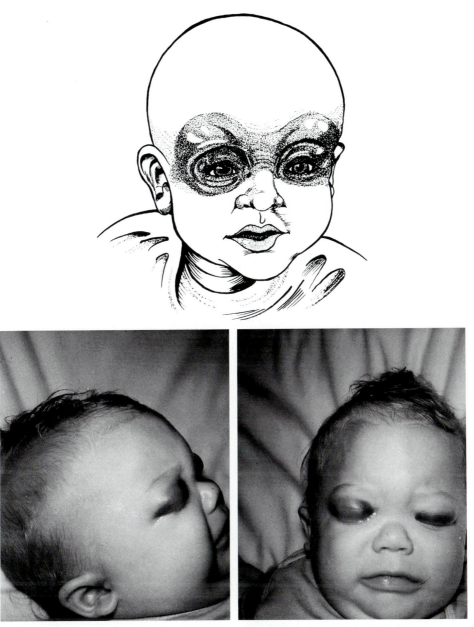

Figure 6–2. The characteristics of classic "raccoon's eyes." The physical changes are from bleeding into the periorbital tissues from fractures of the base of the skull.

child should be admitted to the hospital for observation. Skull films are indicated in a neurologically intact child if any of the following is present:

- Head injury in an infant up to 2 years old
- A history of unconsciousness
- A history of posttraumatic seizure
- Tenderness, ecchymosis, or swelling of the cranium, orbits, or mastoid

Non-contrast-enhanced cranial computed tomography (CT) scanning should be performed in any patient with a focal or global neurologic deficit, including a persistent alteration in the level of consciousness. Drug screening should always be performed in patients with an altered sensorium, regardless of age.

Persistent vomiting following head injury is common in children. Cranial CT may be deferred if the patient is admitted for intravenous hydration and close observation. The persistently vomiting child may be discharged from the hospital *only* after a CT scan has excluded an intracranial lesion. Specific instructions or a "head injury sheet" (Table 6–2) should be given to the parents on discharge. In addition to being given written guidelines, parents should be specifically instructed to return if any decline in neurologic status occurs. The competence and reliability of the parents must be taken into account when discharge of the child is contemplated.

It is our policy to admit *all* children with skull fractures for 24 hours of observation. In infants skull films should be repeated 2 to 3 weeks after discharge to rule out a growing skull fracture (see later discussion of skull fractures).

Table 6–2. Head Injury Sheet Given to Parents of Children Who Have Been Evaluated for Central Nervous System Injuries

---

No medications except Tylenol unless specifically ordered.
Clear liquids for 24 hours.
Contact your doctor or return to the emergency department immediately if anything listed below occurs, even several months from now.
    Persistent vomiting, stiff neck, fever
    Center black circles of eyes unequal in size or disturbed vision
    Unusual headache or drowsiness
    Confusion during waking hours
    Fits or unconsciousness
    Dizziness, stumbling, or other problems with normal use of arms or legs, areas of skin numbness
    Bleeding or drainage from *nose* or *ears*
Awaken the patient every 1 to 2 hours the first night to check for above symptoms and to see if he or she can be aroused.

Continued follow-up films may be necessary to ensure that this complication does not occur.

Severe Neurotrauma

There are two phases of injury to the central nervous system. The first phase is the immediate, or primary, injury. The traumatic impact causes direct or shearing injury to neural structures, resulting in contusion, hemorrhage, or laceration of neural tissues. In addition, shearing injury can cause diffuse axonal injury.[10-12] Bicortical injury or injury to the reticular activating system results in loss of consciousness.[10,13]

The second phase, or secondary injury, of cerebral trauma results from tissue ischemia. Ischemia is a direct result of hypoxia that may be caused by ventilatory depression from primary cerebral injury, hypotension, associated systemic injuries, or cerebral hypertension resulting in decreased cerebral perfusion pressure. Efforts should be directed toward maintaining physiologic, hemodynamic, and intracerebral homeostasis. Treatment of systemic injuries is directed at ensuring adequate oxygenation and ventilation and minimizing loss of red blood cell mass. Rapid identification and surgical treatment of intracranial injury, if indicated, decrease cerebral hypoxia and ischemia resulting from direct effects of mass lesions. A rapid baseline neurologic assessment is performed using the Glasgow Coma Scale score (Table 6–3), and urgent CT scanning is performed as soon as pulmonary and hemodynamic stability is achieved.

Radiographic Evaluation

CT is the most important radiographic tool used in pediatric neurotrauma. The evolution of CT technology has enabled rapid and safe identification of surgically remediable intracranial space-occupying lesions. CT scanning is performed *without* intravenous contrast medium because contused cerebral tissue easily loses its capillary integrity. Intravenously administered contrast material extravasates in areas of contusion and gives a CT appearance of intracranial hemorrhage. This hypertonic extravasation may also exacerbate intracranial hypertension. True intracranial hemorrhage is easily identified on scanning without contrast enhancement because of marked differences in density between blood and neural tissue. Intravenous contrast medium is usually required in abdominal CT scanning for evaluation of intraabdominal injuries. If the injured child requires both CNS and abdominal scanning, the CNS data should be acquired first. As the head CT is being completed, the contrast medium is administered as an intravenous bolus and the abdominal data are acquired in rapid succession. With modern scanners the entire process can be accomplished within 20 minutes.

The use of magnetic resonance imaging (MRI) in the acute phase of traumatic cerebral injury is limited because the signal characteristics of blood

Table 6–3. Glasgow Coma Scale Score

Eye Opening

4 Spontaneous
3 To sound
2 To pain
1 None

Motor Response

6 Follows commands
5 Localizes stimuli
4 Withdrawal
3 Abnormal flexion
2 Abnormal extension
1 No movement

Verbal

5 Oriented
4 Confused conversation
3 Inappropriate words
2 Incomprehensible sounds
1 None

Scores for Eye + Motor + Verbal = Glasgow Coma Scale Score

and surrounding neural structures are similar. The relatively long time required to obtain an adequate study is also a disadvantage in a critically injured, unstable child. MRI is useful, however, in delineating the extent of injuries to brain substance in follow-up examination days to months after the injury.[14]

The child's head is relatively larger, in relation to body size, than the adult's. When a significant violent force is applied to the child, the head acquires a substantial momentum that predisposes to cervical spine injuries. Unconscious children require cervical spine radiography to exclude fracture or dislocation. Cervical films are also indicated in any child with a mechanism of injury associated with a high risk of cervical injury or those with neck pain following trauma. Flexion-extension studies, either passive or under fluoroscopy, may be necessary if ligamentous instability is suspected. Severe paravertebral muscle spasm may result in adequate flexion-extension films and hide ligamentous instability. In this case cervical immobilization may be necessary until the spasm has subsided and adequate flexion-extension studies can be obtained.

SPECIFIC INJURIES
Scalp Injuries

Scalp injury may result in laceration or hematoma. Hematomas may be located within several anatomic layers of the scalp. Subperiosteal accumulations of blood (e.g., cephalhematoma of the newborn) are clinically evident as hematomas that are limited by the cranial sutures (Fig. 6–3). The periosteum adheres to the cranial suture lines and does not allow extravasation of the hematoma beyond them. Cephalhematomas usually resorb spontaneously and rarely require operative intervention. Some cephalhematomas calcify, necessitating surgical removal for cosmetic reasons.

Subgaleal hematomas and scalp lacerations may result in a significant and even life-threatening blood loss, especially in an infant or small child. Subgaleal hematomas are not contained by any anatomic boundaries and thus may reach enormous size. Drainage of the hematoma is not necessary. The child is treated with pressure dressing and fluid support. Immediate action must be taken to control bleeding from scalp lacerations. The laceration should first be digitally explored, and then skull films obtained, to rule out underlying fracture. The laceration is then copiously irrigated with normal saline solution and all foreign debris removed. Galeal closure is essential. Staples or sutures may be used for skin closure. Avulsion injuries may require skin grafts or rotation flaps for closure.

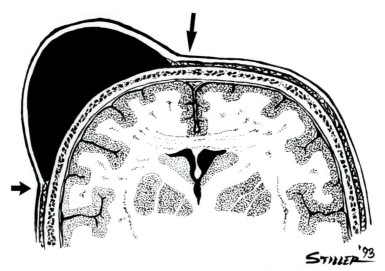

Figure 6–3. Cephalhematoma. Bleeding is subperiosteal and limited by the cranial sutures. The periosteum is adherent to the skull at suture lines and limits extravasation of blood across them *(arrow)*.

Skull Fractures

Approximately 25% of children evaluated in the emergency room for head injuries have an underlying skull fracture.[14] Skull fractures are classified as linear, depressed, compound, and basilar. A linear skull fracture itself may not cause clinically significant problems, but the presence of the fracture indicates a significant traumatic impact to the head. Children suffering skull fractures are at an increased risk for intracranial hemorrhage and should be observed in the hospital. Uncomplicated linear fractures usually heal in 3 to 4 months, but radiographic evidence of the fracture may persist much longer.[16] Linear, non-depressed, closed fractures usually do not require specific treatment. Linear fractures crossing the middle meningeal artery, its tributaries, or major dural sinuses may result in an epidural hematoma. Occasionally, follow-up skull series indicate an enlarging skull fracture. These "growing" skull fractures are typically seen in infants and small children and are believed to result from cerebral tissue or arachnoid membrane herniation through an underlying dural laceration. Seizures and neurologic disability may result from the compromised cerebral tissue within the growing fracture. Therefore neurosurgical intervention is indicated. If a growing skull fracture is evident on serial skull radiographs, cranial CT is performed before surgery.

Depressed fractures from birth trauma are common in the perinatal period (ping-pong fractures) but also may occur throughout childhood as a result of accidental injury (Fig. 6–4). Blunt injury from an unmalleable object is usually the cause. Because of the increasing incidence of violent assaults and child abuse, depressed fractures have become more commonly seen in the emergency center. A child with a fracture depressing the thickness of the skull table requires surgical elevation because damage to the underlying cerebral cortex may lead to seizures. Compound (open) depressed skull fractures require surgical debridement, elevation, and closure. Cosmesis or mass effect on cerebral tissue is also an appropriate indication for elevation of fragments.

Tetanus prophylaxis is essential in all cases of laceration and open fracture. Patients undergoing surgical debridement and elevation of fracture segments may be administered antibiotics such as cephalosporins or vancomycin, although the necessity for antibiotics in all situations is open to debate. Penicillins may lower seizure thresholds and should be used with caution. Antibiotics may be tailored to the individual, considering the mechanism of injury and the environmental location of the trauma.

Basilar skull fractures are clinically manifest as hemotympanum, CSF rhinorrhea, CSF otorrhea, Battle's sign, or raccoon's eyes (see Fig. 6–2). Despite radiographic adjuncts, the diagnosis of basilar fractures is most frequently made on a clinical basis. Cranial nerve dysfunction is frequently associated with skull base injuries. Olfactory and optic nerve injury may be associated with fractures

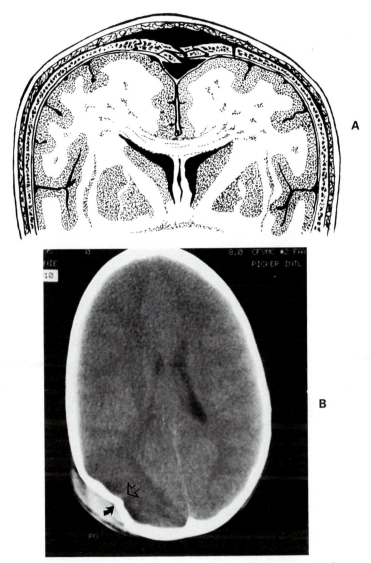

Figure 6–4. Depressed skull fracture. **A,** Depressed skull fractures may be associated with subgaleal bleeding. The subgaleal hematoma is not limited by the periosteum at cranial sutures and therefore crosses anatomic suture lines. Bleeding from this fracture resulted from laceration of the superior sagittal sinus. **B,** The degree of skull fracture depression is best evaluated with CT scan. Depth of depression greater than the width of the skull table usually requires surgical attention. This depressed skull fracture *(closed arrow)* was associated with an underlying contusion *(open arrow)*.

of the frontal fossa. Cribriform plate fractures may be associated with anosmia and CSF rhinorrhea. An oculomotor injury may occur in middle fossa fractures. Facial nerve palsies and vestibular and cochlear nerve injuries are common with petrous bone fractures. Suboccipital fracture and fracture in the region of the foramen magnum may result in injury to the lower cranial nerves, manifest clinically as difficulty with swallowing and phonation. Basilar skull fractures are infrequently seen on plain radiographs and may occasionally be apparent if CT scans are adjusted for bone windows. Pneumocephalus is a frequent accompaniment of basilar skull fractures, especially when a CSF fistula is evident.

Cerebral Injury

Bruising of the brain substance (contusion) is a relatively common phenomenon in cerebral trauma (Fig. 6–5). Cerebral contusions appear as hyperdense lesions on CT scans and are indicative of significant injury to neural tissue. Contusions are frequently found beneath impact or fracture sites, as well as immediately opposite the point of impact. Contrecoup lesions are those occurring immediately opposite the point where the blow to the cranium occurred. For example, an impact to the occipital bone can result in a contrecoup frontal pole contusion. Subfrontal contusions (bruising of the undersurface of the frontal lobes) are also common and result from violent movement of the brain along the floor of the frontal fossa. The tips of the temporal lobes and the occipital poles are especially vulnerable to contusion resulting from traction and impact with surrounding osseous structures. Contrecoup contusions may also occur along parafalcine structures.

Injury to the basal ganglia may be evident as CT-documented hypodensities resulting from stretching and disruption of the lateral perforating vessels of the middle cerebral artery.[17]

Shear injury and penetrating trauma may result in laceration of neural tissue with subsequent hemorrhage and edema. Rapid acceleration-deceleration injuries, as sustained in motor vehicle accidents, may result in diffuse degeneration of white matter from shearing injuries of nerve fibers.[12,14] These patients are generally rendered comatose at the time of impact and remain severely neurologically impaired. The clinical presentation, however, may range in severity from a mild concussive syndrome to significant neurologic devastation. This phenomenon is termed diffuse axonal injury.[12,18,19] In the early stages of injury the lesions are mainly hemorrhagic, but within days axonal retraction bulbs appear throughout the white matter substance. Later, axonal degeneration of the Wallerian type becomes evident.[20] These latter microscopic changes may not be evident on CT scanning in macroscopic form.

Concussion is defined as a transient disturbance in neurologic function following traumatic injury. This produces temporary cerebral dysfunction with-

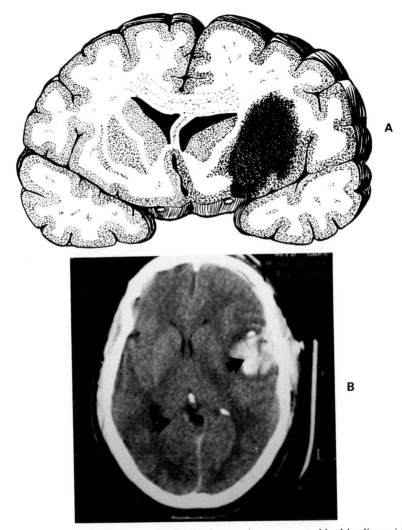

Figure 6–5. Cerebral contusions. **A,** Cerebral contusions are caused by bleeding within the parenchyma of the brain. Such bleeding may cause a mass effect with subsequent alteration of normal architecture such as ventricular size and location. **B,** Cerebral contusions are evident on computed tomographic scan as hyperdense areas in noncontrast studies. This contusion *(arrow)* was caused by blunt trauma to the head. The ventricles are seen to be shifted to the right.

out gross structural lesions. Minor degrees of axonal injury may occur in concussive syndromes.[11]

Intracranial hemorrhage as a result of cerebral trauma is a potentially serious but treatable aspect of neurotrauma. Intraparenchymal hemorrhage may occur in an area of previous contusion or rarely in patients with bleeding dyscrasias or those receiving anticoagulant medications. Intracranial hemorrhages become surgically significant when they contribute significantly to intracranial hypertension or result in neurologic deficits secondary to mass effect.

Subarachnoid hemorrhage is common in neurotrauma and *usually* requires no specific treatment. Erythrocytes within the CSF lyse and resorb with time. Rarely, intraventricular or subarachnoid hemorrhage results in CSF outflow obstruction or resorption abnormalities that require external ventricular drainage or ventriculoperitoneal shunting for hydrocephalus.

Epidural and subdural hematomas are space-occupying lesions that may result in elevations of intracranial pressure. As intracranial pressure increases, the patient may ultimately experience uncal herniation. The pushing of the uncus, located in the medial aspect of the temporal lobe, under the tentorial notch or incisura results in brainstem compression, paralysis, and respiratory arrest. An epidural hematoma accumulates between the inner skull table and the dura mater and occurs in 1% to 3% of children with head injuries.[21,22] On CT, acute epidural hematomas are hyperdense and have a classic lens shape (Fig. 6−6). The most frequent cause of an epidural hematoma is injury or laceration of the middle meningeal artery or one of its tributaries, but it may also occur with injury to a major venous sinus. Arterial epidural hematomas often develop in the patient with a rapidly deteriorating neurologic state and are manifest as a decline in the level of consciousness, followed by motor dysfunction and ultimately coma and death. The patient who "talks and dies" exemplifies this phenomenon. Venous epidural hemorrhages progress more slowly, allowing greater time for evaluation and treatment. Numerous cases of nonoperative management of venous epidural hematomas have been reported, but this may pose greater risk to the patient than the risk associated with surgery (Fig. 6−7).[23]

Subdural hematomas occur when tearing of cortical bridging vessels leads to blood collections between the dura and the brain. They frequently result in a rapidly expanding intracranial mass with shift of cerebral structures and elevation of intracranial pressure. Irritation of the cerebral cortex by hematologic breakdown products may result in seizures and underlying cerebral swelling. These lesions conform to the outline of the cerebral cortex and are crescent shaped (Fig. 6−8). Small (less than 5 mm thick) subdural hematomas without mass effect may be managed by observation in the intensive care setting. Subdural hematomas with mass effect require immediate surgical evacuation.

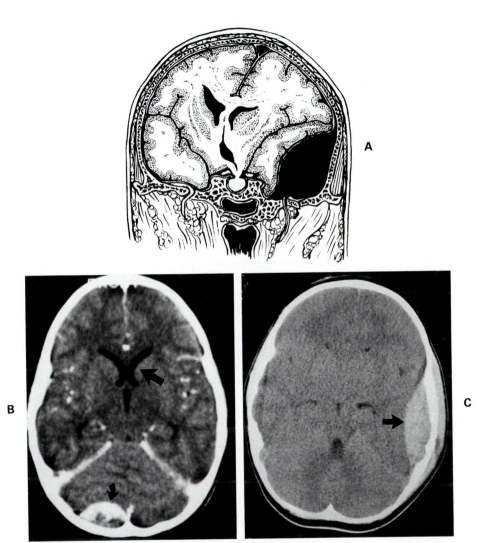

Figure 6–6. Epidural hematoma. **A,** An epidural hematoma is a blood collection between the inner skull table and the dura mater. A progressive increase in size causes shift of midline structures and may ultimately result in herniation. Epidural hematomas may be either venous or arterial. **B,** Computed tomographic (CT) scan of a posterior fossa venous epidural hematoma with obstructive hydrocephalus. The bleeding is lens shaped *(small arrow)* and has resulted in hydrocephalus *(large arrow)* from outflow obstruction of cerebrospinal fluid. **C,** CT scan showing an acute epidural arterial hematoma *(arrow)*. The classic lens shape is again evidenced.

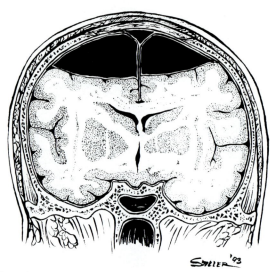

Smiller '93

Figure 6–7. Bilateral venous epidural hematomas. The venous epidural hematoma is a low-pressure bleed between the skull and the dura mater. These hematomas are more insidious in onset than the arterial type and may not be detected until later in the clinical course.

Spine Injuries

Close inspection and directed radiographic investigation of the spinal column must be performed in all children with severe trauma.[24] Conscious children frequently complain of pain and discomfort in the region of a fracture, which helps direct investigation of the appropriate anatomic area. In pediatric spinal trauma, 27% of fractures involve the second cervical vertebra. These fractures include odontoid fractures (types I, II, and III) and hangman's fractures (Fig. 6–9). The tenth thoracic vertebra is involved in 13% of fractures, the seventh thoracic vertebra in 6%, and the first lumbar vertebra in 6%. An unconscious child should be presumed to have a spinal column injury and be treated and investigated accordingly. Spinal column injuries without radiographic evidence of fracture (SCIWORA) occur in as many as 40% of children with spinal trauma. These injuries result from a flexion-extension disruption of spinal ligaments and subsequent displacement of the vertebrae with resulting impact of the vertebral bodies on the spinal cord. Following impact the vertebral column returns to its proper alignment. The initial impact with subsequent vascular compromise, edema, and axonal degeneration is responsible for the observed neurologic deficit. Any question of spinal ligamentous stability can usually be resolved with dynamic passive flexion-extension radiographs or with flexion-extension studies performed under fluoroscopy. The prognosis in complete spinal cord injury is

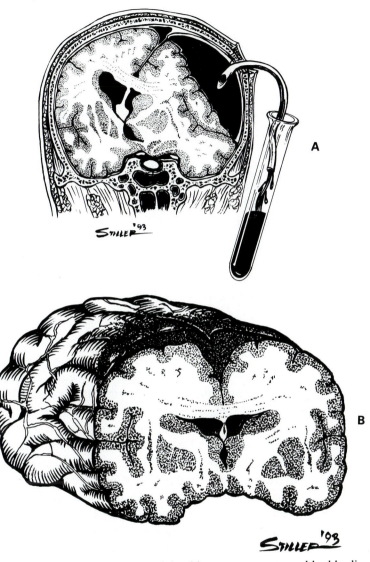

Figure 6–8. Subdural hematoma. **A,** Subdural hematomas are caused by bleeding between the brain and the dura mater. They result in rapidly expanding intracranial masses with a shift of cerebral structures and subsequent elevation of intracranial pressure. These bleeds conform to the outline of the cerebral cortex and are in a crescent configuration. Subdural hematomas with mass effect require immediate surgical evacuation. **B,** Small bilateral subdural hematomas. Small subdural hematomas may be managed nonoperatively if the patient does not demonstrate neurologic changes or exhibit mass effect on a computed tomographic scan. The blood products eventually lyse and are resorbed.

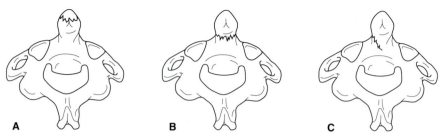

Figure 6–9. The three types of odontoid fracture. **A,** Type I; **B** type II; **C,** type III.

poor. In the patient with an incomplete deficit or neurologic deterioration from spinal trauma, urgent MRI or myelography should be performed in search of a surgically remediable lesion. Traumatic disk ruptures or intraspinal hemorrhage, both intradural and extradural, may be responsible for incomplete spinal cord injury or deterioration in motor or sensory function. These lesions may be amenable to surgical care, which is expected to result in improvement.

PATIENT MANAGEMENT

The management of pediatric neurotrauma is directed primarily toward prevention of secondary injury and maintenance of cerebral homeostasis. Following rapid initial neurologic examination, attention is turned to ensuring adequate oxygen delivery to neural elements. The airway is secured, and oxygen delivery ensured, by intubation and ventilation with 100% oxygen, if required. The concentration of delivered oxygen may be reduced when the patient becomes hemodynamically and neurologically stable. Weaning is guided by serial measurement of blood gases while a PaO_2 greater than 100 mm Hg is maintained.

Adequate cerebral perfusion pressure is necessary to ensure appropriate oxygen delivery to the brain. Cerebral perfusion pressure is determined by the mean arterial pressure (oxygen delivery) minus the intracranial pressure (resistance to oxygen delivery). Cerebral perfusion may be enhanced by elevating systemic blood pressure or by decreasing intracranial pressure. Systemic arterial blood pressure is raised by fluid resuscitation, blood transfusion, and control of hemorrhage. Aggressive treatment of systemic injuries that may be causing hypotension and impaired oxygen content (e.g., viscus disruptions, femur fractures) is crucial to protecting the nervous system from secondary injury.

Following control of the airway, intervention in life-threatening injuries, and hemodynamic stabilization, the patient undergoes CT scanning. Cervical immobilization is maintained until cervical fracture is excluded by a complete cervical spine series. If no surgically remediable lesion is discovered by CT, attention is paid to non-life-threatening systemic, orthopedic, and soft tissue injuries. Intracranial pressure monitoring is considered if the CT scan exhibits signs of elevated intracranial pressure. Intracranial hypertension occurs in as many as 86% of patients with a Glasgow Coma Scale score of 8 or less. Therefore such patients should be considered for placement of an intracranial pressure monitor. A variety of monitoring techniques are available, including intraventricular, intraparenchymal, subarachnoid, and epidural monitors. Intraventricular monitors have the advantage of allowing removal of CSF, which may reduce intracranial pressure by decreasing intracranial volume.

The objectives in treatment of neurologic injuries are to keep intracranial pressure below 20 mm Hg, maintain cerebral perfusion pressure above 50 mm Hg, and minimize oxygen consumption by the brain. Elevation of the head of the bed to 30 degrees provides maximal cerebral perfusion while allowing the most efficient cerebral venous drainage. Sedation and neuromuscular blockade are mainstays of treatment in reducing neural oxygen consumption. Intracranial pressure can be reduced by the use of hyperventilation, maintaining the $Paco_2$ between 25 and 30 mm Hg. The philosophy is thus: The cranium provides a "closed box" in which the brain resides. When the brain is injured, it begins to swell (Fig. 6–10). Swelling elevates the pressure within the box (cranium) and results in increased intracranial pressure. To lower intracranial pressure requires removing volume from the cranium. One aspect that may be varied is the blood perfusing the brain. As the patient is hyperventilated, the decreasing $Paco_2$

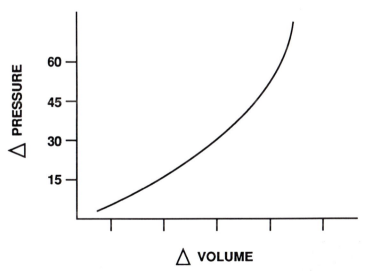

Figure 6–10. The pressure-volume relationship of intracranial tissues. Small increases in intracranial volumes (blood, cerebrospinal fluid, tissue edema) result in dramatic increases in central nervous system pressure.

causes cerebral vasoconstriction in uninjured areas, maintaining cerebral auto-regulation and a linear decrease in cerebral blood flow to those areas. A decrease of $PaCO_2$ from 40 to 25 mm Hg results in a 25% decrease in cerebral blood flow. A decrease in cerebral blood flow decreases the amount of blood to un-injured areas without resultant ischemia. This decrease in hematologic fluid volume helps decrease intracranial pressure. Injured areas have frequently lost autoregulation and may not be affected by hypocarbia-induced vascoconstriction. Hyperventilation to a $PaCO_2$ of 25 mm Hg is relatively safe, but beyond that the degree of vasoconstriction actually decreases oxygen delivery and results in cerebral ischemia. To keep hyperventilation below a $PaCO_2$ of 25 mm Hg, the practitioner should be able to measure oxygen consumption by the brain. This requires placement of a retrograde jugular bulb catheter and should be performed under the direction of a neurosurgeon.

Osmotic diuretics are also important tools used by the physician for the control of intracranial pressure. Diuretics decrease the intravascular and intra-cellular volume and thereby decrease intracerebral pressure. Mannitol may also reduce intracranial pressure by altering the rheologic properties of flowing blood. Mannitol administered as a bolus or rapid drip of 0.5 to 1.5 g/kg body weight usually reduces intracranial pressure; the mannitol dose may be repeated every 15 minutes for a total of four doses. Renal tubular diuretics (furosemide) may also be used as an adjunct to lower intravascular volume. When diuretics are used, serum chemistry and osmolarity must be monitored carefully. After four consecutive doses of mannitol it is appropriate to wait until a serum os-molarity study is obtained before administering more diuretic. Rehydration is performed with 0.9% saline solution to maintain osmolarity at 300 mOsm. A serum osmolarity of 320 mOsm or more precludes the use of additional diuretic therapy, since further therapy has been shown to result in a "rebound effect," actually increasing cerebral edema.

To improve oxygen delivery to the brain, the patient's hematocrit value should be maintained above 30% by transfusion, if necessary.

The requirement for seizure prophylaxis in the neurologically injured pa-tient is controversial. However, because of the risk of additional ischemic injury to already compromised cerebral tissue, we carry out prophylaxis with anticon-vulsant medication for all comatose children. This may be accomplished by the administration of phenobarbital, 15 mg/kg loading dose, followed by 10 mg/kg/day. An alternative regimen is phenytoin, 15 mg/kg for loading and 4 to 7 mg/kg/day for maintenance. Any significant rise in intracranial pressure should prompt immediate reinvestigation with CT. Pentobarbital titrated to electroen-cephalographic burst suppression ("pentobarb coma") should be considered if intracranial pressure cannot be controlled with the preceding methods.

Spinal shock frequently complicates multiple trauma. Acute vasodilation results in hypotension, which may require judicious but aggressive fluid resuscitation. Cervical lesions at C4 or above invariably necessitate ventilatory support. Rigid immobilization should be maintained. Prophylaxis against deep venous thrombosis is essential, as is a bowel regimen consisting of laxatives and stool softeners. Ileus is a common accompaniment of spinal cord injury. All children with spinal cord injury should be started on steroids in high doses, which have been shown to improve long-term outcome. Methylprednisolone (Solu-Medrol) 35 mg/kg over 45 minutes is administered intravenously, followed by a maintenance dose of 5.4 mg/kg/hr for 23 hours. Stabilization with external devices such as haloes, braces, cervical collars, or internal stabilization should be accomplished at the earliest possible time. Early stabilization allows the patient to be mobilized quickly and promotes early rehabilitation.

SUMMARY

Although the prognosis of children with severe neurotrauma is sometimes poor, especially in patients with diffuse cerebral edema or space-occupying intracerebral lesions, their outcomes are frequently better than those of adults with similar injuries.[4,25-27] The mechanical properties of the developing nervous system allow a response to trauma that is unique in comparison with the mature nervous system of adults. Because the ultimate outcome is uncertain, physicians must be aggressive in evaluation and management of the neurotraumatized child. It is critical that neural injury be confined to the primary event. Secondary insult to the nervous system is avoided by maintaining cerebral oxygen delivery and reducing intracranial hypertension.

The multidisciplinary approach to central nervous system trauma is crucial to providing high-quality care of these patients. Pediatric intensivists, pediatricians, pediatric surgeons, urologists, plastic surgeons, neurosurgeons, orthopedists, physiatrists, physical therapists, psychiatrists, and psychosocial and social workers all play integral roles in the successful management of the severely traumatized child.

REFERENCES

1. Annegars JF: The epidemiology of head trauma in children. In Shapiro K (ed): *Pediatric head trauma,* Mt Kisco, NY, 1983, Futura Publishing, pp 1–20.
2. McLaurin RL, Towbin R: *Diagnosis and treatment of head injury in infants and children,* Philadelphia, 1990, WB Saunders, pp 2149–2192.
3. Bruce DA, Schut L: Outcome following severe head injuries in children, *J Neurosurg* 48(5):679–688, 1978.
4. Bergber MS, Pitt LH, et al: Outcome from severe head injury in children and adolescents, *Neurosurgery* 62:194–199, 1978.
5. North AF: When should a child be in the hospital? *Pediatrics* 57:540–546, 1976.

6. Kalsbeck ED, McLauren RL, et al: The national head and spinal cord injury survey: major findings, *J Neurosurg* 53:19–531, 1980.

7. McServy CJ, Towbin R, et al: Radiographic characteristics of skull fractures in child abuse vs accidental injury, *Am J Neurol Radiol* 8:455–457, 1987.

8. Klonoff H: Head injuries in children: predisposing factors, accident conditions, accident proneness and sequelae, *Am J Public Health* 61:2405–2417, 1967.

9. Kraus JF, Rock A, Hemyari P, et al: Brain injuries among infants and children, adolescents and young adults, *Am J Dis Child* 144:684–691, 1990.

10. Graham MB, Adams JH, et al: Pathology of brain damage in head injury. In Cooper P (ed): *Head injury,* Baltimore, 1987, Williams & Wilkins, pp 72–88.

11. Jane JA, Steward O, Gennarelli T: Axonal degeneration induced by experimental non-invasive minor head injury, *J Neurosurg* 62:96–100, 1985.

12. Stritch ST: Shearing of nerve fibers as a cause of brain damage due to head injury: a pathologic study of 20 cases, *Lancet* 2:443–448, 1961.

13. Gade CF, Becker DP, et al: Pathology and pathophysiology of head injury. In Youmans (ed): *Neurological surgery,* Philadelphia, 1990, WB Saunders, pp 1965–2004.

14. Snow RB, Zimmerman RE, Devinsky O: Comparison of magnetic resonance imaging and computerized tomography in the evaluation of head injury, *Neurosurgery* 18:45–52, 1986.

15. Harwood-Nash DC, Hendrick EB, Hudson AR: The significance of skull fractures in children: a study of 1,187 patients, *Radiology* 101:151–155, 1971.

16. Postnatal trauma and injuries by physical agents. In Menkes JH, Till K: *Pediatric neurology,* pp 462–493.

17. Maki Y, Akimoto H, et al: Injuries of basal ganglia following head trauma in children, *Childs Brain* 7:113–123, 1980.

18. Adams JH, Mitchell DE, Enomoto T: Diffuse brain damage of immediate impact type: its relationship to "primary brainstem damage" in head injury, *Brain* 100:489–502, 1977.

19. Zimmerman RA, Bilaniuk LT, Gennaralli T: Computed tomography of shearing injuries of the cerebral white matter, *Radiology* 127:393–396, 1978.

20. Shapiro K, Marmarou A: Clinical application of the pressure volume index in the treatment of pediatric head injuries, *J Neurosurg* 56:819–825, 1982.

21. Dhellemmes P, Lejeune JP, Christiaers JL, Combelles G: Traumatic extradural hematoma in infancy and childhood, *J Neurosurg* 62:861–866, 1985.

22. Hendrick EB, Harwood-Nash DE, et al: Head injuries in children: a survey of 4,465 consecutive cases at the Hospital for Sick Children, Toronto, Canada, *Clin Neurosurg* 11:46–65, 1963.

23. McLaurin RL, Isaacs E, Lewis HP: Results of non-operative treatment in 15 cases of infantile subdural hematoma, *J Neurosurg* 34:753–759, 1971.

24. Ruge JR, Sinson GP, McLone DG, Cerullo LJ: Pediatric spinal injury: the very young, *J Neurosurg* 68:25–32, 1988.

25. Aldrich EF, Eisenberg HM: Diffuse brain swelling in severely head-injured children: a report from the NIH Traumatic Coma Data Bank, *J Neurosurg* 76:450–454, 1992.

26. Graham DI, Ford I, Adams JH, et al: Fatal head injury in children, *J Clin Pathol* 42:18–22, 1989.

27. Levin HS, Aldrich EF, et al: Severe head injury in children: experience of the Traumatic Coma Data Bank, *Neurosurgery* 31(3):435–455, 1992.

7

Abdominal Injury

Kevin D. Halow
Edward G. Ford

The incidence of traumatic abdominal injury in children is third after central nervous system and orthopedic injuries.[1] A separate discussion of intraabdominal injuries is warranted because, even though the incidence is low, a missed intraabdominal hemorrhage or hollow viscous rupture may result in a devastating, if not fatal consequence (expected mortality 3% to 5%).[2] Proper evaluation of the child with a suspected intraabdominal injury includes a careful history of the accident (delineating mechanisms of injury), consideration of the child's subjective complaints, meticulous physical examination, and carefully planned (conservative and invasive) supporting diagnostic evaluations.

The injured child is immediately attended by a multidisciplinary staff of physicians. A cooperative effort including surgical, pediatric, intensive care, and radiographic specialists provides a framework for rapid evaluation and treatment.[2,3] We emphasize the three cardinal rules of pediatric trauma[4]:

- Do not waste time.
- Suspect occult injury.
- Be aware of the anatomic and physiologic differences of the child.

The airway is first protected and secured, intravenous access is established, and the organ systems are supported in a prioritized manner. Central nervous system trauma is usually the first concern in evaluation and treatment, but when abdominal injuries may lead to rapid death, celiotomy may take precedence over all other evaluations and treatment. Children respond to any traumatic event with crying and aerophagia, which combine to cause gastric distention.[5] The air-distended abdomen makes abdominal examination difficult and increases the risks of aspiration and gastric rupture; placement of a nasogastric tube helps to avoid these problems.[5]

This chapter presents a decision scheme for penetrating and blunt abdominal trauma (Figs. 7–1 and 7–2). The algorithms are designed to maximize diagnostic return while minimizing psychologic or physical trauma, delay of

201

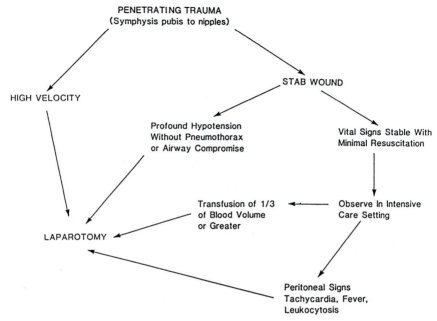

Figure 7–1. Algorithm for diagnosis and treatment of penetrating trauma.

therapeutic intervention, inappropriate use of facility resources, or unnecessary expense.

PENETRATING WOUNDS

There are two types of penetrating wounds: those caused by high-velocity missiles, such as gunshot or shotgun wounds, and those caused by low-velocity penetration, such as stab wounds. Each general type of wound is considered separately here.

High-Velocity Injuries

High-velocity injuries are associated with a "blast effect" (Fig. 7–3).[6] The apparent penetrating wound may be small, but there is a circumferential zone of concussion injury that may disrupt virtually any soft tissue structure. The zone of blast injury may extend for 10 to 40 diameters of the missile (Fig. 7–4).[7] There is no such thing as an "anticipated trajectory" in predicting injuries from firearms. Once a high-velocity missile enters the body, it travels through a variety of tissue densities (skin, subcutaneous tissue, fascia, muscle, viscus, bone), each of which may cause a deflection in trajectory. A single missile entering the thorax may conceivably be deflected enough times to cause a pen-

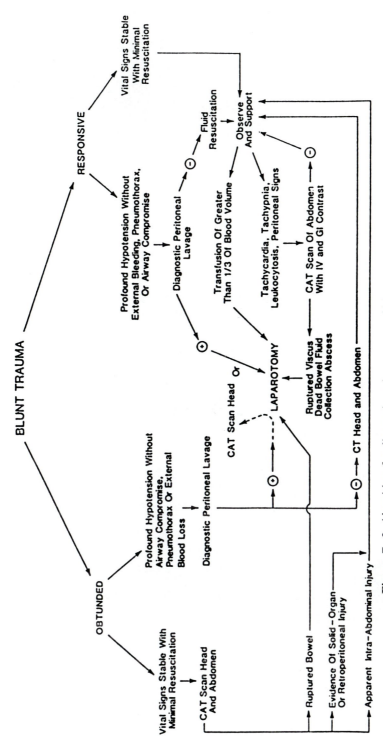

Figure 7–2. Algorithm for diagnosis and treatment of blunt trauma.

203

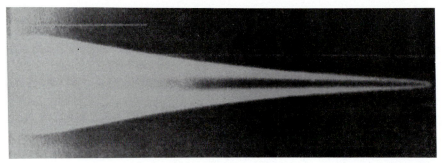

Figure 7–3. Single frame of high-speed motion picture of a steel sphere traveling at high velocity through a container of water (water surface at left of photograph). As the sphere travels through the water density, it generates a zone of concussion (left side of the photograph) many times the diameter of the sphere (right side of photograph). (From Heaton LD, Coates JB Jr, Beyer JC, eds: *Wound ballistics,* Washington, DC, 1962, Medical Department, United States Army, Office of the Surgeon General, p 226.)

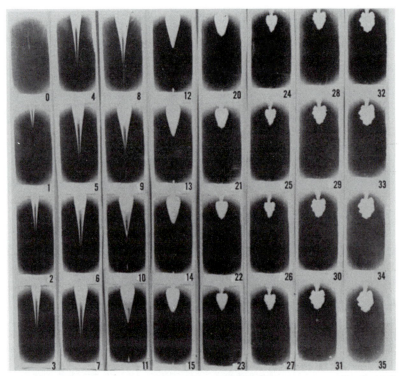

Figure 7–4. High-speed motion picture frames (1920 frames per second) of a 3/16" steel sphere entering water with a velocity of 3160 feet per second. The surface of the water is at the top of the figure. The depth of the water is 55 cm. Of note is the zone of concussion injury noted in Figure 7–3, which creates a sizable cavity in frames 12 and 13. In frames 14 through 27 this cavity is seen to contract progressively. The size of the cavity reaches stability in the subsequent frames, but the final cavity size (frame 35) does not reflect the zone of injury as demonstrated in frames 9 through 14. (From Heaton LD, Coates JB Jr, Beyer JC, eds: *Wound ballistics,* Washington, DC, 1962, Medical Department, United States Army, Office of the Surgeon General, p 154.)

etrating or blast injury to each intraabdominal and intrathoracic organ system. Most intrathoracic injuries may be managed without thoracotomy (see Chapter 9). However, surgical exploration of the abdomen is the only method of ensuring complete evaluation of each intraabdominal organ system.[5]

The abdominal cavity includes regions of the thorax from the nipples to the symphysis pubis (Fig. 7–5). Penetrating high-velocity injuries between these anatomic landmarks dictate fluid resuscitation and celiotomy. Before celiotomy, patients are divided into stable and unstable categories.

The child with a high-velocity penetrating injury to the abdomen, a controlled airway, and profound hypotension unresponsive to a 20 to 50 ml/kg intravenous fluid bolus is evaluated by physical examination supported only by a chest roentgenogram and type and cross-match for blood products. The child is then taken for immediate celiotomy.

The child who is hemodynamically stable should undergo intravenous pyelography to determine the number and position of the kidneys and to evaluate for possible renal pedicle or parenchymal injury. If in the course of roentgenographic evaluation a missile is not identified on abdominal or chest radiograph, further radiographic evaluation of the head, neck, and extremities is undertaken until the missile is found.

During celiotomy the abdomen is carefully and systematically explored. The bowel is visualized from the esophageal hiatus to the peritoneal reflection of the rectum, including complete mobilization of the duodenum. The triangular ligaments of the liver are dissected to allow complete visualization of the diaphragms and the "bare" area of the liver. Diaphragmatic lacerations are repaired with heavy nonabsorbable figure-of-8 sutures. The surgeon should consider the path of the phrenic nerve to prevent iatrogenic diaphragmatic paralysis from improper suture placement. Penetrating wounds of the stomach are resected and primarily repaired.

The gallbladder and common bile duct are fairly well protected beneath the liver, posterior to the costal margin. The gallbladder is the most frequently injured biliary structure, and injuries are managed mainly by cholecystectomy.[8] Cholecystostomy is a rational alternative in the very unstable patient.[8,9] Cholecystorrhaphy is not recommended because of the risk of future stone formation at suture lines and concurrent cholecystitis. The strategy for common bile duct repair depends on the degree of tissue destruction. Primary closure and stenting with a T-tube are performed in clean lacerations. Clean lacerations from blast injuries are extremely rare. Transections of the common duct with 3 to 4 mm of the posterior wall intact may be repaired with autogenous tissue, usually without subsequent stricture formation.[10] If the common bile duct is mobilized from its bed, ischemic stricture formation is invariable. Biliary-enteric bypass, by roux-en-Y cholecystojejunostomy, is preferred when the patient has suffered

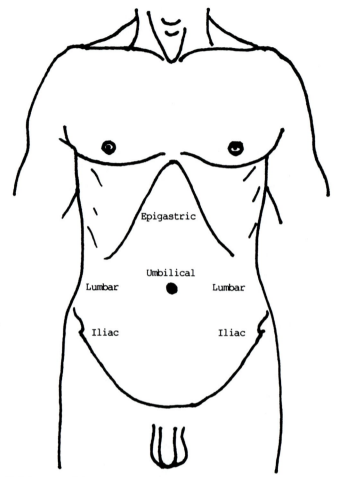

Figure 7–5. Diagram of the anatomic boundaries of the abdomen. The epigastric region is bounded superiorly by the curvature of the diaphragm, which extends approximately to the level of the nipples. The lower extent of the abdominal cavity extends to the pelvis at the level of the pubic symphysis. Lacerations or penetrating injuries between the nipples and the symphysis pubis must be suspect for having injured intraabdominal organs or structures.

a complete traumatic disruption or extensive dissection of the common bile duct.[11]

Infection, with peritonitis, abscess formation, intrahepatic hematomas, traumatic cysts, hematobilia, and biliary obstruction, is a complication that may be expected following bile duct or hepatic injuries.

Penetrating duodenal injury is uncommon in children. Unlike duodenal injuries in adults, the majority of those in children are due to blunt trauma; they are discussed below.

Pancreatic injuries vary with age. In patients greater than 13 years of age the most likely cause is penetrating trauma, whereas in those under 13 years the cause tends to be blunt trauma. Penetrating wounds of the pancreas are best managed with extensive drainage.[5]

Small bowel injuries in children and adolescents are rare but are most likely to be associated with penetrating injuries. In a recent review of the New Orleans experience, 55 of 659 patients with traumatic small bowel injuries were less than 16 years of age (7%).[12] Eight percent of the bowel injuries were the result of high-velocity injuries. Injuries included simple serosal tears, clean lacerations, and blast injuries. Only 27% of the patients with penetrating injuries who underwent celiotomy had such trivial changes that celiotomy might not have been necessary. Segmental resection and reanastomosis were required in an additional 27% of the patients. The small bowel is primarily repaired if the injury is antimesenteric and involves less than 30% of the bowel circumference. For injuries that are greater than 30% of the bowel circumference, mesenteric border wounds, or multiple wounds in a small segment, the small bowel is resected and primarily anastomosed. The morbidity and mortality from small bowel injury relate to the severity of overall injury and the rapidity with which diagnosis is established and treatment is rendered.[12]

Treatment of colon wounds ranges from primary closure (for a minimal wound with no spillage) to resection with colostomy and mucous fistula (for wounds accompanied by a large amount of tissue destruction or fecal spillage). As a rule, stab wounds are closed whereas gunshot injuries (especially to the left colon) are resected or exteriorized or both.

Retroperitoneal hematomas resulting from penetrating injuries are selectively explored in search of vascular or genitourinary injury. The retroperitoneum is divided into three zones to aid intraoperative therapeutic decisions (Fig. 7–6). Severe injury with hypotension occurs in 80% of patients with zone 1 injuries, 28% of patients with zone 2 injuries, and 48% of patients with zone 3 injuries. Zone 1 injuries are routinely explored. Pathologic traumatic changes in zone 1 usually involve the great vascular structures (aorta, vena cava, renal vessels), which are easily repaired. Zone 2 contains the genitourinary organs, and injuries in this zone are explored only when radiographic evaluation suggests a ureteral injury, when the kidney cannot be visualized on intravenous pyelogram, or when a renal parenchymal injury is associated with an expanding hematoma at laparotomy. A full discussion of genitourinary injuries may be found in Chapter 8. Retroperitoneal hematomas originating in the true pelvis (zone 3) are not explored. The most common cause of hematoma in this region is a pelvic fracture with disruption of the pelvic veins. Exploration of such a

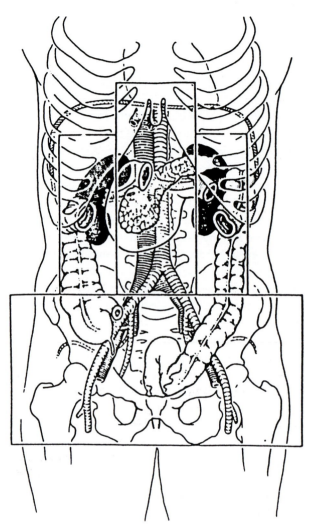

Figure 7–6. Diagram of the retroperitoneum with division into three zones for the purpose of diagnosis and management. Zone 1 injuries involve vascular structures (aorta, vena cava, and renal vessels), are responsible for severe injury, and are routinely explored. Zone 2 injuries involve the genitourinary organs, are less severe, and are explored only if injury is suspected on the basis of radiography or expanding hematoma at laparotomy. Zone 3 injuries involve the true pelvis, represent expanding hematomas, and are not explored.

pelvic hematoma may lead to uncontrolled bleeding and subsequent death. An exception to this rule is the patient with penetrating trauma that obviously traverses the iliac vessels.[13]

Stab Wounds

All children with stab wounds to the abdomen are admitted for observation. Cutaneous stab wounds are usually clean and may be irrigated, debrided, and closed in the emergency center. The need for celiotomy is selectively considered as outlined in Figure 7–1. Hemodynamically stable children are followed with serial physical examinations and serum hematocrit and leukocyte determinations every 4 hours. Anemia requiring a greater than 30 ml/kg transfusion of packed red blood cells, progressive leukocytosis, fever, and peritoneal signs are indications for exploratory celiotomy. Some authors support diagnostic peritoneal lavage (DPL) to determine which patients with stab wounds should undergo celiotomy for surgical exploration. The performance of lavage in a frightened child is no easy task. Furthermore, the procedure provides marginal information about victims of penetrating injury. Therefore our policy is watchful observation in hospital with frequent physical examinations. The development of instability according to the hemodynamic or laboratory indications discussed previously or the development of peritonitis are indications for surgical exploration. This policy is effective *only* if the patient is alert and is compulsively observed and examined.

The child with a stab wound to the abdomen who is hemodynamically unstable (with a patent airway and no evidence of pneumothorax or hemothorax) should spend no more than 15 minutes in the emergency center. The only diagnostic tests required are chest roentgenogram and drawing of a blood specimen for typing. Celiotomy is then performed immediately. Exploration at laparotomy is carried out as discussed previously for high-velocity injuries.

BLUNT INJURY

As with penetrating trauma, children who are victims of blunt injury are evaluated in a systematic fashion (see Fig. 7–2). Children suffering blunt trauma can be divided into two major groups. The first group consists of obtunded children with obvious severe central nervous system injuries, and the second group is children who are minimally mentally impaired and can voice subjective complaints.

The Obtunded Child

The obtunded child provides a diagnostic challenge. Systematic evaluation minimizes missed diagnoses and facilitates rapid and effective treatment (see Fig. 7–2). Obtundation is most commonly a result of hypoxia and acidosis from an insecure airway (e.g., pneumothorax, flail chest, craniofacial trauma, pulmonary contusion). It may also be the result of severe central nervous system injury or severe hemorrhage. We cannot overemphasize the importance of a treatment scheme in which evaluation of the airway is foremost. If a child is not freely moving air, he or she is immediately supported with bag-mask ventilation and expeditiously intubated. Chest roentgenographic examination requires no more than 5 minutes and is efficient in ruling out intrathoracic traumatic changes. The obtunded child in whom the airway has been secured may continue to be hypotensive or may revert to normal vital signs. If the child remains hypotensive despite a secure airway and has no apparent external source of hemorrhage, evaluation of the abdomen takes precedence over treatment of the central nervous system. In these patients the most efficient means of quickly diagnosing intraperitoneal hemorrhage is DPL. Although DPL is associated with complications, it is an important adjunct to rapid clinical evaluation. The majority of deaths occurring in children in the emergency department are a direct result of intraabdominal injury and hemorrhage.[14] Numerous authors have noted that the diagnosis of abdominal injury can be in doubt in up to 25% of cases of pediatric trauma.[15] In patients who are obtunded and profoundly hypotensive, the benefits of data acquired from DPL, leading to rapid celiotomy, far outweigh the risk of complications from the procedure.

The accuracy of DPL for blunt injury has been proved in a number of reviews. In a study of 1465 adult and child victims of trauma, DPL had an overall accuracy of 98.8% in identifying patients with intraperitoneal disease.[16] In selected children (14 years of age and under) and adolescents (15 and 16 years of age) evaluated by open DPL, the overall accuracy for detection of injury was as high as 95.5%.[17]

The technique and findings of DPL are well established.[18] The child is sedated, and the stomach and bladder are decompressed. An open technique is used via an infraumbilical midline incision. The catheter is directed toward the pelvis, and the peritoneum and fascia are closed. Lactated Ringer's solution is infused at a volume of 10 ml/kg (up to 1 L) over 10 minutes and is then recovered by gravity drainage. Positive and indeterminate findings are listed in Table 7–1. In patients with an indeterminate lavage the catheter is left in place and the lavage repeated in 2 hours.[18]

DPL has been criticized, not so much because of the occasional false-positve result (leading to an unnecessary celiotomy) as because of the false-negative rates (missing the presence of surgically correctable injury). Critics argue that DPL is inaccurate in detecting injuries to retroperitoneal viscera such as the second and third portions of the duodenum, the pancreas, and the kidneys; significant retroperitoneal bleeding; and diaphragmatic injuries.[19] Proponents of DPL cite its usefulness in the rapid triage of children with blunt abdominal

Table 7–1. Criteria for Interpreting Peritoneal Lavage

Criteria for positive lavage (need only one)
Free aspiration of greater than 10 ml of blood
Grossly bloody lavage fluid
Passage of lavage fluid out of Foley or chest tube
RBC > 100,000/mm³
WBC > 500/mm³
Amylase > 175 u/dl
Criteria for indeterminant lavage (need only one)
RBC > 50,000/mm³ and < 100,000/mm³
WBC > 100/mm³ and < 500/mm³
Amylase > 75 u/dl and < 175 u/dl
Dialysis catheter fills with blood
Positive lavage → exploration
Indeterminant lavage → leave catheter in place and repeat in 2 hours
Negative lavage → remove catheter

From Drew R, Perry JF, Fischer RP: *Surg Gynecol Obstet* 145:885–888, 1977. By permission of *Surgery, Gynecology & Obstetrics.*

injury. In the University of Colorado experience a review of celiotomy performed because of positive DPL in children less than 14 years old showed that only 37.5% of the operations were "necessary." The remaining patients had injuries that probably could have been managed nonoperatively.[20] A selective management protocol was then instituted. The protocol included immediate celiotomy after a positive DPL in conjunction with hemodynamic instability, selective celiotomy (based on transfusion requirement) after a positive DPL in a stable patient, and mandatory celiotomy after a DPL positive by criteria other than blood. With these criteria the unnecessary celiotomy rate was reduced to 18%.[20] The rapidity of DPL evaluation combined with its accuracy and low procedural morbidity make it an important part of evaluation of the obtunded hypotensive child.

If the unresponsive, hypotensive child is found to have a positive DPL by the Denver criteria, he or she is taken for immediate celiotomy. After control of intraabdominal injury the patient is taken from the operating suite to the radiology department for a computed tomographic (CT) scan of the head and if necessary is returned to the operating suite for a definitive neurosurgical procedure. Transport to the radiographic site occurs with the patient still under general anesthesia and with the anesthesiologist and surgeon in attendance.

The hypotensive patient with central nervous system injury, with a secure airway, without external hemorrhage, and with a negative DPL probably has a transtentorial herniation. This patient is taken to the radiology suite for CT examination of the head and abdomen. The abdomen is included in the evaluation because of the rare possibility of hypotension resulting from a large retroperitoneal hemorrhage or subcapsular hematomas of the liver or spleen.

The obtunded child who has suffered blunt abdominal trauma but is hemodynamically stable is differentiated from the child who is hemodynamically unstable. DPL is used only for the unstable child. The abdomen of the hemodynamically stable child is best evaluated with CT scanning. DPL in the obtunded but hemodynamically stable child is performed only if CT scanning is not available *and* the patient has neurologic or orthopedic injuries requiring general anesthesia for management.[5]

Although many authors believe that CT scanning is the "gold standard" for detecting intraabdominal injury in children, it is important to realize that the routine CT evaluation of all trauma patients is inappropriate. CT evaluation of patients with thoracic trauma is time consuming. Most injuries within the chest cavity are nonoperative and best identified by plain roentgenograms (see Chapter 9). The initial chest roentgenogram readily identifies most acute intrathoracic injuries such as rib fractures, pneumothorax, hemothorax, or ruptured diaphragms. Plain films may also suggest associated injuries of the esophagus (mediastinal emphysema) or great vessels (mediastinal widening).

Use of CT scanning is best suited for patients who are initially stable and have the following[5,21]:

- The likelihood of intraabdominal injury because of the mechanism of injury
- Declining hematocrit value
- Continued fluid requirements
- Hematuria

The routine use of abdominal CT scanning in patients with neurologic injury has been challenged by some authors. They argue that although the risk of abdominal and thoracoabdominal injury is higher in patients with neurologic injury, the yield of abdominal CT is low in patients who are not strongly suspected to have intra-abdominal injury.[21] Most authors, however, support neurologic injury as an indication for abdominal CT scanning because of the following[5,14,15,22,23]:

- The high association of abdominal and thoracoabdominal injury in patients with neurologic injury
- The unreliability of physical examination in obtunded patients
- The expediency with which concomitant abdominal CT scanning can be performed
- The significant mortality associated with missed intraabdominal injury

CT scanning has been compared to other abdominal imaging techniques such as nuclear scintigraphy and ultrasonography for the evaluation of blunt abdominal trauma.

Kaufmann and associates[24] reported on 100 consecutive children with serious blunt abdominal trauma requiring celiotomy. Twenty percent were found to have liver injuries, 25% had splenic injury, and 12% had renal injuries. CT scanning was superior to nuclear scintigraphy in identifying liver and splenic injuries with fewer false-negative and false-positive findings. CT scanning and ultrasonography were equal in their ability to diagnose liver and renal injury, but ultrasonography was markedly inferior to CT in diagnosing splenic trauma, with a false-negative rate of 50%.[24] Ultrasonography is attractive in that it does not use ionizing radiation, may be performed at the bedside, assesses vascular pulsations, provides information concerning adjacent organs, and accurately shows free intraabdominal fluid.[24]

Nuclear scintigraphy offers the advantages of being easier to perform than CT, being less affected by patient motion, requiring less patient cooperation or sedation, and not requiring intravenous or oral contrast media. However, scintigraphy may take as long as, or longer than, CT scanning, the observed radiation dose to the liver and spleen is slightly greater than that with CT, scanning may be difficult in the patient who cannot be moved, and numerous successive scans may be required for injury identification.[24]

Proponents of CT scanning argue that CT has the following advantages[22,24]:
- It is as good as or better than nuclear imaging in detecting hepatic and splenic injuries.
- It is as good as ultrasonography in detecting hepatic and renal injuries and better at detecting splenic injuries.
- It is able to identify and evaluate other intraperitoneal structures.
- It is able to identify retroperitoneal injuries.
- It is noninvasive.
- It obviates the need for multiple diagnostic studies.
- It is relatively fast and available.

CT scanning does have some disadvantages, including the following[5,23]:
- Expense
- Amount of time necessary to perform the study (with older machines)
- Lack of a definitive difference in CT appearance between liver and spleen injuries and a subsequent need for celiotomy

We perform our study with intravenous contrast material only. The diagnostic yield of acute CT scanning for hollow viscus abdominal injuries is low, and we consider the risk of hypertonic contrast aspiration in head-injured patients or patients with nasogastric tubes to be significant enough that we do not use oral contrast medium.

The Responsive Child

The second major subset of children with blunt abdominal trauma is those who are responsive and able to answer questions regarding suspected abdominal injuries. Responsive patients who have profound hypotension (without obvious external hemorrhage) and who remain hemodynamically unstable despite fluid resuscitation undergo an immediate DPL as previously described. Children with intraabdominal hemorrhage may or may not have abdominal complaints. Whole blood in the abdomen is not a peritoneal irritant and may not lead to physical signs of intraperitoneal injury (guarding, rebound, loss of bowel sounds) until the red blood cell membrane is disrupted and the hemoglobin molecule itself irritates the peritoneum. The patient with a positive DPL is taken for immediate celiotomy. The patient with a negative DPL is taken for CT scanning of the abdomen to detect retroperitoneal hemorrhage or subcapsular hematomas. The patient is then taken to the pediatric intensive care unit (PICU) and supported with blood products and fluids, as required.

The responsive patient who remains hemodynamically stable, maintains stable vital signs with a minimum of fluid resuscitation, and has a history of significant trauma is also observed in the PICU. Patients with indications as listed previously are taken for CT scanning.

Children observed in the intensive care unit are monitored closely. Evaluations include hourly assessment of vital signs, frequent physical examinations, and frequent hemoglobin, hematocrit, and white blood cell count determinations. Patients with radiographic evidence of intraabdominal or retroperitoneal organ fracture are given transfusions as required for a hematocrit value less than 30%. If the transfusion requirements exceed 20% of the patient's blood volume in 24 hours (approximately 30 ml/kg), the patient is considered to have ongoing and life-threatening hemorrhage and is taken for exploratory celiotomy.[25] If tachycardia, fever, leukocytosis, or peritoneal signs develop, the patient is taken for CT of the abdomen with intravenous and gastrointestinal contrast enhancement. The patient with a negative CT returns to the PICU for continued observation. The patient with CT evidence of fluid collections, free air, necrotic bowel, or intraperitoneal abscess undergoes expeditious celiotomy, drainage of fluid, and tissue resection, as necessary.

Early detection of intraabdominal organ injury does not mandate immediate celiotomy. CT is useful for detecting the extent and location of injury; however, the decision for celiotomy should be based not on the CT findings of injury, but on the physiologic condition of the child.[23,26] The term "nonoperative" does not mean "nonsurgical"; the pediatric surgical team should always be included in the patient's management. With close observation in the PICU, many children with intraabdominal injury can be managed nonoperatively, with a subsequent reduction in anesthetic risk, infection, and postsplenectomy sepsis.[27]

SPECIFIC ORGAN SYSTEM INJURIES
Liver

Liver injuries are a major cause of death in children with blunt trauma, but not all liver injuries require surgical repair. In one review of children suffering blunt abdominal injury, 28% had liver or biliary tract injuries or both.[28] Only 8% required emergency celiotomy for exsanguinating hemorrhage. The mortality rate in the immediate celiotomy group was 50%, with all deaths attributed to hepatic vein injuries. Of the 92% of patients who did not require immediate operation for hemorrhage, 8% subsequently had complications, but only 4% required surgical exploration with repair of the biliary tree. In this study the diagnosis of hepatobiliary injury was made based on CT scanning in 92% of patients.[28] In a separate study of 106 pediatric trauma victims, factors that predicted the need for early celiotomy included the following[29]:

- Significantly lower Pediatric Trauma Score
- Transfusion requirement within the first 2 hours of hospitalization
- Total transfusion volume of greater than 30 ml/kg
- Twenty-five percent or greater lobar disruption on CT scan
- Large amounts of intraperitoneal fluid on CT scan

Some authors advocate the use of transaminase levels to predict liver injury.[28,30,31] Aspartate aminotransaminase and alanine aminotransaminase levels are sensitive but not specific for liver injury, so we believe that patients with enzyme elevations should still undergo abdominal CT scanning to document the presence of liver injury.

Following the diagnosis of liver injury by CT in the hemodynamically stable patient, expectant therapy is judicious, safe, and effective management of even extensive lacerations.

Large liver injuries are associated with large blood losses. As the blood loss is replaced, the child's total body temperature becomes depressed, leading to impairment of clotting cascades.[32] Impaired clotting associated with a large raw fractured liver surface presents to the operating surgeon a frustrating and at times impossible clinical problem. Simple lacerations of the liver surface are easily controlled with large mattress sutures through Glisson's capsule.[33] Fractures of lateral segments of the liver may be found with already adequate hemostasis and only a small isthmus of remaining attached tissue. These patients may be adequately managed with completion resection.[34] The difficult patient is the one who has large lacerations through the midportions of the liver. An immediate Pringle maneuver (occlusion of the portal triad) aids in hemostasis. For the cold, hypotensive patient with intractable bleeding, hepatic artery ligation and packing of the liver have been suggested. When ligating the right hepatic artery, the surgeon must remember that the cystic artery is usually a distal branch. To avoid necrosis of the gallbladder, the ligature should be placed above the cystic artery or the gallbladder should be removed.[34] The patient is then transported to the intensive care unit for resuscitation. When the patient becomes warmer and is fluid resuscitated (usually in 24 to 48 hours), he or she is returned to the operating suite for removal of packs. These patients have a high incidence of postoperative intraabdominal abscesses. The presence of foreign bodies (celiotomy pads) within the abdominal cavity that mix with blood (an excellent bacterial culture medium) in the presence of contaminated bile leads to infection.[33]

Alternatively bleeding points within the large liver fracture may be ligated under direct vision and the liver laceration drained.

In a few patients we have achieved excellent results with a liver wrap (Fig. 7–7). The triangular ligament on the side of the injury is dissected to allow a circumferential approach to the injured area. The laceration is explored, and bleeding points are controlled with direct suture ligature. If the patient continues

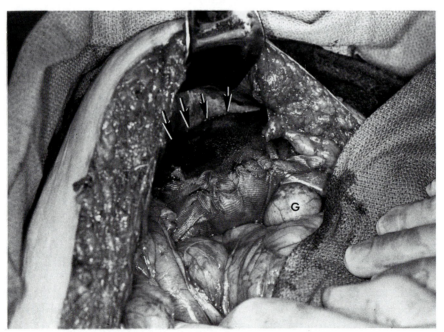

Figure 7–7. Intraabdominal photography of a hepatic laceration that has been treated with a Vicryl mesh wrap. The falciform ligament has been incised and the Vicryl wrapped around the right lobe of the liver. The wrapped right hepatic lobe is outlined by solid arrows. This wrap was accomplished lateral to the gallbladder *(G)*. Had the injury been more medial, the gallbladder would have been removed. The wrap is prevented from slipping laterally by tacking to the falciform ligament medially.

to bleed, several sheets of Dexon or Vicryl mesh are sewn together to form a long cloth. This material is wrapped around the injured side of the liver and tightened to close the liver laceration and apply circumferential pressure to the injured lobe. We have found this method to achieve excellent hemostasis in difficult cases. To prevent the wrap from sliding laterally from the liver, we tack its superior aspect to the falciform ligament and posteriorly to the leaf of the diaphragm. Before the right side of the liver is wrapped, the gallbladder must be removed to prevent compression with subsequent necrosis and perforation.

Biliary Tract

Isolated biliary tract injuries from blunt injury are rare. Unless there is a large bile leak, biliary tract injuries may be missed for several days following injury. Injuries usually involve the extrahepatic bile ducts or the common bile ducts. If the bile leak is small and the duct is able to seal itself without stricture, the injury may be missed entirely. The usual disease course is a symptom-free interval followed by fever, right upper quadrant pain, and jaundice several days after an injury.[28] Radionuclide imaging is a reliable diagnostic modality for identifying common duct disruption.[35] An important distinction must be made between extrahepatic biliary tract disruption and posttraumatic hepatic insufficiency. Posttraumatic hepatic insufficiency occurs after massive resuscitation for major trauma and is associated with an episode of hypotension and progressive respiratory failure, renal insufficiency, and sepsis that parallel periods of peak metabolic response.[36]

Blunt injuries to the portal structures usually cause disruption of the common bile duct with shearing of the portal vein. The hepatic artery is tortuous and not fixed, allowing a moderate degree of motion of the portal structures without disruption. The common bile duct is fixed at the pancreaticoduodenal junction and at the bifurcation of hepatic ducts.[11,37] These are the characteristic areas of shear injury.

Pancreas

Pancreatic injury is uncommon. One report showed 13 pancreatic injuries out of 300 injuries in patients evaluated with CT scanning for abdominal trauma.[38] In this study 11 of 13 cases were correctly diagnosed with CT, but two injuries were missed on early scans. Pancreatic fractures and CT findings of other pancreatic trauma may be subtle in the first few hours after injury. Scanning requires adequate bowel contrast, gastric decompression, sedation, and repeat scans if initial images are not satisfactory.[38]

Because of the pancreas's close association with other organs and vascular structures, it is not surprising that injury to the pancreas is often associated with injury to any or all neighboring vital structures. Outlining a standardized approach to pancreatic injury, however, is impossible because of the variability of injuries to the pancreas and the associated tissues. Several authors have reported small series of pancreatic injuries and their management. Their suggestions cannot be construed as standard treatment because the series are usually small and the number of patients followed up is even smaller or the follow-up is incomplete.

Our approach to surgery for pancreatic injuries is conservative, even when conservative management requires large tissue resection.

Simple pancreatic lacerations, not involving major ductal structures, are oversewn and drained. In all instances of drainage of a lesion, we use active drains, such as Hemovac or Jackson-Pratt drains alone, rather than passive drains, such as Penrose drains, or active plus passive drains.

Pancreatic injuries that involve the tail of the pancreas (lateral to the superior mesenteric vessels) and that are extensive or involve the major ductal structures are most conservatively managed by distal pancreatectomy. If the tail of the pancreas can be safely dissected from the splenic vessels, it is resected, leaving the spleen in place. If the dissection cannot be undertaken safely, or if there is thrombosis of the splenic vein, the spleen is removed en bloc with the tail of the pancreas. Resection of the spleen necessitates consideration of prophylaxis against overwhelming postsplenectomy sepsis.

Lacerations of the head of the pancreas that do not involve major ductal structures are oversewn and drained. Injuries that involve major ductal structures, or a large amount of tissue injury, are treated by roux-en-Y pancreaticojejunostomy. Surgical management of more extensive pancreatic injuries or injuries associated with other regional organs or organ systems must be individualized. When possible, we attempt to restore continuity of the normal anatomy and minimize tissue resection. When repairs are tenuous or of questionable reliability, the risk of pancreatic enzymatic activity on major vascular structures is substantial and we resect the gland and restore the anatomy to as close to normal as possible. We find uncontrolled pancreatic fistulas much easier to manage than uncontrolled retroperitoneal proteolytic processes and freely place drains in regions of retroperitoneal injury.

Spleen

When splenic injury is identified on x-ray evaluation, the stable patient is usually managed nonoperatively. When the child meets criteria for ongoing blood loss (see previous discussion), he or she is taken for celiotomy. Up to 50% of actively bleeding spleens may still be preserved by splenorrhaphy.[39-41] Exceptions are spleens that are pulverized, are severely fragmented, or have fractures deep into the hilum. We prefer to wrap the fractured spleens (as described for the liver). The circumferential wrap pressure provides superior hemostasis, and use of the technique avoids further trauma from needle and suture lacerations. Preservation of the spleen is emphasized because of the risk of overwhelming postsplenectomy sepsis. This is the syndrome of septicemia, meningitis, or pneumonia that is caused by encapsulated organisms and follows splenectomy.[27] The mechanism is multifactorial; the syndrome may occur from decreased clearance of bacteria, decreased immunoglobin production, and decreased opsonin production. The most common organisms are pneumococcus, meningococcus, *Escherichia coli, Haemophilus influenzae, Staphylococcus,* and *Streptococcus.* The most susceptible children are those less than 2 years of age. If splenectomy is necessary, therapeutic considerations include the following:

- Use of Pneumovax and immunizations for encapsulated organisms
- Lifetime antibiotic prophylaxis with penicillin
- Educating the parents concerning risks of infection

Intestine

Perforation of the intestine occurs in less than 2% of children evaluated for significant blunt trauma. The initial history, physical examination, and laboratory analysis have not been reported as helpful in identifying children with hollow viscus injury. Free air is not evident on abdominal films in up to 60% of patients, and contrast studies are also not helpful in the initial evaluation. Rarely a ruptured viscus is diagnosed on initial CT examination because free intraperitoneal air is detected. Serial abdominal examinations in the alert patient have proved most reliable in determining the need for operative intervention.[12,42,43] The suspected causes of hollow viscus rupture following blunt trauma include bursting of the bowel when fluid-filled loops are subjected to sudden increases in intraluminal pressure, compression of loops against the vertebral column, and tangential forces acting at fixed points of adhesion. Viscus perforations have been reported in abused children. Any injured child with an unclear history and properly diagnosed abdominal tenderness must be considered a possible victim of abuse. Similarly, if child battering is suspected, trauma to the abdomen must be considered and carefully evaluated.

The current experience leads to the following conclusions[44,45]:

- The major etiologic factors in childhood blunt trauma are motor vehicle accidents and child abuse.
- Abused children must be recognized and properly evaluated for abdominal injury.
- Accurate and rapid diagnosis of intestinal perforation by objective emergency center criteria is difficult.
- A child with stable vital signs at admission and no life-threatening injuries has an excellent prognosis in spite of a 12- to 24-hour delay in diagnosis of the ruptured viscus.

- Peritoneal lavage should be performed when diagnostic difficulties exist.
- The patient with a ruptured viscus should undergo immediate celiotomy.

Children are relatively hypermetabolic when compared with adults, and because of their small size they have relatively lower nutritional substrate stores. Severe trauma may increase the child's metabolic rate by as much as 100% to 200%, and the child may quickly enter a state of acquired malnutrition. We begin nutritional support within the first 48 hours after injury. The recognition and prevention of posttraumatic malnutrition are discussed in Chapters 14 and 15.

REFERENCES

1. Mayer T, Walker M, Johnson DG, Matlak ME: Causes of morbidity and mortality in severe pediatric trauma, *JAMA* 245(7):719–721, 1981.
2. Nihoul-Fekete C, Juskiewenski S: Diagnostic and therapeutic strategy in severe abdominal trauma in children with multiple trauma, *Intensive Care Med* 15:57–60, 1989.
3. Harris BH, Barlow BA, Ballantine TV, et al: American Pediatric Surgical Association principles of pediatric trauma care, *J Pediatr Surg* 27(4):423–426, 1992.
4. Blair GK: Update on pediatric trauma, *Can J Surg* 33(6):443–446, 1990.
5. Haller JA, Pokorny WJ: Pediatric trauma. In Mattox K, Moore E, Feliciano D, eds: *Trauma*, ed 2, Norwalk, Conn, 1992, Appleton-Century-Crofts.
6. Harvey EN, McMillen JH, Butler EG, Puckett WO: Mechanism of wounding. In Heaton LD, Coates JB Jr, Beyer JC, eds: *Wound ballistics*, Washington, DC, 1962, Medical Department, United States Army, Office of the Surgeon General.
7. French RW, Callender GR: Ballistic characteristics of wounding agents. In Heaton LD, Coates JB Jr, Beyer JC, eds: *Wound ballistics*, Washington, DC, 1962, Medical Department, United States Army, Office of the Surgeon General.
8. Beart RW, Mroz CT: Cholecystectomy for noninflammatory disease, *Am J Surg* 141:342–343, 1981.
9. Soderstrom CA, Kazuhiko M, Dupriest RW: Gallbladder injuries resulting from blunt abdominal trauma: an experience and review, *Ann Surg* 193:60–66, 1981.
10. Belzer FO, Watts JM, Ross HB: Auto-reconstruction of the common bile duct after venous patch graft, *Ann Surg* 162:346–355, 1965.
11. Busuttil RW, Kitahama A, Crrise E: Management of blunt and penetrating injuries to the porta hepatis, *Ann Surg* 162:346–355, 1965.
12. Reilly A, Marks M, Nance F, et al: Small bowel trauma in children and adolescents, *Am Surg* 51(3):132–135, 1985.
13. Selivanov V, Chi HS, Alverdy JC, et al: Mortality in retroperitoneal hematoma, *J Trauma* 24(12):1022–1027, 1984.
14. Williams RD, Zollinger RM: Diagnostic and prognostic factors in abdominal trauma, *Am J Surg* 97:575–581, 1959.
15. Bivins BA, Jona JZ, Belin RP: Diagnostic peritoneal lavage in pediatric trauma, *J Trauma* 16(9):739–742, 1976.
16. Engrav LH, Benjamin CI, Strate RG, et al: Diagnostic peritoneal lavage in blunt abdominal trauma, *J Trauma* 15:854–859, 1975.

17. Dupriest RW, Rodriguez A, Shatney CH: Peritoneal lavage in children and adolescents with blunt abdominal trauma, *Am Surg* 48(9):460–462, 1982.

18. Drew R, Perry JF, Fischer RP: The expediency of peritoneal lavage for blunt trauma in children, *Surg Gynecol Obstet* 145:885–888, 1977.

19. Feliciano DV: Diagnostic modalities in abdominal trauma, *Surg Clin North Am* 71(2):241–256, 1991.

20. Rothenberg S, Moore EE, Mark JA, et al: Selective management of blunt abdominal trauma in children—the triage role of peritoneal lavage, *J Trauma* 27(10):1101–1106, 1987.

21. Taylor GA, Eichelberger MR: Abdominal CT in children with neurologic impairment following blunt trauma, *Ann Surg* 210(2):229–233, 1989.

22. Mohamed G, Reyes HM, Fantus R, et al: Computed tomography in the assessment of pediatric abdominal trauma, *Arch Surg* 121:703–707, 1986.

23. Peitzman AB, Makaroun, Slasky BS, Ritter P: Prospective study of computed tomography in initial management of blunt abdominal trauma, *J Trauma* 26(7):585–592, 1986.

24. Kaufman RA, Towbin R, Babcock DS, et al: Upper abdominal trauma in children: imaging evaluation, *AJR* 142:449–460, 1984.

25. Hoelzer DJ, Brian MB, Balsara VJ, et al: Selection and nonoperative management of pediatric blunt trauma patients: the role of quantitative crystalloid resuscitation and abdominal ultrasonography, *J Trauma* 26(1):57–62, 1986.

26. Taylor GA, Fallat ME, Potter BM, Eichelberger MR: The role of computed tomography in blunt abdominal trauma in children, *J Trauma* 28(22):1660–1664, 1988.

27. Schiffman MA: Nonoperative management of abdominal trauma in pediatrics, *Emerg Med Clin North Am* 7(3):519–535, 1989.

28. Oldham KT, Guice KS, Ryckman F, et al: Blunt liver injury in childhood: evolution of therapy and current perspective, *Surgery* 100(3):542–549, 1986.

29. Moulton SL, Lynch FP, Hoyt DB, et al: Operative intervention for pediatric liver injuries: avoiding delay in treatment, *J Pediatr Surg* 27(8):958–963, 1992.

30. Coant PN, Kornberg AE, Brody AS, Edwards-Holmes K: Markers for occult liver injury in cases of physical abuse in children, *Pediatrics* 89(2):274–278, 1992.

31. Hennes HM, Smith DS, Schneider K, et al: Elevated liver transaminase levels in children with blunt abdominal trauma: a predictor of liver injury, *Pediatrics* 86(1):87–90, 1990.

32. Svoboda JA, Peter ET, Dang CV, et al: Severe liver trauma in the face of coagulopathy: a case for temporary packing and re-exploration, *Am J Surg* 144:717–721, 1992.

33. Pachter HL, Spencer FC, Hofstetter SR, et al: Significant trends in the treatment of hepatic trauma: experience with 411 injuries, *Ann Surg* 215(5):492–500, 1992.

34. Reed RL II, Merrell RC, Myers WC, et al: Continuing evolution in the approach to severe liver trauma, *Ann Surg* 216(5):524–538, 1992.

35. Popovsky J, Wiener FB, Felder PA, et al: Liver trauma, *Arch Surg* 108:184–186, 1974.

36. Champion HR, Jones RT, Trump BF, et al: Post-traumatic hepatic dysfunction as a major etiology in post-traumatic jaundice, *J Trauma* 16:650–657, 1976.

37. Fish JC, Johnson GL: Rupture of the duodenum following blunt trauma: report of a case with avulsion of the papilla of Vater, *Ann Surg* 162:917–919, 1965.

38. Jeffrey RB, Federle MP, Crass RA: Computed tomography of pancreatic trauma, *Radiology* 147:491–494, 1983.

39. Kakkasseril JS, Stewart D, Cox JA, Gelfand M: Changing treatment of pediatric splenic trauma, *Arch Surg* 117:758–759, 1982.

40. Norby II, Max MH: Splenorrhaphy in patients with abdominal trauma, *South Med J* 79(12):1503–1505, 1986.
41. Mishalany H: Repair of the ruptured spleen, *J Pediatr Surg* 9(2):175–178, 1974.
42. Schenk WG, Lonchyna V, Moylan JA: Perforation of the jejunum from blunt abdominal trauma, *J Trauma* 23(1):54–56, 1983.
43. Cobb LM, Vinocur CD, Wagner CW, Weintraub WH: Intestinal perforation due to blunt trauma in children in an era of increased nonoperative treatment, *J Trauma* 26(5):461–463, 1986.
44. Kirks DR: Radiological evaluation of visceral injuries in the battered child syndrome, *Pediatr Ann* 12(12):888–893, 1983.
45. O'Neill JA, Meacham WF, Griffin PP, Sawyers JL: Patterns of injury in the battered child syndrome, *J Trauma* 13(4):332–339, 1973.

8

Urinary Tract Injuries

Joseph N. Corriere, Jr.

Traumatic injuries to the genitourinary system are second in frequency only to injuries involving the central nervous system.[1] Pediatric trauma is characteristically blunt in nature, usually resulting from vehicular and pedestrian accidents. Most pediatric genitourinary injuries are relatively minor (renal contusions), but a recent dramatic increase in violent crime within the pediatric population is increasing the frequency of penetrating, usually severe, genitourinary injury. This chapter focuses on genitourinary injuries unique to children and explores and updates current controversies in the management of the more complex urologic injuries.

RENAL INJURIES

Authors generally agree that minor renal injuries are amenable to conservative, nonoperative management and that major renal parenchymal and vascular lesions require immediate surgical repair. Controversy surrounds the proper treatment of renal injuries needing intermediate intervention.[2–5]

Etiology

Approximately 80% of renal injuries are due to blunt trauma, usually the result of motor vehicle accidents, falls, sports, or fights.[6,7] The most common penetrating injuries, which comprise the other 20% of renal injuries, are gunshot wounds. About 8% of penetrating abdominal injuries involve the kidneys; associated visceral injuries are present in 80% of these patients. Although the kidneys are apparently well protected by the ribs, vertebral bodies, and heavy lumbar muscles, traumatic injuries to the kidneys are common. The kidney is more susceptible to injury in children than in adults for the following reasons:

- The kidney is less well protected because of reduced amounts of perinephric fat, weaker abdominal muscles, and a less ossified thoracic cage.
- The kidney is relatively larger in proportion to abdominal size.
- Rapid deceleration may cause excessive movement of the kidneys with

223

stretching of the renal hilar vessels and arterial intimal tearing with subsequent thrombosis.

Diagnosis

Patients who have upper abdominal trauma and a high probability of renal injury usually have hematuria and abdominal or flank tenderness. Occasionally contusions or abrasions are seen over the flanks. Plain films of the abdomen may reveal fractures of the lower ribs or vertebrae. The kidneys receive 25% of the cardiac output, so a severe renal injury may lead to a rapidly expanding retroperitoneal hematoma manifest as an abdominal mass or shock early in the disease process.

Hematuria. The urine contains blood in more than 90% of patients with significant renal injuries. The presence and degree of hematuria are inconsistent with the degree of injury. Severe renal pedicle or parenchymal injuries may be present without hematuria, whereas gross hematuria may occur with relatively minor renal damage.[8-10]

Radiographic examination. An intravenous urogram (IVU) is indicated in pediatric patients who have sustained significant upper abdominal or flank trauma, have *any* degree of hematuria (in contrast to adults), have a fracture of the eleventh or twelfth rib, or have fractures of the transverse processes of lumbar vertebrae. If the IVU findings are normal, no additional radiographic studies are necessary.[11-13] If a kidney is nonfunctioning, a renal vascular injury should be suspected and ruled in or out by computed tomography (CT) or arteriography.[14,15] If a functioning kidney is seen on urography but the architecture of the kidney is distorted or extravasation is present, CT scanning is performed to define fully the extent of parenchymal or collecting system injury.[16,17]

Classification and Therapy

Renal contusion. Renal contusion is manifest on IVU as a functioning kidney with decreased perfusion, an intact renal outline, and no evidence of contrast extravasation. Bed rest and conservative nonoperative support are all that are necessary for these children. Ambulation is allowed if the results of frequent urinalysis indicate a resolution of the hematuria. Contact sports are prohibited for 3 to 4 weeks. The patient's blood pressure should be routinely checked for up to 1 year to exclude the development of renin-mediated hypertension (so-called Page kidney).

Renal laceration. Renal lacerations are suspected when the IVU shows an indistinct renal outline, an area of decreased perfusion, contrast extravasation, or a retroperitoneal mass. CT is then used to identify the extent of renal parenchymal injury, as well as the presence of an intrarenal or perirenal hematoma. Most lacerations may be treated with bed rest and observation.[18,19] The following are indications for surgical exploration of the kidneys following blunt injuries[20,21]:

- Expanding or uncontained hematoma
- Presence of major segments of nonviable renal parenchyma
- Ureteropelvic junction disruption

Less than 10% of renal injuries should fall into this category. However, penetrating wounds should be explored. If the patient is to be explored, a CT scan is not necessary but IVU must be performed to be sure the uninvolved kidney is normal.

A midline transabdominal incision is used for renal exploration. Associated injuries of the liver, spleen, and bowel are corrected before a retroperitoneal hematoma is opened. The traditional literature recommends medial control of the vascular pedicle before the retroperitoneal hematoma is entered, but unless there are both a wound and a hematoma over the renal vessels, it is easier and quicker merely to reflect the colon laterally along the white line of Toldt, aspirate the hematoma, and correct the injury.[6]

Intrarenal hematomas should be evacuated, the wound debrided by guillotine incision, and the individual arteries and veins suture ligated with 5-0 absorbable suture. The calyces are closed with a running 5-0 absorbable suture and made as watertight as possible. If sufficient capsule is present to cover the defect, it should be closed to tamponade persistent vessel oozing. If the capsule has been destroyed, pedicle grafts of omentum or free peritoneal patch grafts may be used to cover the renal defect. A polyglycolic mesh "wrap" may also be employed and sewn into a pocket to support the organ. Retroperitoneal drains are always placed near the injured kidney and are brought out of the abdominal wall through a separate stab wound.

If renal artery thrombosis is present, the injured segment of artery must be removed and circulation reestablished with interposition vein or artery grafts.[15] Suitable autogenous grafts in children include saphenous vein, internal jugular vein, or hypogastric artery. Autotransplantation should be considered before the surgeon resorts to nephrectomy.[22] Small (polar) arterial occlusions may be left alone without fear of complication. Venous injuries are repaired with 5-0 vascular suture. The renal venous system has unique intrarenal anastomoses so that injured segmental veins may be safely ligated.

Postoperative Care and Complications

Complications peculiar to renal injuries are delayed bleeding and hypertension.[23,24] While as much renal parenchyma as possible is preserved intraoperatively, there are times when devitalized tissue may be left in situ. Tissue slough may occur 10 to 14 days after the injury with subsequent bleeding or urinary extravasation.

Arteriovenous fistulas or aneurysms may develop in association with stab wounds or following percutaneous renal biopsy.

Renal arteriography is the most sensitive and specific method for identifying the source of ongoing or delayed hemorrhage following either blunt or penetrating renal trauma. Intravascular, radiographically controlled, transarterial embolization techniques may be used to treat such bleeding problems.[25]

Early-onset hypertension may be caused by transient renal vessel or parenchymal compression. The hypertension usually resolves in a matter of weeks as the hematoma liquefies and is reabsorbed. If significant perirenal fibrosis with renal vascular compression results, a Page kidney may be induced and prolonged renin-mediated hypertension may result.

Patients who have sustained a significant renal injury should undergo follow-up IVU 3 to 6 months after injury. These patients are also followed closely with blood pressure evaluations for at least a year.

URETERAL INJURIES

Ureteral injury is relatively uncommon in childhood. When ureteral integrity is compromised, urinary extravasation occurs and may result in a retroperitoneal urinoma or urinary ascites. If an associated injury has occurred in contiguous structures (vagina, skin, bowel), a fistulous communication with those structures may develop. If the extravasated urine is infected, life-threatening sepsis may result.

Etiology

Ureteral injuries are generally divided into two etiologic classifications: those caused by external violence (blunt or penetrating trauma) and iatrogenic injuries (surgical misadventure, late complication of radiation therapy, migrating foreign bodies).

In adults the vast majority of injuries are related to iatrogenic trauma, usually surgical misadventure. In children external violence is the usual source of injury. Gunshot wounds account for more than 95% of these injuries; knife wounds are the next most common.[26-36] Rarely, patients fall and become impaled on a spike or suffer a crushing blow that results in a bone fracture and a sharp bone fragment injury. Ureteral avulsion caused by blunt trauma is rare but primarily affects children.[37] The mechanism of injury is thought to be compression of the renal pelvis and upper ureter against the lower thoracic cage or upper lumbar transverse processes, or stretching of the ureter by sudden, extreme extension of the trunk. Ureteral avulsion probably occurs more commonly in children because of their hyperextensible and hypermobile spine.[38-40] The diagnosis of ureteral injury in children is often delayed, with less than half diagnosed on the day of injury.[41]

Diagnosis

IVU is indicated in the trauma patient who has had one of the following[27]:

- Penetrating injury of the abdomen, retroperitoneum, or pelvis in the area of the urinary tract
- A fracture of the eleventh or twelfth rib, a transverse lumbar process, or the bony pelvis
- Hematuria in association with significant abdominal or pelvic trauma

IVU is the best screening test for ureteral injury. The injury is manifest as urinary extravasation or a decrease in collecting system visualization or both.

If at surgical exploration the path of the ureter is in proximity to the path of a penetrating wound, the ureter should be dissected from its bed and examined. If injury cannot be excluded on direct visualization, one vial (5 ml) of indigo carmine should be injected intravenously. Within 7 to 10 minutes the dye is seen leaking into the periureteral tissues from an occult laceration.

If the patient does not meet the criteria for surgical exploration but uncertainty remains concerning ureteral integrity, the most definitive study is a retrograde ureterogram. In many situations this is not feasible. CT with intravenous contrast is the next best diagnostic aid for demonstrating extravasation.

Classification

If a missile passes close to the ureter but does not penetrate it, a contusion may result. If the missile penetrates the ureter, a partial laceration, complete laceration, or avulsion from the ureteropelvic junction results.

Therapy

Contusion. No ureter-specific therapy is necessary in patients with ureteral contusion. If the wound was caused by a high-velocity bullet (over 2500 ft/sec), there is a risk of late necrosis of the ureter from concussion injury. In this instance, placement of an internal ureteral stent and a drain in the area of the injury should be considered. High-velocity wounds are seen more often in military conflicts than in civilian practice; with the recent change in the magnitude and character of violent assaults, we will be seeing more and more patients with these injuries.[42-45]

Laceration. If a partial laceration is present and the ureter that is still in continuity is viable, placement of an indwelling "double-pigtail" stent and primary closure of the wound with interrupted 4-0 or 5-0 absorbable sutures provides the best reconstructive results.[27,34] Some authors advocate a running closure of the wound and elimination of all stents.[46] Before the advent of the totally indwelling stent, this was clearly a better way to handle minor lesions because the placement of a transcutaneous stent and formal nephrostomy increased the risk of complications and extended the scope of the procedure.[47]

However, with the development and use of totally indwelling stents, urine drainage from the repair is found to be minimal and patients can be discharged at an early date. All devitalized tissue must be debrided, and a separate drain must be placed at the site of the repair and brought out through a separate stab wound.

If the remaining intact ureter is of questionable viability or the ureter is completely lacerated, all devitalized tissue must be excised before the technique of reconstruction is selected. The procedure with the lowest complication rate is ureteroneocystostomy. This repair is largely limited to patients with an injury below the level of the iliac vessels. The kidney may be mobilized and lowered to decrease the gap between the ureter and bladder, allowing a tension-free repair. A bladder flap may also be constructed to bridge the gap from the bladder to the ureter. At times, merely suturing the bladder to the psoas fascia (psoas hitch) minimizes tension on the repair. A nonrefluxing reimplantation is most desirable but cannot always be performed.

If the injury is too high to permit a ureteroneocystostomy, a ureteroureterostomy should be performed. Most authors advocate the use of a double-pigtail catheter to stent the repair. A Penrose drain should be placed adjacent to the ureteroureterostomy site and brought externally via a separate stab wound.

If a major length of ureter is lost, consideration should be given to a transureteroureterostomy or a cutaneous ureterostomy for later definitive repair. Autotransplantation adds significantly to the operative time and risk to the patient, but in the patient with a solitary kidney the procedure may be lifesaving.

Avulsion injury. An avulsion injury is essentially a complete laceration that requires debridement and definitive repair with stenting, as described previously.

Surgical injuries. Surgical injuries are exceedingly rare in children. Three basic types of injuries are discussed: crush injuries, laceration injuries, and ligation injuries.

Crush injuries are managed in several ways. The crushed segment may be excised and either a ureteroneocystostomy or a ureteroureterostomy with internal stenting performed. If the surgeon chooses not to resect the damaged segment, placement of an indwelling stent may be accomplished by intraoperative cystotomy. Drain placement is not mandatory in this instance. Endoscopic placement in a small child, especially a boy, is difficult and hazardous and should be avoided.

When the ureter has been completely severed by avulsion or transection and this is recognized intraoperatively, a repair by any of the previously mentioned techniques is employed. If the injury is not recognized intraoperatively and diagnosis is delayed, two options are available. Initially, retrograde ureteral catheterization may be attempted. Unfortunately, this is not usually successful, especially in the patient with a complete avulsion. If it is successful, however, a double-J stent is inserted and the patient is observed for resolution of the extravasated urine. As a second alternative a percutaneous nephrostomy tube may be placed. When the urinoma resolves, surgical reconstruction may be attempted. This is usually months later. Surgical exploration and immediate reconstruction are the best therapeutic choice if the injury is only a few days old.[48,49] In the first few postoperative days, primary repair should be considered. If the injury is discovered later, a formal nephrostomy tube is placed and the urinoma is drained. Repair 3 to 6 months later is then planned.

When large segments of ureter are injured and lost, an ileal ureter may be constructed. Ileal replacement has been used less often with the increasing popularity and success of autotransplantation. In some instances (e.g., a seriously ill child with a normal contralateral kidney), nephrectomy is the best treatment alternative.

When complete ureteral obstruction is thought to be the result of inadvertent surgical ligation, it is tempting to return to the operating room and remove the ligature. Although this is a reasonable treatment option in the first few days, it is hazardous a week or 10 days postoperatively because it may lead to delayed necrosis and fistula formation. The more conservative approach is to place a percutaneous nephrostomy tube and to attempt antegrade catheterization past the obstruction.[50–52] Retrograde stenting is almost invariably unsuccessful. If stenting is successful, balloon dilation to disrupt the suture may be attempted but is not necessary.[53] If the obstruction is caused by chromic suture, it usually resolves in 3 to 4 weeks.[51] Polyglycolic acid suture may take 6 to 8 weeks to resorb. If the obstruction has not resolved in 4 to 6 months, formal repair is indicated.

Radiation injury. Radiation injuries of the ureter are rare and usually discovered months to years after the radiation therapy has been completed. Ureteral stricture and fibrosis are often present, and repair is difficult. Permanent internal stenting is an option reserved for chronically ill children with a poor prognosis. Urinary diversion into an isolated bowel conduit, using both ureter and bowel from outside the irradiated field, may be employed. Occasionally, reconstructive procedures using irradiated tissue wrapped in omentum are successful.[54] Nephrectomy may be considered for a debilitated child with adequate contralateral renal function.

Postoperative care and complications. Indwelling ureteral stents may be left in place for up to 2 months without fear of complications. If a drain has been placed, it should be removed when the drainage stops or at least in 5 days, even if the stent remains for a longer time. Most children may be discharged from the hospital with plans to remove stents in the outpatient clinic or through day surgery.[34]

Stents should be left in place for at least 4 to 6 weeks. When they are removed, a pullout ureterogram or IVU is performed to ensure that the ureter is intact. Once all foreign materials have been removed, the patient should be treated with antibiotics for 7 to 10 days to sterilize the urinary tract. Follow-up excretory urography is performed 3 to 6 months after the repair.

BLADDER INJURIES

The bladder is an abdominal organ in the child and therefore is vulnerable to external trauma. As the bony pelvis grows, the bladder eventually becomes a pelvic organ and is protected from injury, especially when empty of urine.

When the bladder is distended or the pelvis is fractured, the normal protective influence of the intact pelvic ring is lost and shearing forces tear the bladder at its moorings. A spicule of bone may also lacerate the organ. A direct blow to the abdomen may result in rupture of the bladder dome without a pelvic fracture. Missiles may always find the bladder despite its position or its level of urinary distention.

Etiology

Penetrating trauma to the bladder from external violence is most commonly due to gunshot wounds.[55–58] Overall, however, the most common cause of bladder injuries in children is blunt trauma to the abdomen. Blunt injury most commonly occurs in motor vehicle accidents but may also result from falls, crushing injuries to the bony pelvis, or blows to the abdomen.

The full bladder is especially vulnerable to a deceleration injury.[55] Deceleration injuries are most commonly seen in restrained passengers involved in motor vehicle accidents. The force of the collision is focused on the abdomen at the level of the lap belt. The full bladder is ruptured between the belt and the pelvis or vertebral column.

In our experience with 111 bladder injuries over a 7-year period, 86% were due to blunt trauma; 90% of those blunt injuries followed motor vehicle accidents. Eighty-nine percent of the blunt injuries were associated with pelvic fractures. Conversely, 9% of patients with pelvic fractures have a concomitant bladder injury.[56,57]

Diagnosis

Signs and symptoms. The signs and symptoms of bladder rupture are usually nonspecific. The child may complain of suprapubic pain or inability to urinate. Commonly the discomfort of a concomitant fractured pelvis or other organ system injury overshadows the pain from the disrupted urinary tract. Bowel sounds may be absent, especially with intraperitoneal rupture. If recognition of an intraperitoneal injury is delayed, uroascites may develop and cause marked respiratory distress and even lower limb venous occlusion, especially in a neonate.[59] Peritoneal signs of tenderness and rebound eventually develop, and if the urine is infected, frank peritonitis may result.[60]

Hematuria is a hallmark of bladder injuries. In our experience, gross hematuria occurs in more than 95% of patients, with microscopic hematuria present in the remaining cases.[55,61]

Radiographic examination. The static cystogram is the only radiographic study that accurately and consistently identifies a ruptured bladder.[62,63] In a male with a pelvic fracture, blood at the urethral meatus, a high-riding prostate gland on rectal examination, or marked ecchymosis and edema of the perineum, scrotum or penis, a retrograde urethrogram must be obtained before attempted urethral catheterization for cystography. If a ruptured urethra is identified, urethral catheterization may be contraindicated and a suprapubic cystostomy performed. If the cystostomy is placed percutaneously, static cystography must still be performed to rule out a concomitant bladder injury.

Therapy

Penetrating injuries. All patients with high-velocity penetrating injuries of the abdomen should undergo surgical abdominal exploration. The missile tract is followed from the entrance wound to the exit wound. The peritoneal cavity is opened, and the intraabdominal viscera and major vasculature are examined for damage, even if the injury is thought to be entirely extraperitoneal. The bladder and ureters are closely inspected for injury. All devitalized tissue and debris (e.g., bullets, bone spicules, clothing) are removed from the abdomen and bladder.[55] If the ureteral orifices are involved in the injury, or if the integrity of the ureters is in question, 5 ml of indigo carmine is injected intravenously. In 7 to 10 minutes the blue dye should appear in the bladder. The retroperitoneum is examined for extravasation and the ureters are intubated with 5F whistle-tip catheters if there is any concern that they have been damaged.

If the patient has a large pelvic hematoma, it is best left undisturbed. The integrity of the bladder neck, ureters, and vasculature in these patients must be established by proper radiography.

During abdominal exploration the bladder should be entered through its peritoneal surface at the dome and thoroughly inspected for injury. After injury debridement, any extraperitoneal bladder defects are closed with a one-layer, running suture of 3-0 chromic or polyglycolic suture from the inside of the bladder. Extensive mobilization of the retroperitoneal bladder to ensure a watertight closure or to place the knots on the outside of the bladder usually results in increased bleeding. If closing the extraperitoneal defects is impossible, they should not be disturbed. With adequate bladder drainage through the Foley catheter and suprapubic catheter, extraperitoneal lacerations will eventually heal without difficulty. A suprapubic cystostomy tube is inserted into the bladder through a separate stab wound. At least a 20F tube should be used to ensure egress of blood clots. The intraperitoneal bladder incision is closed with a double layer of 3-0 chromic or polyglycolic suture in a running watertight fashion. One–inch Penrose drains are placed near the suture lines and brought through the abdominal wall via separate stab wounds.

Bladder contusions. Bladder contusion is an injury of the bladder mucosa or muscularis without loss of bladder wall continuity. Extravasation of contrast medium is not seen on the static cystogram. These injuries are considered minor and usually require only a few days of Foley catheter drainage, if any therapy at all. When the patient has an associated major sacral injury and cannot urinate, cystometrography should be performed to ensure that the sacral nerve roots innervating the bladder have not been damaged.

Interstitial ruptures. Interstitial ruptures are either incomplete bladder wall ruptures or small, full-thickness ruptures that seal themselves with clot or omentum. These injuries are treated with 10 days of bladder catheter drainage, as is done with the complete but unrepaired extraperitoneal ruptures. Cystography is performed before catheter removal.[56]

Intraperitoneal rupture. Intraperitoneal rupture of the bladder occurs following a sudden rise in intravesical pressure resulting from a blow to the pelvis or lower abdomen (seat belt injury). The increased pressure ruptures the dome of the bladder, which is the weakest and most mobile part of the organ. Contrast material from static cystography is seen to fill the cul-de-sac, outline loops of bowel, and eventually extend into the paracolic gutter. Intraperitoneal ruptures are common in children because of the normal intraperitoneal location of the bladder. Intraperitoneal bladder ruptures account for one third of bladder injuries in children and are about equal in incidence to extraperitoneal ruptures.

Patients with intraperitoneal bladder ruptures must undergo formal surgical repair.[56,57] The peritoneal cavity is opened, and all urine and blood are evacuated. The viscera and vasculature are inspected for injury, and appropriate therapy for associated injuries is instituted. The bladder characteristically has a 5 cm or greater laceration in the dome. The laceration is opened to allow thorough inspection of the bladder interior. Concomitant extraperitoneal lacerations are closed from inside the bladder. Devitalized tissue is excised, and after a suprapubic tube has been placed, the dome wound is closed with absorbable suture material. The suprapubic tube is brought through a separate stab wound, and an extraperitoneal drain is brought through the abdominal wall via a second separate stab wound.[55,60,61]

A few scattered reports describe treatment of intraperitoneal bladder injuries with simple Foley catheter drainage.[64,65] When the literature is carefully reviewed, it is clear that most of these authors are discussing iatrogenic transurethral bladder perforations and not wounds caused by external violence. Most patients with intraperitoneal bladder ruptures caused by abdominal blows or a fractured pelvis have large, gapping lacerations and marked uroascites. These patients must undergo prompt surgical repair or they will rapidly deteriorate.[55,60]

Extraperitoneal rupture. Extraperitoneal bladder ruptures are seen almost exclusively in association with pelvic fractures. The bladder is usually sheared on its anterior lateral wall, near the bladder base, by soft tissue distortion associated with pelvic ring disruption. Occasionally the bladder is lacerated by a sharp, bony spicule. On cystography such injuries are evident by flame-shaped areas of extravasation that are confined to the perivesical soft tissues.[62,66] Extravasation may extend into the thigh via the obturator foramen, to the scrotum via the inguinal canal, along the anterior abdominal wall, or retroperitoneally as high as the kidneys. If the associated pelvic hematoma is large, the bladder may be compressed into a "teardrop deformity."

Isolated extraperitoneal bladder ruptures are easily and safely managed by 10 days of Foley catheter drainage.[57,65,67,68] Some authors suggest treating small, extraperitoneal ruptures with catheter drainage and formally closing large ruptures. It is impossible to relate the extent of the injury to the amount of contrast extravasation.[55,62,67] Extravasation is related both to the size of the injury and to the amount of contrast medium instilled. In our experience even extravasations extending into the pelvis, down the inguinal canal to the scrotum, or up the retroperitoneum as high as the kidneys can be successfully treated with catheter drainage.

If the patient with an extraperitoneal bladder rupture is explored for associated injuries and is not gravely ill, appropriate therapy is opening the dome of the bladder, not disturbing the pelvic hematoma, repairing the rupture intravesically, closing the bladder, and inserting a suprapubic tube as previously described. If the pelvic hematoma is opened for another reason, a drain should be placed. If it is not opened, no drain is necessary.

Postoperative Care and Follow-up

The bladder heals remarkably quickly. If good surgical repair was achieved, the suprapubic tube or Foley catheter may be removed within a week. Cystography is performed before tube removal. If extravasation is present, the catheter is left in place for further drainage and cystography is repeated on the tenth postoperative day.

When the patient is voiding normally and urine has not leaked from the drainage site for 24 hours, the drain may be removed. Routine antibiotics are not necessary, but once the catheter has been removed, the urine should be cultured and appropriate antibiotics given to the patient. If the urine is infected at the time of the injury, antibiotics should be administered preoperatively and continued for at least a week.

In the patient with an extraperitoneal injury treated with Foley catheter drainage alone, cystography is performed on the tenth postoperative day. In our experience more than 85% of the bladders are healed by that time and the catheter may be removed. Virtually all injuries treated in this fashion are healed with less than 3 weeks of catheter drainage. In the rare male patient who has persistent extravasation, a percutaneous suprapubic tube may be placed in the bladder to prevent urethral complications from prolonged intubation.

Complications

The most serious complications of bladder rupture follow delays in diagnosis. When urine leaks into the peritoneal cavity, the electrolytes equilibrate with serum. Therefore peritoneal fluid analysis for creatinine and urea is not helpful in differential diagnosis. If uroascites becomes marked, respiratory difficulty develops, especially in infants.[59] Emergency paracentesis in these patients may be lifesaving.

Sepsis from infected intraperitoneal urine is a major threat to the patient. If the intraperitoneal rupture is not recognized, generalized peritonitis or loculated abscesses may develop. The laceration must then be closed, the urine diverted, all purulent collections surgically drained, and appropriate antibiotic therapy instituted.

The mortality rate of patients with bladder ruptures is approximately 12%.[55,57] The cause of death is usually associated visceral or vascular injuries. Patients should never die from a bladder wound that has been properly diagnosed and treated.

Injuries to the bladder neck, urethra, and vagina may result in incontinence or fistula or stricture formation if not promptly and properly repaired. In patients with delayed diagnosis, definitive reconstruction may have to be delayed for months to allow edema, infection, and induration to resolve. A neuropathic bladder may accompany severe pelvic fractures, and voiding may become impossible. Intermittent self-catheterization then becomes necessary.

URETHRAL INJURIES

The urethra in a man can be divided anatomically into (1) the prostatic urethra, (2) the membranous urethra, (3) the bulbous urethra, and (4) the penile, or pendulous urethra. For the purpose of determining appropriate therapy, injuries to the uretha in male patients can be divided into posterior urethral injuries (those of the prostatic and membranous urethra, above and including the urogenital diaphragm) and anterior urethral injuries (those of the bulbous and penile, or pendulous, urethra below the urogenital diaphragm).[69]

In women the urethra is short and rarely injured.[70] When damage occurs, it is usually accompanied by a severe bony pelvic disruption with concomitant injury to the bladder neck and vagina. Female urethral injuries are more common in children than adults.[64,71-74]

Etiology

Posterior urethral injuries. Almost all injuries of the posterior urethra in males occur in conjunction with fracture of the bony pelvis.[75,76] Ninety percent of these injuries are due to motor vehicle accidents involving automobiles, motorcycles, or pedestrians. Falls from a height, industrial crushing injuries, and sporting accidents cause the other 10% of pelvic fractures. Urethral injury is caused by shearing forces of the bony disruption. The prostate gland, attached by the puboprostatic ligaments, is pulled in one direction while the membranous urethra, attached to the urogenital diaphragm, is pulled in another.

Penetrating wounds of the posterior urethra from external violence are uncommon but occur occasionally.

Anterior urethral injuries. Most injuries of the anterior urethra are due to blunt trauma to the perineum.[77-79] The bulbous urethra is crushed against the pelvic arch as the patient falls astride an object. Common causative events include falling from a height, straddling a fence, having a foot slip from the rung of a ladder, being kicked in the perineum, or hitting a bump in the road while riding a bicycle and coming down hard on the seat or the crossbar.

Diagnosis

Signs and symptoms. Urethral injuries should be suspected in male patients with a history of trauma to the perineum or in patients who have a fracture of the bony pelvis. The patient may be unable to void or may relate a sensation of voiding with no urine coming out of the urethra. The majority of patients with a ruptured urethra have blood at the urethral meatus and ecchymosis of the penis, scrotum, or perineum. Rectal examination may reveal the prostate gland to be in a higher position than usual. This "high-riding prostate" is caused by disruption of the urethra with elevation of the prostate gland from its normal position by a large associated pelvic hematoma. The soft, boggy hematoma is felt where the prostate gland is normally found. Patients who are able to urinate have gross or microscopic hematuria.

Radiographic examination. Any patient with a suspected urethral injury according to the preceding criteria must undergo retrograde urethrography.[66,80,81] Under no circumstances should an attempt be made to catheterize the urethra until the urethrogram delineates the anatomy and injury. Injudicious catheterization of the injured urethra risks converting a partial urethral laceration into a complete urethral disruption. There is also the risk of infecting a sterile periurethral or pelvic hematoma.

Sometimes, desperately ill patients who may have urethral injuries are taken to the operating room for abdominal exploration before radiographic examination. These patients should not be studied intraoperatively; instead a suprapubic tube should be inserted into the dome of the bladder so that the lower tract can be studied in the postoperative period. If the tube is not needed, it is easily removed.

Classification and Therapy

The classification of posterior urethral injuries is based on urethrographic appearances of the injury. Three patterns of posterior urethral injuries are described:

- Type I: The posterior urethra is stretched because of rupture of the puboprostatic ligaments. A hematoma collects in the pelvis, resulting in dislocation of the bladder base from the pelvis. Although stretched, the posterior urethra is intact.
- Type II: The urethra is disrupted at the membranoprostatic junction above the urogenital diaphragm. Urethrography reveals extravasation of contrast medium into the pelvic extraperitoneal space above an intact urogenital diaphragm.
- Type III: The membranous urethra is disrupted, and the injury extends into the proximal bulbous urethra or the urogenital diaphragm itself is disrupted, or both. Urethrography demonstrates contrast extravasation both above and below the urogenital diaphragm.

Prepubertal children sustaining blunt pelvic trauma associated with posterior urethral disruption have several distinct anatomic sites of injury that are not seen in adults and postpubertal patients. These include complete avulsion of the bladder neck from the prostate gland and transprostatic urethral lacerations. These injuries are classified as type II. Boone and associates retrospectively reviewed their pediatric experience with prepubertal posterior urethral disruptions. They found that 17% (4/24) of patients with posterior disruptions sustained prostatovesicle avulsion, 17% had transprostatic laceration, and 66% (16/24) experienced disruption of the prostatomembranous urethra.

Management

Type I posterior urethral injury. The patient with a large pelvic hematoma compressing the urethra may have difficulty voiding. This injury is treated with bladder catheter drainage. Once the child has recovered sufficiently that urine output monitoring is no longer necessary, the catheter is removed. Patients with a severe pelvic disruption, especially those with a sacral injury, may be unable to urinate because of a neurologic defect. If multiple trials of voiding fail, the patient should be taught clean, intermittent self-catheterization while awaiting return of detrusor function.

Partial posterior urethral rupture, types II and III. The patient with a minimal partial urethral rupture may be treated with urethral catheter drainage for 14 to 21 days but is best managed by placement of a suprapubic cystostomy. A follow-up voiding cystourethrogram is used to document healing of the injury.[83] If the urethral injury is extensive, catheterization should not be attempted because it might convert a partial rupture to a complete disruption. The patient should undergo suprapubic cystotomy, and cystography must also be performed to rule out a concomitant bladder rupture.

The most conservative way to manage partial urethral disruptions is to place a suprapubic cystotomy and not attempt urethral instrumentation. A voiding cystourethrogram via the cystotomy tube is obtained 14 to 21 days after the injury. If extravasation is no longer present and the urethra is of normal caliber, or if only a minimal stricture is present at the site of the injury, the suprapubic tube may be removed and the patient allowed to void.[81] If a significant stricture is present, an immediate visual internal urethrotomy should be performed. If urethral occlusion is present and the stricture is long, suprapubic drainage should be continued for 4 to 6 months and delayed open repair performed.

Complete posterior urethral rupture, types II and III. There are two management options in patients with a complete rupture of the posterior urethra: (1) immediate surgical realignment or (2) suprapubic cystotomy and delayed surgical repair.

Immediate surgical realignment is the procedure of choice for a stable patient who is undergoing pelvic exploration for a concomitant vascular or rectal injury. If a major bladder neck laceration or prostatic fragmentation is present, immediate repair is mandatory.[84–89] Intraoperatively, a catheter is passed into the urethral meatus and advanced through the urogenital diaphragm into the prevesical space. The bladder is opened, and another catheter is passed through the bladder neck into the prostatic urethra and then into the perivesical space. The catheters are then tied together, the bladder catheter is used to guide the urethral catheter into the bladder, and the catheter is fixed to the abdominal wall. The prostate gland and bladder may then be easily repositioned without tension against the urogenital diaphragm. A suprapubic tube is placed into the bladder, and a drain is placed in the perivesical space. Vest sutures from the prostate gland to the perineum help to stabilize the repair, but can be placed only in a postpubertal child with a well-developed prostate gland.

Delayed surgical repair is the procedure of choice if the patient is medically unstable or if the surgeon is unskilled in performing major urethral reconstructive surgery.[1,89–94]

Anterior urethral contusions. Anterior urethral contusions are seen in straddle injuries. The urethrogram shows no abnormality, but there is hematuria at the beginning or end of voiding. The patient is usually able to void normally, and the hematuria promptly clears. No special therapy is necessary for patients with this injury.

Partial anterior urethral rupture. If anterior urethral extravasation on the urethrogram is minimal or contained by Buck's fascia, and urethral continuity is good, the patient has suffered a partial urethral disruption. There are two management options in these patients: allowing the patient to void or placing a urethral catheter into the bladder for a few days. If the injury is extensive or extends outside Buck's fascia, a suprapubic tube should be placed into the bladder and a voiding cystourethrogram obtained in 10 to 14 days.

Periodic measurement of urinary flow rates and urethrography are important follow-up measures in patients with partial anterior urethral ruptures to identify strictures resulting from healing. Therapy should be the same as for partial posterior urethral ruptures.

Complete anterior urethral rupture. Complete urethral disruption is evidenced on urethrogram by extensive extravasation or loss of urethral continuity or both. This condition is managed with a suprapubic cystostomy. When the skin of the genitalia and perineum is intact and at least 14 days has elapsed since the injury, a voiding cystourethrogram and retrograde urethrogram are obtained to delineate the extent of residual injury. A stricture of some magnitude will probably have developed. If urethral continuity has been maintained, panendoscopy and visual urethrotomy may be all that are required to incise and open the stricture.[95,96] In most patients complete occlusion of the urethra by a very short stricture will have developed. In these patients suprapubic drainage is continued for 4 to 6 months to allow complete healing before definitive reconstruction is attempted.[97–100]

Penetrating anterior urethral injury. Penetrating injury of the anterior urethra requires prompt attention. Clean knife wounds should undergo minimal debridement, closure of the defect with absorbable sutures, and suprapubic catheter drainage for 2 to 3 weeks.

Dirty wounds with extensive tissue destruction and foreign material in the wound (e.g., metal pellets, oil, grease, hair, clothing) are thoroughly cleansed with antiseptic solutions and copious irrigation. Debridement of devitalized tissue is important, but contused corpus spongiosum tissue is hemorrhagic and ecchymotic and may appear necrotic when it is only badly bruised. If debridement is vigorous, more urethra than is necessary may be removed and discarded, making eventual repair a formidable task.

Suprapubic diversion is instituted until the perineum has healed. This may take weeks to months. Radiographic studies demonstrate the extent of residual strictures, which may be managed by formal urethroplasty.

Postoperative Care and Complications

The progress of urethral injury is followed up by measurement of voiding flow rates at 3-month intervals for at least a year. A significant decrease of flow suggests development of a stricture, the extent of which is further evaluated by a retrograde urethrogram.

Patients with neurologic bladder injury may not be able to void and may have to be taught intermittent self-catheterization. Patients with bladder neck damage or denervation may require alpha-adrenergic medications to become continent.

Patients treated with primary realignment have a much higher long-term complication rate than do patients treated with delayed operative repair, despite the technique employed. The stricture recurrence rate with primary repair is approximately 70% (range 30% to 100%), the impotence rate is 44% (range 20% to 50%), and the incontinence rate is 20% (range 2% to 44%).[56] Boone's report included the incidence of various complications resulting from traumatic posterior urethral disruptions in prepubertal patients followed into the post-pubertal period.[101] He found that the frequency of impotence, intractable strictures, and incontinence was significantly higher in patients who sustained injuries proximal to the prostatomembranous region (impotence 75% versus 31%, strictures 75% versus 12%, urinary incontinence 25% versus none). In all patients in the reported series with injuries proximal to the prostatomembranous junction, the urethra was repaired by primary realignment.

With the delayed procedures it is the rare patient who has a long-term stricture problem, the impotence rate is only 11% (range none to 56%), and the incontinence rate is 2% (range none to 5%).[102]

GENITAL INJURIES

Injuries to the scrotum and its contents are not uncommon. Testicular injuries and scrotal skin injuries are discussed in the following sections.

Testis Injury

Injury to the testicle may occur when the child forcibly straddles an object. The testis is forced against the pubic ramus, tearing the investing tunica albuginea.[103] Injuries of this type are relatively rare in infants and young boys because the testicles are small and hypermotile.[104] Traumatic testicular injuries are usually sustained by adolescents who are hit in the scrotum during sporting events or are kicked during fights. Rarely these injuries are associated with motor vehicle accidents.

The patient with a testicular injury has a swollen, ecchymotic, tender scrotum. Examining the testis is often difficult because of pain and hematocele or hematoma formation. Sonography is the diagnostic evaluation of choice.[105,106] The contralateral testis is evaluated for comparison with the injured testis.

The best long-term results are achieved when the patient undergoes early scrotal exploration. The hematoma or hematocele is decompressed, extruded necrotic seminiferous tubules are excised, and the laceration of the tunica albuginea is closed with absorbable suture. Broad-spectrum antibiotic coverage is also employed.

Scrotal Skin Injuries

Scrotal skin laceration, with or without testicular extrusion, is relatively uncommon in pediatric patients. Significant skin loss is usually related to machinery accidents. Burns, zipper injuries, and animal bites have all been reported as etiologic factors in children.

Treatment of scrotal skin injuries depends on the severity of injury and the degree of contamination. Clean, simple lacerations are treated with primary closure. Even in patients with significant skin loss, testicular coverage can usually be attained because of the elastic nature of the scrotal skin. When the patient has suffered major avulsion of the scrotum, the testes should be left in place and treated with daily applications of warm saline solution after minimal debridement. When granulation tissue covers the testes, either the regenerated scrotum can be used for closure or split-thickness skin grafting may be undertaken.

Penile Injuries

Circumcision and associated complications are the most common cause of pediatric penile injuries. Zipper injuries are also common, especially in uncircumcised boys. These injuries occur when the child zips up his pants quickly after voiding, entrapping the redundant prepuce.[107] The entrapped skin may be released by using bone-cutting instruments to cut the small bridge or "diamond" of the sliding portion of the zipper. This may be accomplished in the emergency room without anesthesia.

Occasionally, infants have a tourniquet injury from bands, rings, or even human hair. A fine hair, concealed within the diaper, lodges in the coronal groove, cutting into the shaft of the penis. The degree of laceration may eventually cause urethral or corporal damage. The initial diagnosis in these infants is often balanitis, cellulitis, or paraphimosis.[108]

Degloving injuries of the penis are unusual in children. These occur when the penis and clothing are caught in roller-type machinery (e.g., garden or farming tools). Degloving injuries are repaired by skin debridement with excision of all the distal skin to the level of the coronal sulcus. The defect is then covered with a split-thickness skin graft, placed proximally to the level of intact body skin. A thickness of approximately 0.15 mm is important to allow for normal expansion of the healed penis during erection.[109]

Corpus cavernosum injuries, exceedingly rare in children, should be surgically repaired. The hematoma is evacuated, and hemostasis and closure of the tunica albuginea are achieved with absorbable suture.[108] This aggressive treatment approach decreases the incidence of corporal fibrosis and subsequent curvature of the penis.

Penile amputations are repaired microsurgically if feasible. Total penile loss as a complication of circumcision necessitates sex reassignment.

Any genital injury in a young child should raise the suspicion of child abuse.

REFERENCES

1. Allen TD: The transpubic approach for strictures of membranous urethra, *J Urol* 114:63, 1975.
2. Cass AS, Ireland GW: Comparison of the conservative and surgical management of the severe degrees of renal trauma in multiple injured patients, *J Urol* 109:8, 1973.
3. Evins SC, Thomason WB, Rosenblum R: Nonoperative management of severe renal lacerations, *J Urol* 123:24, 1980.
4. Mogensen P, Agger P, Ostergaard AH: A conservative approach to the management of blunt renal trauma, *Br J Urol* 52:338, 1980.
5. Wein AJ, Arger PH, Murphy JJ: Controversial aspects of blunt renal trauma, *J Trauma* 17:662, 1977.
6. Corriere JN Jr, McAndrew JD, Benson GS: Intraoperative decision-making in renal trauma surgery, *J Trauma* 31(10):1390–1392, 1991.
7. Young LW, Wood BP, Linke CA: Renal injury from blunt trauma in childhood, *Ann Radiol* 18:359–376, 1975.
8. Bright TC, White K, Peters PC: Significance of hematuria after trauma, *J Urol* 120:455, 1978.
9. McAninch JW: Acute renal artery thrombosis from blunt trauma, *Urology* 6:6, 1975.
10. Stables DP, Fouche RF, de Villiers von Niekirk JP, et al: Traumatic renal artery occlusion: 21 cases, *J Urol* 115:229, 1976.
11. Griffen WO Jr, Belin RP, Ernst CB, et al: Intravenous pyelogram in abdominal trauma, *J Trauma* 18:387, 1978.
12. McDonald EF, et al: The role of emergency urography in evaluation of blunt abdominal trauma, *Am J Radiol* 126:739, 1976.
13. Taddei L, Dalla Palma F, Della Selva A Jr: The role of urography in blunt trauma of the kidney, *Diagn Imag* 48:305, 1979.
14. Lang EK: Arteriography in the assessment of renal trauma, *J Trauma* 15:553, 1975.
15. Stables DP: Unilateral absence of excretion at urography after abdominal trauma, *Radiology* 121:609, 1976.
16. McAninch JW, Federle MP: Evaluation of renal injuries with computed tomography, *J Urol* 128:456, 1982.
17. Sandler CM, Toombs BD: Computed tomographic evaluation of blunt renal injuries, *Radiology* 141:461, 1981.
18. Peters PC, Bright TC: Blunt renal injuries, *Urol Clin North Am* 4:17, 1977.

19. Wein AJ, Murphy JJ, Mulholland SG, et al: A conservative approach to management of blunt renal trauma, *J Urol* 117:425, 1977.

20. Schoenberg HW, Gregory JG: Delayed flank approach to isolated renal trauma in children, *J Pediatr Surg* 10:525–530, 1975.

21. Scott R Jr, Carlton CE, Ashmore AJ, et al: Initial management of non-penetrating injuries: clinical review of 111 cases, *J Urol* 90:535, 1963.

22. Guttman FM, Homsy Y, Schmidt E: Avulsion injury to the renal pedicle: successful autotransplantation after "bench surgery," *J Trauma* 18(6):469, 1978.

23. Kassow AS: Hypertension complicating blunt trauma, *Urology* 16:84, 1980.

24. Spark RF, Berg S: Renal trauma and hypertension, *Arch Intern Med* 136:1097, 1976.

25. Easlam JA, Wilson TG, Larsen DW, Ahlering TE: Angiographic embolization of renal stab wounds, *J Urol* 148(2):268–270, 1992.

26. Bright TC III, Peters PC: Ureteral injuries due to external violence: 10 years' experience with 59 cases, *J Trauma* 17:616, 1977.

27. Corriere JN Jr: Ureteral injuries. In Gillenwater JY, Grayhack JT, Howards SS, Duckett JW, eds: *Adult and pediatric urology,* vol 1, Chicago, 1987, Year Book, pp 436–443.

28. Eickenberg H, Amin M: Gunshot wounds to the ureter, *J Trauma* 16:562, 1976.

29. Fischer S, Young DA, Malin JM Jr, et al: Ureteral gunshot wounds, *J Urol* 108:238, 1972.

30. Holden S, Hicks CC, O'Brien DP III, et al: Gunshot wounds of the ureter: a 15 year review of 63 consecutive cases, *J Urol* 116:562, 1976.

31. Liroff SA, Pontes JES, Pierce JM Sr: Gunshot wounds of the ureter: 5 years of experience, *J Urol* 118:551, 1977.

32. Pitts JC III, Peterson NE: Penetrating injuries of the ureter, *J Trauma* 21:978, 1981.

33. Rusche F: Injury of the ureter due to gunshot wounds, *J Urol* 60:63, 1948.

34. Steers WD, Corriere JN Jr, Benson GS, et al: The use of indwelling stents in managing ureteral injuries due to external violence, *J Trauma* 25:1001, 1985.

35. Stone HH, Jones JH: Penetrating and nonpenetrating injuries to the ureter, *Surg Gynecol Obstet* 114:52, 1962.

36. Walker JH: Injuries of the ureter due to external violence, *J Urol* 102:410, 1969.

37. Walling E, DeSy W, Fonteyne E: Blunt ureteral trauma with peritoneal fistulization: review of the literature, *J Urol* 114:942, 1975.

38. Ambiavager R, Nambiar R: Traumatic closed avulsion of the upper ureter, *Injury* 11:71, 1979.

39. LaBerge I, Homsy YL, Dadour G, et al: Avulsion of ureter by blunt trauma, *Urology* 13:172, 1979.

40. Palmer JM, Drago JR: Ureteral avulsion from non-penetrating trauma, *J Urol* 125:108, 1981.

41. Liune PM, Gonzalez ET: Genitourinary trauma in children, *Urol Clin North Am* 12(1):53–65, 1985.

42. Cass AS: Ureteral contusion and delayed necrosis from gunshot injury, *Urology* 12:195, 1978.

43. Christenson PJ, O'Connell KJ, Clark M, et al: Ballistic ureteral trauma: a comparison of high and low velocity weapons, *Contemp Surg* 23:45, 1983.

44. Rohner TJ Jr: Delayed ureteral fistula from high velocity missiles: report of 3 cases, *J Urol* 105:63, 1971.

45. Stutzman RE: Ballistics and the management of ureteral injuries from high velocity missiles, *J Urol* 118:947, 1977.

46. Carlton CE Jr, Scott R Jr, Guthrie AG: The initial management of ureteral injuries: a report of 78 cases, *J Urol* 105:335, 1971.

47. Weaver RG: The effect of large caliber splints on ureteral healing, *Surg Gynecol Obstet* 103:590, 1956.

48. Hock WH, Kursh ED, Persky L: Early aggressive management of intraoperative ureteral injuries, *J Urol* 114:530, 1975.

49. Mendez R, McGinty DM: The management of delayed recognized ureteral injuries, *J Urol* 119:192, 1978.

50. Dowling RA, Corriere JN Jr, Sandler CM: Iatrogenic ureteral injury, *J Urol* 135:912, 1986.

51. Hursman MW, Pollack HM, Banner MP, et al: Conservative management of ureteral obstruction secondary to suture entrapment, *J Urol* 127:121, 1982.

52. Lang EK, LaNasa JA, Garrett J, et al: The management of urinary fistulas and strictures with percutaneous ureteral stent catheters, *J Urol* 122:736, 1979.

53. Kaplan JO, Winslow OP Jr, Sneider SE, et al: Dilatation of a surgically ligated ureter through a percutaneous nephrostomy, *Am J Radiol* 139:188, 1982.

54. Underwood PB Jr, Lutz MH, Smoak DL: Ureteral injury following therapy for carcinoma of the cervix, *Obstet Gynecol* 49:663, 1977.

55. Carroll PR, McAninch JW: Major bladder trauma: mechanisms of injury and a unified method of diagnosis and repair, *J Urol* 132:254, 1984.

56. Corriere JN Jr: Trauma to the lower urinary tract. In Gillenwater JY, Grayhack JT, Howards SS, Duckett JW, eds: *Adult and pediatric urology,* vol 1, Chicago, 1987, Year Book, pp 444–466.

57. Corriere JN Jr, Sandler CM: Management of the ruptured bladder: 7 years of experience with 111 cases, *J Trauma* 26:830, 1986.

58. Johnson PA: Rectal impalement with perforation of the bladder, *Br Med J* 2:748, 1971.

59. Dmochowski RR, Crandell SS, Corriere JN Jr: Bladder injury and uroascites from umbilical artery catheterization, *Pediatrics* 77:421, 1986.

60. Culp OS: Treatment of ruptured bladder and urethra: analysis of 86 cases of urinary extravasation, *J Urol* 48:266, 1942.

61. Hayes EE, Sandler CM, Corriere JN Jr: Management of the ruptured bladder secondary to blunt abdominal trauma, *J Urol* 129:946, 1983.

62. Carroll PR, McAninch JW: Major bladder trauma: the accuracy of cystography, *J Urol* 130:887, 1983.

63. Sandler CM, Harris JD, Corriere JN Jr, et al: Posterior urethral injuries after pelvic fracture, *Am J Radiol* 137:1233, 1981.

64. Parkhurst JD, Coker JE, Halverstadt DB: Traumatic avulsion of the lower urinary tract in the female child, *J Urol* 126:265, 1981.

65. Richardson JR Jr, Leadbetter GW Jr: Nonoperative treatment of the ruptured bladder, *J Urol* 114:213, 1975.

66. Sandler CM, Phillips JM, Harris JD, et al: Radiology of the bladder and urethra in blunt pelvic trauma, *Radiol Clin North Am* 19:195, 1981.

67. Brosman SA, Paul JF: Trauma of the bladder, *Surg Gynecol Obstet* 143:605, 1976.

68. Mulkey AP Jr, Witherington R: Conservative management of vesical rupture, *Urology* 4:426, 1974.

69. Aubert J, Court B: Traumatic ruptures of the urethra in children, *Eur Urol* 1:122, 1975.

70. Buxton RA: Rupture of the urethra in a female child with a fractured pelvis: a case report, *Injury* 9:209, 1978.

71. Garrett RA: Pediatric urethral and perineal injuries, *Pediatr Clin North Am* 22:401, 1975.

72. Merchant WC, Gibbons MD, Gonzales ET: Trauma to the bladder neck, trigone and vagina in children, *J Urol* 131:747, 1984.

73. Persky L: Childhood urethral trauma, *Urology* 9:603, 1978.

74. Williams DI: Rupture of the female urethra in childhood, *Eur Urol* 1:129, 1975.

75. Devine PC, Devine CJ Jr: Posterior urethral injuries associated with pelvic fractures, *Urology* 20:467, 1982.

76. Palmer JK, Benson GS, Corriere JN Jr: Diagnosis and initial management of urological injuries associated with 200 consecutive pelvic fractures, *J Urol* 130:712, 1983.

77. Blumberg N: Anterior urethral injuries, *J Urol* 102:210, 1969.

78. Kiracofe HL, Pfister RR, Peterson NE: Management of non-penetrating distal urethral trauma, *J Urol* 114:57, 1975.

79. Macleod DAD: Anterior urethral injuries, *Injury* 8:25, 1976.

80. Corriere JN Jr, Harris JD: The management of urologic injuries in blunt pelvic trauma, *Radiol Clin North Am* 19:187, 1981.

81. Haller JC, Kassner EG, Waterhouse K, et al: Traumatic strictures of the prostatomembranous urethra in children: radiologic evaluation before and after urethral reconstruction, *Urol Radiol* 1:43, 1979.

82. Glassberg KI, Talete-Velcek F, Ashley R, et al: Partial tears of prostatomembranous urethra in children, *Urology* 13:500, 1979.

83. DeWeerd JH: Immediate realignment of posterior urethral injury, *Urol Clin North Am* 4:75, 1977.

84. Malek RS, O'Dea MJ, Kelalis PO: Management of ruptured posterior urethra in childhood, *J Urol* 117:105, 1977.

85. Myers RP, DeWeerd JH: Incidence of stricture following primary realignment of the disrupted proximal urethra, *J Urol* 107:265, 1972.

86. Patterson DE, Barrett DM, Myers RD, et al: Primary realignment of posterior urethral injuries, *J Urol* 129:513, 1983.

87. Turner-Warwick R: A personal view of the management of traumatic posterior urethral strictures, *Urol Clin North Am* 4:111, 1977.

88. Webster GD, Mathes GL, Selli C: Prostatomembranous urethral injuries: a review of the literature and a rational approach to their management, *J Urol* 130:898, 1983.

89. Badenoch AW: A pull-through operation for impassable traumatic stricture of the urethra, *Br J Urol* 22:404, 1950.

90. Brock WA, Kaplan GW: Use of the transpubic approach for urethroplasty in children, *J Urol* 125:496, 1981.

91. Kramer SA, Furlow WL, Barrett DM, et al: Transpubic urethroplasty in children, *J Urol* 126:767, 1981.

92. Malloy TR, Wein AJ, Carpiniello VL: Transpubic urethroplasty for prostatomembranous urethral disruption, *J Urol* 124:359, 1980.

93. Waterhouse K: The surgical repair of membranous urethral strictures in children, *J Urol* 116:363, 1976.

94. Waterhouse K, Laungani G, Patel U: The surgical repair of membranous urethral strictures: experience with 105 consecutive cases, *J Urol* 123:500, 1980.

95. Katz AS, Waterhouse K: Treatment of urethral strictures in men by internal urethrotomy: a study of 61 patients, *J Urol* 105:807, 1971.

96. Waterhouse K, Selli C: Technique of optical internal urethrotomy, *Urology* 11:407, 1978.
97. Blandy J, Singh M, Tresidder GC: Urethroplasty by scrotal flap for large urethral strictures, *Br J Urol* 40:261, 1960.
98. Devine PC, Fallon B, Devine CJ Jr: Free full thickness skin graft urethroplasty, *J Urol* 116:144, 1976.
99. Gibbons MD, Koontz WW Jr, Smith MJV: Urethral strictures in boys, *J Urol* 121:217, 1979.
100. Leadbetter GW Jr, Leadbetter WF: Urethral strictures in male children, *J Urol* 87:409, 1962.
101. Boone TB, Wilson WT, Husmann DA: Postpubertal genitourinary function following posterior urethral disruptions in children, *J Urol* 148:1232–1234, 1992.
102. Gibson GR: Impotence following fractured pelvis and ruptured urethra, *Br J Urol* 42:86, 1970.
103. Zivrovic SM, Janjir G: Traumatic rupture of the testis and epididymis, *J Pediatr Surg* 15:287, 1980.
104. Nagerajan VP, Pranikoff R, Imabori SC, et al: Traumatic dislocation of the testis, *Urology* 22:521, 1983.
105. Anderson KA, McAninch JW, Jeffrey RB, et al: Ultrasonography for the diagnosis and staging of blunt scrotal trauma, *J Urol* 130:933, 1983.
106. Finkelstein MS, Rosenberg HK, Snyder HM, Duckett JW: Ultrasound evaluation of the scrotum in pediatrics, *Urology* 27(1):1–9, 1986.
107. Kaplan GW: Complications of circumcision, *Urol Clin North Am* 10:43, 1983.
108. Livne PM, Gonzales ET: Genitourinary trauma in children, *Urol Clin North Am* 12(1):62, 1992.
109. Peters PC, Sagalowsky AI: Genitourinary trauma. In Walsh PC, Retik AB, Stamey TA, Vaughan ED Jr, eds: *Campbell's urology,* Philadelphia, 1992, WB Saunders, p 2591.

C H A P T E R

9

Thoracic Injury in Children

Douglas E. Paull

Nearly half of childhood deaths in the United States are a result of accidents.[1,2] Chest injuries are present in 7.9% to 58% of pediatric trauma admissions.[3–6] The mere presence of a thoracic injury is a marker for an increased mortality in the range of 7% to 26%.[2–8] Chest injuries directly affect the perfusion and tissue oxygenation in the critically injured child and therefore must be diagnosed and rectified early in the child's care. Educating parents and children about accident prevention may be the best policy to save lives, since nearly half of children who die of chest trauma never reach the hospital alive.[2–4,9]

Chest trauma in children is strikingly different from that in adults. Blunt injuries account for 41% to 97% of thoracic trauma in children.[7,10,11] Gunshot and stab wounds are much less frequent than in adults, but these differences become less pronounced in adolescents and in urban areas.[9,11] Whereas the majority of blunt chest injuries in adults are the result of motor vehicle accidents in which the victim is a driver or passenger, children are more commonly injured as pedestrians struck by moving vehicles.[2–4,11] The mechanism of chest injury varies with the specific age group of the child and includes motor vehicle–pedestrian accidents, motor vehicle accidents, bicycle accidents, falls, penetrating trauma, and child abuse (Fig. 9–1).[3,7] The younger the victim with a chest injury, the greater the likelihood of mortality (Fig. 9–2). Males are more likely to be victims in childhood accidents by a ratio of 2.8:1, a predominance further exaggerated for penetrating injuries with a ratio of 5:1.[1,7] Children less than 5 years of age with a chest injury may have a mortality rate of 25%.[5,6] When child abuse is the cause of thoracic injury, the overall mortality rate may increase to 50%.[1,4]

Approximately 61% of children with chest injuries have multiple associated injuries, and the overall Injury Severity Score is higher among children with chest injuries.[1,4,7,12] Associated injuries are usually impressive, and their need for immediate attention may distract the health care team and delay the diagnosis of a potentially life-threatening chest injury. Head injuries and bleeding from

246

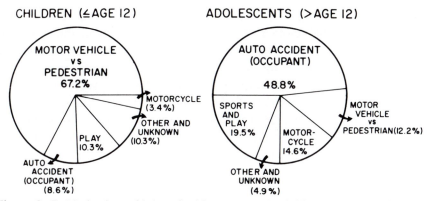

Figure 9–1. Mechanism of injury for blunt trauma in children. (From Sinclair MC, Moore FC: *J Pediatr Surg* 9:156, 1974.)

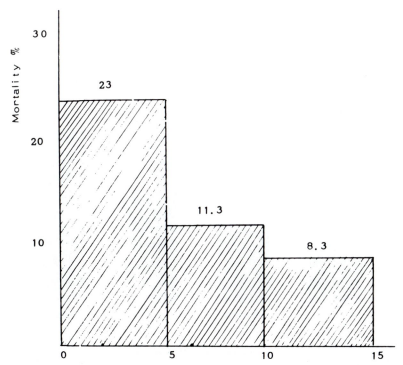

Figure 9–2. Age versus mortality in pediatric trauma. (From Smyth BT: *J Pediatr Surg* 25:964, 1990.)

associated injuries account for the majority of deaths in these children.[4,7,12] The mortality rate among children with chest injuries and two additional system injuries may be as high as 58% (Fig. 9–3).[2,3] The frequency of concomitant injuries further underscores the necessity for thorough, sequential evaluation of the chest-injured child by a well-trained team.[13,14] Strict adherence to the ABCs of trauma care helps to avoid confusion and missed injuries when the trauma team is confronted by an impressive array of injuries in a small child. A thorough knowledge of the types of chest injury and a high index of suspicion are prerequisites for the team leader caring for the injured child.

Anatomic and physiologic differences between children and adults lead to differences in the frequency of specific types of chest injury. For example, children's ribs are less mineralized and more flexible, and they transmit significantly more energy to the intrathoracic organs on impact. Pulmonary contusion is twice as common in children as in adults, accounting for 48% to 61% of chest injuries.[3,4,7] For similar reasons the presence or absence of a rib fracture may not always be a reliable guide to significant underlying intrathoracic injury in children. Only 52% of major intrathoracic injuries are accompanied by a rib fracture.[7]

The majority of blunt thoracic injuries in children are effectively managed nonoperatively, with only 3.8% to 15% requiring thoracotomy.[4,7,10] This further

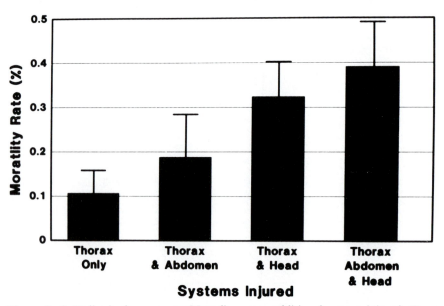

Figure 9–3. Pediatric chest trauma. Mortality versus additional systems injured. (From Peclet MH, Newman KD, Eichelberger MR, et al: *J Pediatr Surg* 25:964, 1990.)

Table 9–1. Thoracic Injuries in Children

Injury	No./7.5 Years
Immediately Life Threatening	
Airway obstruction	15*
Tension pneumothorax	9
Open pneumothorax	0
Massive hemothorax	14
Flail chest	1
Cardiac tamponade	2
TOTAL	41
Potentially Life Threatening	
Pulmonary contusion	56
Myocardial contusion	3
Aortic transection	1
Diaphragmatic hernia	2
Esophageal disruption	0
TOTAL	62

From Nakayama DK, Romauopsky ML, Rowe MI: *Surg Clin North Am* 61:1187, 1989.
*During 1987, 2 of 605 patients admitted to the trauma service had airway obstruction.

emphasizes the importance of a well-trained trauma team initially caring for the child with a chest injury, since many life-threatening injuries are readily treated with simple procedures, such as tube thoracostomy, in the emergency department. Again, these relatively simple treatments are predicated on recognition of the injury.

Thoracic injuries in children have been divided into those that are immediately life threatening, which are diagnosed and treated during the primary survey, and serious injuries that are potentially life threatening, which are diagnosed in the secondary survey (Table 9–1). In this chapter each specific injury is discussed in detail.

IMMEDIATELY LIFE-THREATENING INJURIES
Pneumothorax

Establishment of an effective airway should be the first priority in treating the child with chest injury.[6] The unique anatomic aspects of the pediatric airway are discussed in Chapter 1. Once an airway is ensured, decreased breath sounds in a child with evidence of ventilatory and circulatory compromise should suggest the diagnosis of a tension pneumothorax. In this situation the lung injury has a ball-valve effect, in which air leaks from the damaged lung but is trapped in the pleural cavity. As intrapleural pressure rises above atmospheric pressure, the lung collapses, the mediastinum shifts away from the injury and compresses the contralateral lung, the inferior vena cava is kinked, impeding venous return to the heart, and circulatory collapse ensues. In addition to absent or diminished breath sounds, signs and symptoms of a tension pneumothorax include evidence of tracheal shift, hyperresonance to chest percussion, subcutaneous emphysema, cyanosis, and hypotension. Immediate treatment consists of placing a 14- to 18-gauge needle into the second intercostal space in the midclavicular line on the affected side. This decompresses the pleural space and converts the tension pneumothorax to a simple pneumothorax. Needle thoracentesis is then followed by tube thoracostomy in the fourth intercostal space in the midaxillary line. The chest tube is placed on continuous underwater suction at -20 cm H_2O (Fig. 9–4). The chest tube should remain in place until the air leak ceases, drainage is minimal, and the patient's clinical condition and chest x-ray studies stabilize, generally in several days. A high-volume air leak or failure to reexpand the lung suggests a diagnosis of tracheobronchial injury.

Pneumothorax is one of the more common blunt pediatric thoracic injuries, occurring in 37% of patients with chest injury. Pneumothorax is often, but not always, associated with rib fractures.[2,7] In a study of 45 pediatric patients with rib fractures, 15 (33%) had a pneumothorax.[3] Even in children with *isolated* chest trauma, associated pneumothorax may carry a mortality rate of up to 15%.[4]

The asymptomatic child with an incidental, small (less than 15%) pneumothorax may be carefully observed in the hospital with serial examinations and chest x-ray studies. In children who have respiratory symptoms, those with a large pneumothorax (greater than 15%), or those who require general anesthesia, such as for laparotomy, a prophylactic tube thoracostomy should be performed to prevent a tension pneumothorax.

Unfortunately, the clinical situation is often complex, with the pneumothorax coexisting with other thoracic injuries, such as pulmonary contusion or hemothorax, as well as nonthoracic injuries. The chest tube becomes only one aspect of overall care in these patients. Rib fractures are the common cause of pneumothorax, but the diagnostician must remember other potential causes of intrapleural air such as esophageal rupture or perforation or tracheobronchial injury.

In part because of the relatively fewer penetrating chest injuries in children, an open pneumothorax, or the "sucking chest wound," is extremely rare.[10] Treatment includes covering the chest wall defect with petroleum jelly–impregnated gauze dressing and inserting a chest tube. A particularly extensive wound may require operative debridement and reconstruction for closure.

Iatrogenic injuries have become an important source of chest trauma, especially pneumothorax.[5] In neonatal intensive care units, pneumothorax, usually

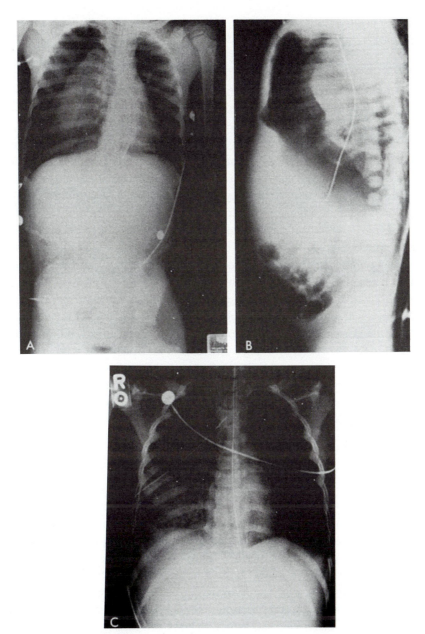

Figure 9–4. A and **B,** Chest radiographs demonstrating large right tension pneumo-thorax. There is contralateral mediastinal shift. **C,** Resolution of pneumothorax following chest tube insertion. (From Eichelberger MR, Randolph JG: *Surg Clin North Am* 61:1187, 1981.)

caused by positive end-expiratory pressure, develops in 30% of infants receiving mechanical ventilation. Treatment is similar to that described previously.

Hemothorax

Hemothorax occurs in 13.3% of childhood thoracic injuries and may be the result of blunt or penetrating trauma.[7] Bleeding is often from an intercostal artery that has been lacerated by a fractured rib, but bleeding may also be due to a pulmonary parenchymal injury or to a major vascular injury such as a transected aorta. Hemothorax is particularly detrimental to children, since a child's chest cavity can easily contain his or her entire blood volume. Because the total blood volume is a relatively greater percentage of total body weight in children than in adults, blood loss in a hemothorax can quickly lead to hypotension.[6] The combination of bleeding, hypoxic respiratory embarrassment, and compressed lung from pleural blood and clot makes hemothorax a life-threatening injury. In one study the mortality rate was as high as 57% in pediatric trauma associated with a significant hemothorax.[4] Symptoms include shock, flat neck veins, and diminished breath sounds. Chest x-ray examination shows opacification of the hemithorax. A chest tube should be inserted in the fifth intercostal space in the posterior axillary line. Although most intrathoracic bleeding does not require thoracotomy, bleeding in excess of 1 to 2 ml/kg/hr is an indication for immediate thoracotomy.[2] Failure to evacuate blood from the pleural cavity can lead to an infected hematoma-empyema or a trapped lung–fibrothorax.[5] These preventable complications may necessitate thoracotomy and decortication to reexpand the lung.

Cardiac Tamponade

Cardiac tamponade results from the accumulation of blood or air in the pericardial space. The pericardium is a relatively nonexpansile sac. Progressive pressure is placed on the heart as air or fluid accumulates between the pericardium and the heart. Diastolic filling of the ventricles becomes impaired, cardiac output falls, and shock ensues. The diagnosis of cardiac tamponade is suggested by the presence of hypotension and distended neck veins. Bleeding into the pericardium may follow a stab wound, gunshot wound, or blunt trauma of the heart. In infants, pneumopericardium may also develop from positive-pressure ventilation. When the clinical situation permits, the diagnosis can be confirmed by measurement of an elevated central venous pressure (greater than 15 cm H_2O) or by echocardiography. In a hemodynamically compromised patient, emergency pericardiocentesis is indicated. An 18-gauge needle and catheter attached to an electrocardiographic electrode is directed from a subxiphoid point of entry and aimed toward the left shoulder at a 45-degree angle to the frontal plane. Aspiration of nonclotting blood, without an electrocardiographic current of injury, may lead to rapid clinical improvement. A catheter with a stopcock may be left in place for repeated aspiration to facilitate safe transfer to the operating room. The patient should be taken immediately to the operating room for median sternotomy and repair of the cardiac injury.

A gunshot wound of the heart is generally fatal. A stab wound or blunt cardiac injury results in slower accumulation of blood within the pericardium and may allow survival until the patient arrives in the emergency room. Even then, pediatric injuries of the heart carry a mortality rate of about 75%. This high mortality rate is due both to the pump insult and to the high incidence of associated injuries.[4] The neonate with pneumopericardium and tamponade can be treated with pericardiocentesis and appropriate tube thoracostomy to decompress the pleural space.

The immediately life-threatening injuries (tension pneumothorax, massive hemothorax, and cardiac tamponade) may be diagnosed within minutes of the pateint's arrival in the emergency room and are readily treated. The airway is secured, and the chest is auscultated for adequacy of ventilation. Diminished or absent breath sounds in the presence of clinical instability necessitate needle thoracentesis and tube thoracostomy. Intravenous fluid resuscitation is initiated. Distended neck veins and shock necessitate emergency pericardiocentesis. These lifesaving procedures can be performed by emergency room and trauma team physicians within minutes, stabilizing the patient's condition and allowing transport to the operating room for definitive operation by more specialized members of the trauma team.

POTENTIALLY LIFE-THREATENING INJURIES
Foreign Body Aspiration

Foreign body aspiration (FBA) leads to the deaths of 500 to 3000 children a year in the United States.[15–17] FBA accounts for 7% of accidental deaths in children less than 4 years of age and is most prevalent from 6 months to 3 years of age.[15,16,18–20] Boys outnumber girls in nearly all studies, for unclear reasons.[15,20] A choking episode occurs in 90% of patients.[18,21] Other symptoms include cough, wheezing, hemoptysis, cyanosis, and cardiorespiratory arrest.[15,16,19,21] Symptoms depend on the location of the object in the tracheobronchial tree. A patient with a tracheal foreign body, rare at only 6% of FBA, demonstrates inspiratory and expiratory wheezing and sternal retractions.[21] Patients with the more common mainstem bronchial location, 67% of FBA, cough.[15] Unlike adults, in whom FBA is primarily via the right mainstem bronchus, FBA in children is equally divided between left and right sides because of a more symmetric carinal angle.[15,20]

A significant delay may occur in diagnosis of FBA. Twenty-one percent of patients have had symptoms for over 2 weeks by the time of diagnosis.[16] Failure to diagnose FBA in a timely fashion may result in chronic complications, including pneumonia, lung abscess, bronchiectasis, erosion of blood vessels, mediastinitis, and tracheoesophageal fistula. In one study the complication rate was 27% when FBA was diagnosed within 24 hours of ingestion, but 67% when diagnosis was delayed.[21] Viral bronchitis, croup, and asthma have similar symptoms and are more common diseases in this age group, making the diagnosis of FBA difficult unless a high index of suspicion is maintained.

Physical examination of the child suffering FBA usually shows unilateral decreased breath sounds and wheezing.[15,20] Chest x-ray studies demonstrate unilateral hyperexpansion, atelectasis, or an infiltrate in 81% of cases.[16] However, the chest x-ray findings may be normal in 58% of cases of laryngotracheal FBA.[21] Dynamic studies such as forced expiratory techniques and fluoroscopy demonstrate air trapping and mediastinal shift. The majority of foreign bodies are radiolucent.[19]

The key to early diagnosis and treatment of FBA is a high index of suspicion and early bronchoscopy. When a history of sudden choking is combined with suggestive findings on physical examination and radiologic studies, the child should undergo rigid bronchoscopy under general anesthesia in the operating room. Appropriate supportive equipment and measures include temperature monitor and heat lamps, blood pressure cuff, pulse oximetry, electrocardiographic monitoring, oxygenation, and intravenous access. A tracheostomy set should also be available.

A ventilating rigid bronchoscope with a 4 mm outside diameter is used for infants, and up to a 6.2 mm outside diameter is used for older children.[16,22] Zero- and 30-degree Hopkins rod telescopes allow excellent visualization of the foreign body in the tracheobronchial tree. A variety of forceps, both optical grasping forceps and forceps placed through the working channel of the bronchoscope, can be used to remove the foreign body. Occasionally an embolectomy balloon catheter is inflated distal to the foreign body and used to pull the object to the tip of the bronchoscope. The balloon, foreign body, and bronchoscope are then removed as a unit.[18] Foreign bodies in the laryngotrachea may be removed with McGill forceps. Exceedingly large objects have been occasionally removed through a tracheostomy using the rigid bronchoscope, avoiding the narrow subglottic area.[23] A negative rigid bronchoscopy rate of 9% to 15% is reasonable to decrease the chance of missing the diagnosis of FBA.[18]

Complications following successful early rigid bronchoscopy, although common, are relatively minor. In several series almost no deaths have occurred.[15,16,20] Complication rates are higher for tracheal FBA, a delay in diagnosis, and retained foreign bodies.[21] Fever, pneumonia, respiratory failure, and pneumothorax may follow FBA. Bronchodilators are useful postoperatively. Preoperative steroid use to decrease airway edema is controversial, since pneumonia may be more common following steroid administration.[15] The usual hospital stay is several days.

In less than clear-cut cases of FBA, flexible bronchoscopy has been used as a diagnostic procedure.[24] Nineteen percent of patients with suspected FBA but no radiographic abnormalities have a foreign body detected by flexible bronchoscopy. Once the foreign body is visualized, preparations are made for removal by rigid bronchoscopy.

As is the case for pediatric chest trauma in general, prevention is important. Children less than 3 years of age should not be given food that is difficult to chew and should not be allowed to eat while running and playing. Small objects should be kept away from infants and toddlers.

Tracheobronchial Rupture

Tracheobronchial rupture (TBR) occurs in 0.7% to 2.2% of all patients with chest injuries.[25] It is more common in younger adults and children, and males greatly outnumber females.[25-29] TBR poses two problems: the immediate threat to ventilation and the long-term complication of stenosis of the healed or repaired bronchus. The mortality rate is high (30%), which is due in part to the high prevalence (50%) of associated injuries.[25-27,30] Diagnosis is sometimes difficult, leading to costly delays in proper management.

Most TBRs result from violent, high-speed automobile accidents, falls, or crushing chest injuries. Several mechanisms, alone or in combination, appear to produce TBR. Sudden compression of the sternum toward the vertebral column increases the transverse thoracic diameter, placing lateral disruptive forces on the tracheobronchial tree by the lungs remaining in contact with the chest wall. This mechanism may account for the higher incidence of TBR among children, who have much more compliant chest walls. Another mechanism is the sudden increase in airway pressure that occurs when crushing chest forces are applied against a closed glottis. Shearing forces from sudden deceleration, as in a high-speed crash, may also be important.[25,26]

Nearly 80% of TBRs occur within 2 cm of the carina, and 15% occur in the more proximal trachea; both sides appear to be affected equally.[26-28] Injuries may be of two types.[25] A tracheal laceration or transection may be associated with intact peribronchial connective tissue. Since there is no pleural communication, these patients may not have pneumothorax and the TBR may go undetected. The second type of TBR communicates with the pleural space, leading to air leak and pneumothorax (Fig. 9–5). This presentation usually is clinically evident, allowing early diagnosis and permitting early bronchoscopy and subsequent repair.

Improvements in emergency medical transport and the increased number of high-speed motor vehicle accidents has led to an increase in the number of

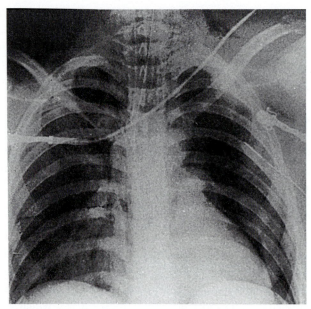

Figure 9–5. Chest radiograph in a patient with a ruptured left bronchus. Mediastinal and subcutaneous emphysema is present. (From Mahoubi S, Ohara AE: *Pediatr Radiol* 10:135, 1981, Figure 3A. Copyright Springer-Verlag.)

patients with TBR arriving in the emergency room alive. The clinical presentation may be dominated by associated major injuries. Pneumothorax is present in 80% of cases of TBR and may be bilateral (5%) or on the side opposite the bronchial injury.[25,28,30,31] A large air leak or failure of the lung to reexpand completely after chest tube placement for a pneumothorax should immediately suggest TBR.[28] Subcutaneous emphysema occurs in 65% of patients and may yield Hamman's crunch on physical examination.[25] Other symptoms include dyspnea, cyanosis, hemoptysis, and respiratory distress. Rib fractures are by no means universal, especially in children.[26,27] In one study, four of five patients had no rib fractures on the affected side.[27] Chest x-ray findings associated with TBR include pneumothorax, pneumomediastinum, deep cervical emphysema, and atelectasis. The "fallen lung sign" occurs as the atelectatic lung falls away from the mediastinum instead of toward it because of the loss of normal bronchial integrity.[25] A high index of suspicion is necessary to make the diagnosis of TBR.[25,26] Seventy percent of TBRs are diagnosed within 24 hours of admission and 40% after 1 month. This is not an insignificant point, since 50% of the 30% associated mortality occurs within the first hours after injury.[27,28]

In nearly all cases a preoperative diagnosis of TBR is confirmed by bronchoscopy.[26–28,30,31] Bronchoscopy allows careful assessment of the location and extent of the injury, which then dictates the operative approach. The majority of patients with TBR require surgery. The *unusual* patient with TBR is one in whom less than one third of the circumference of the bronchus is injured and who has full expansion of the lung without an air leak. Such a patient may be successfully treated nonoperatively.[26] The patient with TBR and stable ventilatory status but massive intraabdominal hemorrhage may undergo laparotomy before thoracotomy.[30]

Immediate management of the patient with TBR includes establishment of an airway, relief of pneumothorax with a chest tube, and intravenous resuscitation for associated injuries. If massive air leak or atelectasis threatens ventilation, a single-lumen tube may be inserted into the contralateral "good" mainstem bronchus.[29] Alternatively, a polyvinyl double-lumen tube may be used to permit selective ventilation before and during operative repair. The bronchoscope allows proper positioning of these tubes. High-frequency ventilation is helpful in supporting the patient with TBR.[29]

Intrathoracic tracheal, right mainstem, and proximal left mainstem injuries are approached through a right posterolateral thoracotomy. More distal left mainstem injuries are approached via a left thoracotomy.[28] The injured area is debrided, and an end-to-end anastomosis is performed with a single-layer, interrupted, nonabsorbable, monofilament suture having knots on the outside.[25,26,28,30,32] The repair is wrapped with a pleural, pericardial, or muscle flap. The chest is drained with several chest tubes, the lung is reexpanded, and the chest is closed. A single-lumen endotracheal tube is placed in the trachea. Ninety percent of survivors with repaired TBR have a satisfactory long-term result.[25,26] The major long-term complication is bronchial stenosis, which may lead to distal lung suppuration and require eventual pulmonary resection.

Delayed treatment of TBR is more difficult. The majority of patients may still have lung parenchyma–sparing operations in which an affected bronchial segment is resected and an anastomosis performed. Unfortunately, long-standing obstruction and lung infection require pulmonary resection, lobectomy, or pneumonectomy in 25% of patients.[25,28]

Traumatic Rupture of the Diaphragm

Traumatic diaphragmatic rupture (TDR) occurs in 5% of patients who undergo laparotomy for blunt trauma.[33] Five percent or less of TDRs occur in children.[34] TDR has a mortality rate of 7% to 50%, which is due almost exclusively to complications of severe associated injuries.[33-40] Associated injuries may make the diagnosis of TDR difficult, and a delayed or missed diagnosis may occur in as many as 69% of cases.[36] Failure to make a timely diagnosis may allow chronic diaphragmatic herniation, incarceration, or strangulation of an intraabdominal viscus with a high associated mortality.

TDR is usually the result of a high-speed motor vehicle accident or a motor vehicle–pedestrian accident. Penetrating injuries of the diaphragm are the most common diaphragmatic injuries in urban centers and are considered separately.[35] Breath-holding at the moment of thoracoabdominal crash impact leads to rupture of the posterolateral muscular attachments of the diaphragm.[33] Left-sided injuries predominate (56% to 95% of patients),[33,34,36,40] but right-sided TDRs are being increasingly reported.[41,42] The theory that the liver "buffers" the right hemidiaphragm has been challenged.

Owing to the severity of associated injuries, 41% to 52% of patients with blunt TDR are in shock when initially examined.[35,37] Nearly 100% of patients have associated injuries.[33–40] Skeletal fractures (especially pelvic fractures), intraabdominal bleeding, and brain injuries occur in 68%, 59%, and 27% of patients, respectively.[33] In 59% of patients the diagnosis of TDR is first made during urgent laparotomy for intraabdominal bleeding.[36] Physical examination is nonspecific, insensitive, and usually dominated by the associated injuries. Borborygmi, bowel sounds over the chest on auscultation, are specific but rare.[38] Decreased breath sounds and a scaphoid abdomen suggest the presence of TDR in children.[34] Chest x-ray findings in blunt TDR are frequently abnormal, but only in 32% to 41% of patients are the findings even suggestive of TDR.[33,36,37] X-ray findings may include rib fractures, hemothorax, contusion, and an elevated hemidiaphragm. Chest x-ray examination showing intrathoracic viscera allows a specific preoperative diagnosis; the finding of a nasogastric tube curled in the stomach in the left chest is pathognomonic (Fig. 9–6). Diagnostic peritoneal lavage (DPL), although useful in detecting intraabdominal bleeding from associated injuries, is notoriously inaccurate in diagnosing TDR.[35,36] DPL fluid emanating through a chest tube would be diagnostic but once again is unusual. Radionuclide scanning is particularly helpful in diagnosing right-sided TDRs because it shows a "ring of compression" of the diaphragm on the herniated liver.[41] CT scanning, ultrasound, and thoracoscopy have been variously used in diagnosis. The key to diagnosis is a high index of suspicion.

More than 80% of TDRs may be repaired through a midline laparotomy.[33,36,40] This is a matter of necessity in some patients, who require laparotomy for bleeding from associated intraabdominal injuries, especially spleen and liver laceration. Even if the diagnosis of TDR is established preoperatively in a stable patient, the majority of TDRs should be approached transabdominally to allow management of the frequently associated intraabdominal injuries. Herniated viscera are reduced from the chest, and the defect is primarily closed with one or two layers of interrupted or running sutures with heavy suture material.[36,38,41] Rarely, the large size of the diaphragmatic defect necessitates muscle flap transposition or incorporation of synthetic materials for adequate closure. Some authors advocate a right thoracotomy for acute right-sided TDR, which they

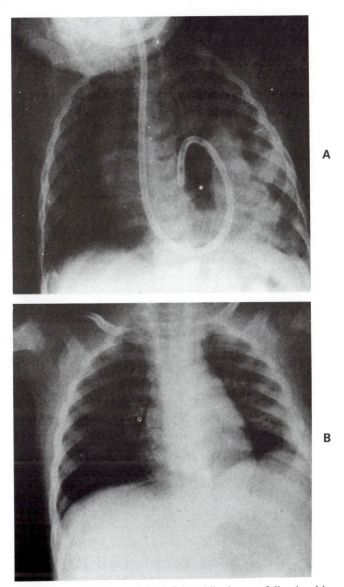

Figure 9–6. A, Traumatic rupture of the left hemidiaphragm following blunt trauma. Nasogastric tube position is pathognomonic. **B,** Chest radiograph after repair. (From Melzig EP, Swank MS, Salzberg AM: *Arch Surg* 111:1010, 1976. Copyright 1976, American Medical Association.)

claim improves exposure and ease of dealing with frequency-associated retrohepatic caval injuries.[41] A chest tube is necessary preoperatively or postoperatively in up to 90% of patients.[36,40]

The mortality rate associated with TDR is 7% to 50%. Right-sided TDR has a higher mortality than left-sided lesions.* Isolated TDR, which is rare, has a low mortality. Patients with more than four associated injuries have an overall mortality of 51%.[35] Deaths are usually due to hemorrhage, multiple organ failure, sepsis, and central nervous system injuries. Other complications include atelectasis, pneumonia, empyema, and intraabdominal abscess. Ventilator support averages 4.5 days and hospital stay 16 days.[36]

If a TDR is not diagnosed during the acute phase, the patient may proceed to a latent phase, followed by an obstructive phase of injury years after the accident.[40] The negative intrathoracic pressure and intraabdominal/pleural pressure gradient favors herniation of viscera into the chest. Stomach, colon, small intestine, and omentum may become incarcerated and strangulated. The operative approach to chronic TDR is via a thoracotomy, necessitated by multiple characteristic adhesions from the viscera to intrathoracic structures. The mortality rate for chronic TDR with strangulation is 36%.[43]

Gunshot and stab wounds of the diaphragm are becoming more common in adolescents, especially in urban areas. Gunshot wounds affect both sides equally; stab wounds are more likely to injure the left hemidiaphragm, since most assailants are right handed.[35] Most patients with gunshot wounds to the lower chest and abdomen are routinely explored and the diaphragmatic defect is diagnosed and repaired during laparotomy. The key to effective treatment is prompt diagnosis by inspection of the diaphragm during the abdominal exploration.

A stab wound to the left lower chest, below the fourth intercostal space anteriorly, causes isolated diaphragmatic injury in up to 50% of all cases.[44] Such injuries may be accompanied by normal chest x-ray and physical examination findings. DPL is inaccurate for the diagnosis of isolated diaphragmatic injury. Routine laparotomy may be the best policy for stab wounds to the lower chest to prevent the development of chronic diaphragmatic hernia and incarceration. These complications occur in 18% of such patients with TDR and have a mortality of up to 36%.[43,44] Unfortunately, the negative laparotomy rates may approach 35% with such a policy; however, a negative laparotomy should be associated with minimal morbidity and no mortality.

Pulmonary Contusion and Flail Chest

Pulmonary contusion is the most common injury in pediatric patients with chest trauma, occurring in up to 73%.[45] Pulmonary contusion is the result of

---

*References 33, 35, 36, 38, 40–42.

a motor vehicle accident in 86% of cases, the majority of children having been struck by a vehicle as pedestrians.[46,47] The compliant chest wall of the child transmits tremendous energy to the pulmonary parenchyma without causing rib fracture. Whereas 70% of adults with pulmonary contusion have rib fractures, only 40% of children with pulmonary contusion have a rib fracture.[47] Multiple extrathoracic injuries, including skeletal fractures, head injury, and splenic injury, are common in children.[45,46] Additional intrathoracic injuries, including pneumothorax and hemothorax, occur in 57% of patients.[47] Overall mortality for pulmonary contusion is 22% to 30%.[46,48,49] Flail chest, for reasons already given, is extremely rare in children, but if present it adversely affects survival.[47,48]

Physical findings of rib fractures, tachypnea, and decreased breath sounds may be absent in more than 50% of patients.[47] The characteristic radiographic findings of pulmonary contusion are a result of localized interstitial edema and alveolar hemorrhage, which may be delayed by 24 to 48 hours. The pulmonary contusion is generally present on the admission chest radiograph, although an associated hemothorax or pneumothorax may develop later and worsen the patient's respiratory status (Fig. 9–7).[45,47] An associated pleural effusion or pneumothorax requires tube thoracostomy. Most patients with pulmonary contusion exhibit hypoxemia on arterial blood gas (ABG) analysis.[47] Chest x-ray examination characteristically underdiagnoses and underestimates the severity of pulmonary contusion when compared with CT scanning.[48]

The majority of patients (82%) do not require mechanical ventilation.[45] Mechanical ventilation is more likely to be required for hyperventilation management of an associated head injury than for respiratory failure. Patients should be managed in an intensive care unit with oxygenation, fluid restriction, pulmonary hygiene, analgesics (including epidural catheters), and monitoring of serial arterial blood gases. Factors that increase the mortality of a pulmonary contusion include shock, Glasgow Coma Scale score less than 7, Injury Severity Score greater than 40, PaO_2/FIO_2 less than 300, and blood transfusion.[48,49] Pneumonia may develop in 47% of patients; this percentage approaches 100% in ventilated patients.[49]

The hypoxemia associated with pulmonary contusion is a result of ventilation-perfusion mismatch. The decreased compliance of the injured lung often causes hyperinflation of the opposite lung. Increased intraalveolar pressure ultimately reduces capillary perfusion to the normal lung. This process may be further aggravated by traditional mechanical ventilation. The normal physiologic hypoxic vasoconstriction response to the injury counteracts this phenomenon to a certain extent and reduces blood flow to the injured, nonventilated parenchyma.[50] In patients with pulmonary contusion who have hypoxemia and respiratory failure refractory to traditional mechanical ventilation, synchronized independent lung ventilation (SILV) has been used with encouraging results.[51] This requires placement of a double-lumen endotracheal tube.

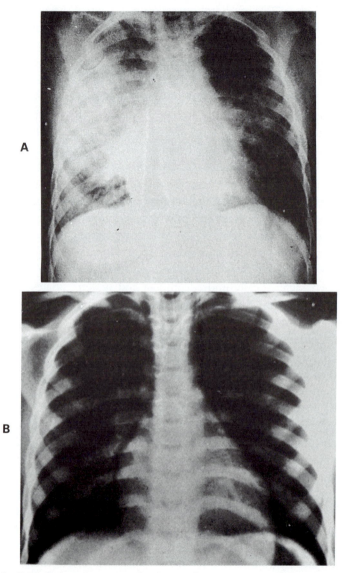

Figure 9–7. A, Pulmonary contusion. **B,** Follow-up chest radiograph. (From Haller JA: *Pediatr Ann* 5:78, 1976.)

Rib Fractures

Rib fractures, although rare in children, are a marker of increased severity of injury and, when unexplained, are a marker for child abuse.[52,53] Only 1.6% of children admitted for trauma have rib fractures. Of the 5.9% of pediatric trauma patients suffering thoracic trauma, 31.7% have a rib fracture and 88% have multiple injuries.[52] Nearly all rib fractures are a result of blunt trauma. In older children involvement in motor vehicle accidents, especially as pedestrians, predominate as the cause of rib fractures.[52,54] Child abuse is the leading cause in children less than 3 years of age.[52] Overall mortality is high, 42%, but is even greater among patients with multiple rib fractures and rib fractures associated with head injury. Fractures of the first rib are a particular concern because of the high frequency of associated major vascular injury.[54] Aortography should be performed in any child with first rib fractures, pulse deficits, or a discrepancy in blood pressure between arms. Rib fractures as a result of cardiopulmonary resuscitation are rare in children. Multiple rib fractures, especially of the posterior rib neck, in various stages of healing should immediately suggest the diagnosis of child abuse.[53,55]

Traumatic Rupture of the Thoracic Aorta

Traumatic rupture of the aorta (TRA) is less common in children than in adults. TRA accounts for 1% to 2.1% and 12% to 30% of all deaths following blunt trauma in children and adults, respectively.[56–58] There are several reasons for this disparity. Children are usually injured as pedestrians struck by a motor vehicle and are unlikely to suffer a steering wheel chest crush injury. The force of impact to the child is spread over the entire body, whereas in adults the force of impact of the steering wheel or dashboard is concentrated on the chest.[56,57] Forty-six percent of TRAs in children are due to pedestrian–motor vehicle collisions, while 38% are seen in passengers in motor vehicle accidents. Children at the highest risk for TRA are those who are unrestrained passengers in vehicles traveling faster than 55 mph.[56]

The majority of TRAs occur at the ligamentum arteriosum, just distal to the left subclavian artery.[56,59,60] The severity of the impact and decelerative forces leads to shearing stresses on the aorta where it is relatively fixed at the ligamentum.[57] In one study 77% of children with TRA died at the scene of the accident, 16% died in the emergency room, and only 7% survived.[56] This is lower than the overall adult survival of 14%. The lower incidence of TRA in children may lead to a less heightened index of suspicion and delay or to failure to make an early diagnosis.

Nearly all TRAs are accompanied by multiple, severe, life-threatening injuries, including intraabdominal bleeding, pulmonary contusion, skeletal fractures, head injuries, and myocardial contusion.[56,59–61] Symptoms and signs of

TRA include shock, coma, hypertension, pseudocoarctation, dyspnea, chest and back pain, hoarseness, dysphagia, paraplegia, stridor, decreased femoral pulses, murmur, and visible chest wall injury.[58,59] Specific clues to aortic injury such as back pain, decreased pulses, and murmurs are rare.[59] Once again, the key to early diagnosis is a high index of suspicion.[57,58] Suggestive radiographic signs of TRA include mediastinal widening (ratio greater than 0.28 mediastinum/chest at aortic knob), a prominent aortic knob, obliteration of aortic outline, tracheal deviation, depression of the left mainstem bronchus, hemothorax, deviation of nasogastric tube to the right, rib fractures, or an extrapleural cap.[57,58,61,62] Children with TRA may not have rib fractures. Arteriography is nearly 100% specific and should be performed in any patient in whom the diagnosis of TRA is suspected (Fig. 9–8).[57,58,61] The majority of patients undergo prompt left thoracotomy and repair.[61] Some hemodynamically stable patients with TRA who have other associated severe injuries (e.g., head injury requiring craniotomy, intraabdominal bleeding requiring laparotomy) may be temporarily managed with intraarterial monitoring of blood pressure and control of dP/dT with beta blockers and nitroprusside.[59,61] Twenty-two percent of patients with TRA require another operation before left thoracotomy.[59]

Since 77% to 97% of TRAs occur at the ligamentum of the descending

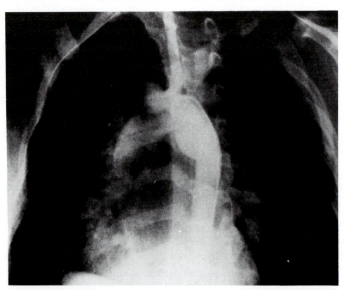

Figure 9–8. Aortogram demonstrating traumatic disruption of the descending thoracic aorta at the level of the ligamentum arteriosum. (From Ali IS, Fitzgerald PG, Gillis DA, et al: *J Pediatr Surg* 27:1282, 1992.)

thoracic aorta, the operative approach is through a posterolateral left thoracotomy in the fourth intercostal space.[56,62] In older children a double-lumen endotracheal tube permits collapse of the left lung and improves exposure. Proximal and distal control of the aorta is initially obtained without disturbing the hematoma. The proximal aortic clamp is usually placed between the left carotid and subclavian arteries. The hematoma is opened, exposing the separated edges of the transected aorta. Primary repair with a running Prolene suture or Dacron graft interposition is usually accomplished in 14 to 47 minutes of aortic cross-clamp time.[57–63]

The most feared complication of TRA is paraplegia, which occurs in 5.4% to 15% of patients.[57,59–62] The duration of aortic cross-clamp time is in part responsible, with the incidence of paraplegia less than 5% if cross-clamp time is less than 45 minutes.[61] Unfortunately, other factors out of the surgeon's control (presence of preoperative shock, degree of intercostal artery involvement in the injury) may be responsible for the paraplegia.[59,63] Up to 31% of patients have paresis or paraplegia preoperatively.[59] A variety of techniques have been used to prevent spinal ischemia during aortic clamping. These include femoral-femoral cardiopulmonary bypass, Gott shunts, and left atrial-femoral bypass with centrifugal pumps.[57,64,65] It is controversial whether any of these adjuncts actually decreases the rate of paraplegia when compared with the "clamp and sew" technique alone.[61,63] For those who insist on using a bypass modality, left atrial-femoral bypass with a Biomedicus pump has certain benefits. It provides distal organ and spinal perfusion, decreases left ventricular afterload, does not require heparinization, and is technically easier than performing a Gott shunt.[64,65]

Mortality in those fortunate few patients surviving to reach the hospital appears to be bimodal. Early deaths are usually due to exsanguination, often before the patient reaches the arteriography suite or operating room, while late deaths are often due to the multiple associated injuries.[59] Overall hospital mortality is 15.7% to 39%.[59–62,66] Additional postoperative complications include pneumonia, adult respiratory distress syndrome, sepsis, renal failure, intraabdominal abscess, empyema, ischemic bowel, and recurrent nerve injury.[60] Late complications include graft infection or pseudoaneurysm formation in 0.8% to 3.6% of patients.[60]

Blunt injuries to the ascending aorta and arch vessels are less common.[67,68] Most of these are injuries to the innominate artery.[68] The operative approach includes median sternotomy with neck incision in many of these injuries. Although repair using partial occluding clamps on the ascending aorta may be possible, complex arch injuries may require cardiopulmonary bypass, deep hypothermia, and circulatory arrest.

Cardiac Injury

No single, specific, reliable diagnostic test is available to confirm myocardial contusion after blunt trauma, nor is there a test to predict the development of arrhythmia or pump failure in patients with myocardial contusion following blunt injury. As a result the incidence of myocardial contusion following blunt injury is variable, 9% to 76%, depending on whether electrocardiographic changes, creatine phosphokinase MB (CPK MB) isoenzyme concentrations, echocardiography, pyrophosphate scanning, and multiplegated acquisition (MUGA) scanning alone or in combination, were used to establish the diagnosis.[69–71] In one study of 39 children suffering blunt injury, 8% (3/39) had elevated CPK MB levels, 56% (22/39) had nonspecific electrocardiographic changes, and 34% (12/35) had abnormal isotope scans.[71] Only 5% (2/39) of those patients required antiarrhythmic therapy, and pump failure did not develop in any patient. Using a combination of electrocardiographic changes and scans, an incidence of myocardial contusion of 23% was estimated among patients with blunt injury. Another study of 41 children with blunt injury to the chest showed electrocardiographic abnormalities in 36%, elevated CPK MB levels in 31%, and an abnormal scan in 14%, but only 10% (4/41) had more than one of these positive studies.[69] No patient suffered an arrhythmia or cardiac failure.

Electrocardiographic abnormalities associated with myocardial contusion include inverted T waves, elevated ST segments, atrioventricular conduction delay, and bundle branch block. Cardiac enzyme levels may be either falsely positive because of skeletal muscle damage or falsely negative. Autopsy series have shown patients to have myocardial contusion despite normal isoenzyme levels. Pyrophosphate scans generally are diagnostic for only 72 hours after injury and the equipment is not portable, limiting their usefulness in early diagnosis. MUGA scans may be more useful for timely diagnosis.[72] Echocardiography is becoming increasingly important in the management of blunt cardiac injury. Echocardiographic abnormalities include regional wall motion abnormalities, pericardial effusion, and valvular insufficiency.[69–71,73] Combined with other studies, the echocardiogram provides a means of risk stratification and triage for patients with blunt chest trauma and suspected myocardial contusion. Patients with myocardial contusion diagnosed by a regional wall motion abnormality have more associated injuries, a higher Injury Severity Score, and higher CPK MB levels than patients with a normal echocardiogram and suspected myocardial contusion. The echocardiogram is also useful for follow-up.[71] Late sequelae of myocardial contusion such as ventricular septal defect (VSD), aneurysm, and valvular insufficiency are readily diagnosed by echocardiogram.

Patients with suspected myocardial contusion, especially those with a conduction abnormality on admission electrocardiogram, should be placed in a monitored setting. Only 4% will be expected to have an arrhythmia.[74] Generally, associated injuries have already dictated monitoring in an intensive care unit. Patients with myocardial contusion, when well monitored, can safely undergo operations for other injuries.

Rarely, blunt injury produces serious mechanical injury to cardiac structures, including rupture of a cardiac chamber with tamponade or exsanguination, disruption of cardiac valves, VSD, and aneurysms.[70] Patients with congestive heart failure may have suffered a VSD or valvular insufficiency as a late sequela.[71] Echocardiography and cardiac catheterization, when necessary, confirm the diagnosis before definitive repair. An asymptomatic VSD with a left-to-right shunt of less than 1.5 : 1 and with normal pulmonary artery pressures may be closely followed nonoperatively. Larger VSDs require Dacron patch closure.

The aortic valve is the most commonly injured cardiac valve in blunt injury. Valvular involvement may include leaflet tears, avulsion of commissural attachments, and aortic tears. The development of congestive heart failure or left ventricular hypertrophy is an indication for subsequent valve replacement or repair.[75] Rarer still, blunt trauma to the heart can cause death without structural injury. Commotio cordis may occur in Little League baseball when a pitched ball strikes a child's chest. Sudden ventricular fibrillation can be quite unresponsive to therapy.[76]

Penetrating cardiac wounds may outnumber blunt cardiac wounds in urban trauma centers, especially among adolescents. Injuries may be due to gunshot or stab wounds; patients with the latter are more likely to reach the hospital alive. In one study 78 of 90 patients who lived long enough to undergo cardiorrhaphy in the operating room ultimately survived.[77] Most of the deaths from penetrating cardiac trauma occur in the prehospital phase. Treatment of a patient with suspected penetrating cardiac injury includes aggressive fluid resuscitation, transfusion, pericardiocentesis, and prompt operation.[78] The majority of such patients are explored through a median sternotomy, although an anterolateral thoracotomy is occasionally used. The right ventricle is most frequently involved.[78] Cardiopulmonary bypass is not usually required during the initial lifesaving operation. However, a VSD, valvular insufficiency, or fistula requiring later intracardiac repair develops in 5.4% of patients.[78]

Infants and children may suffer iatrogenic cardiac perforation from temporary pacing wires and central venous lines.[79–81] Infants are at greatest risk. Perforation of the right ventricle during a cardiac catheterization occurs in 2% of infants, but in only 0.5% of children over 1 year of age.[79] Unfortunately, signs of tamponade may not be apparent for 12 hours after injury. Only a small amount (40 ml) of pericardial blood is necessary to cause a tamponade.[80] Prevention is the best policy; this includes keeping central lines in the superior vena cava rather than to the right atrium and obtaining frequent chest radiographs to ascertain line position. Treatment of iatrogenic cardiac perforation includes pericardiocentesis, removal or repositioning of the offending catheter, and possibly operation.

Traumatic Asphyxia

Traumatic asphyxia is a syndrome of cervicofacial cyanosis, subconjunctival hemorrhages, venous engorgement, and petechiae of the head and neck, generally resulting from blunt injury.[82] This syndrome is rare, occurring in only 1 of 18,500 hospital trauma admissions.[83] The cause is a sudden, severe, anteroposterior compression of the chest. Most children with traumatic asphyxia have been run over or pinned by a motor vehicle. Although variable, the crushing weight is usually 300 to 2000 pounds and the duration of application is 2 to 5 minutes. A crush over five times the body weight for greater than 10 minutes is fatal.[83] The clinical findings of traumatic asphyxia are due to a sudden, severe increase in intrapulmonary pressure and superior vena cava venous pressure. The "fear response" in the victim just before impact consists of maximal inspiration and closure of the glottis. These protective mechanisms set the stage for traumatic asphyxia as the compressive chest force is then delivered.[82-84] Blood is forced from the right atrium into the valveless jugular venous system. Venous pressure may be increased as much as eightfold.[83]

Neurologic symptoms of traumatic asphyxia include agitation, disorientation, and occasionally seizures. In the absence of associated head injuries a CT scan is usually normal. The neurologic manifestations usually clear within 24 hours, and long-term sequelae are unusual.[85] Visual loss may occur secondary to retinal hemorrhages, which on rare occasion is permanent.[86] Pulmonary signs and symptoms are common and include pulmonary edema, hemorrhage, contusion, and pneumothorax.[82,84,85] Management may require endotracheal intubation and mechanical ventilation.

Isolated traumatic asphyxia, although rare, has a greater than 90% survival rate.[85] Associated injuries are common and are responsible for most of the expected mortality. In one study 37.5% of patients with traumatic asphyxia had blunt cardiac injury and one patient died of right ventricular rupture.[87]

Treatment of traumatic asphyxia includes admission to an intensive care unit, administration of oxygen, elevation of the head, serial arterial blood gas studies, eye examination, and at times endotracheal intubation.[82,84-86] The use of steroids is controversial. Despite the often moribund appearance of patients, the prognosis for traumatic asphyxia is good.[83,85]

Esophageal Perforation

Corrosive injury to the esophagus, an extremely important topic in pediatric trauma, is discussed in Chapter 10. This chapter focuses on the diagnosis and management of esophageal perforation in children. The esophagus lacks a serosa and is surrounded by loose areolar tissue. Perforation quickly leads to medias-tinitis, sepsis, and death.[88] Most studies demonstrate that the earlier esophageal perforation is diagnosed and treated, the better is the prognosis.[89,90] Treatment strategies vary according to the duration of the perforation, site of injury, un-derlying esophageal disease, and age of the patient. Treatment may range from the nonoperative management of most neonates with esophageal perforation to nearly universal surgical exploration in minimally symptomatic older children or adults.[89,91]

Swallowed foreign bodies are a common problem in younger children; 70% of cases occur in children less than 4 years of age.[92] Coins are the most commonly swallowed object. Usually natural peristalsis allows spontaneous pas-sage, but when lodged, generally in the cervical esophagus, foreign bodies can usually be removed with esophagoscopy. Perforation of the esophagus, however, can occur, especially when the swallowed coin has gone undetected and erodes through the esophagus over a period of time. Coins are responsible for 8.4% of esophageal perforations caused by foreign bodies.[92] Children may have ex-cessive salivation, painful swallowing, vomiting, refusal to eat, or wheezing.[93] The coin may actually be found in an extraluminal position in the chronic stages of swallowed foreign bodies. The foreign body readily appears on neck and chest radiographs. Esophagography or esophagoscopy may not visualize the extraluminal coin. Removal requires cervical exploration or thoracotomy and dissection of the coin from extensive surrounding granulation tissue. Usually no esophageal mucosal defect remains. Unfortunately, undetected esophageal foreign bodies may lead to death from aortoesophageal fistulas.[92,93]

With the advent of neonatal critical care units, iatrogenic neonatal esoph-ageal perforation has become a significant problem. Premature infants are at the highest risk. The injury is usually caused by endotracheal intubation or placement of orogastric tubes. The clinical presentation may mimic esophageal atresia, or there may be a right pneumothorax with the offending feeding tube found in the right side of the chest.[94,95] Nearly all perforations occur in the upper esophagus. Esophagograms demonstrate a double esophagus (true and false lumens).[94,95] Treatment includes removal of the offending tube, insertion of a chest tube, intravenous antibiotics, and peripheral nutrition. Nine of 11 such treated infants survived in one study.[94] Operation in neonates is usually not necessary. Deaths are usually unrelated to the esophageal perforation and are usually due to an intraventricular hemorrhage.[94,95]

Lower esophageal rupture following misplacement of gastrostomy Foley balloons has also been reported.[96] These injuries occur when a gastrostomy tube is replaced with a Foley catheter. The Foley catheter is inadvertently inserted through the gastric fistula and up into the distal esophagus. When the balloon is inflated, the esophagus is ruptured. These larger ruptures require thoracotomy, repair, and drainage. Barotrauma is also a source of esophageal perforation in childhood. Such peculiar injuries can occur if an unsuspecting child bites an inflated inner tube or twists the cap of a carbonated beverage off with his or her teeth.[97–99] Approximately 5 to 10 PSI is necessary to perforate the esophagus.[97,98] The injury is usually pharyngoesophageal, occurring near the cricopharyngeus muscle, but may be located in the thoracic esophagus. Patients have respiratory distress, neck pain, and subcutaneous emphysema. Esophagograms and esophagoscopy delineate the location and extent of injury. Exploration, repair, and drainage are curative. Several children with small perforations have been successfully treated nonoperatively.[99]

Esophageal perforation in older children and adults may be the result of either intraluminal or extraluminal causes. Intraluminal causes include iatrogenic instrumentation or spontaneous rupture of the esophagus. Extraluminal causes include gunshot and stab wounds and blunt trauma. In one study 48% of esophageal perforations were iatrogenic, 33% were traumatic, and 12% were spontaneous.[89] In urban trauma centers, external trauma may be as common as or more common than instrumentation as a cause of esophageal perforation.[100] Regardless of the cause, certain management principles apply. A high index of suspicion is necessary for early diagnosis. Early diagnosis and treatment are the ultimate keys to clinical success. In one study patients whose esophageal perforation was diagnosed within 24 hours had a 92% survival compared with only a 67% survival for patients with perforations diagnosed after 24 hours.[89]

Eighty-three percent of external traumatic esophageal perforations occur in the cervical esophagus; penetrating trauma is a more common cause than blunt trauma.[89] Nearly all patients with external traumatic esophageal perforation have associated injuries, and 64% have concomitant tracheal injuries.[90] In up to 46% of patients the esophageal perforation is found during routine mandatory neck exploration for penetrating neck trauma.[100] Patients may have subcutaneous and mediastinal air, neck hematoma, or positive nasogastric aspirate. In the trauma setting, where patient cooperation is not optimal, a Gastrografin contrast study may fail to show extravasation.[90,100] Endoscopy and thorough esophageal inspection during neck exploration may reduce missed injuries. Treatment is generally by primary two-layer closure and drainage. Concomitant tracheal repairs should be separated from esophageal and arterial repairs using sternohyoid muscle flap interposition to prevent subsequent tracheoesophageal fistula and tracheoinnominate artery fistulas.[101] The mortality rate of esophageal repair is 15%; death is generally due to an esophageal leak or tracheoinnominate artery fistula and exsanguination.[90] Thoracic esopageal perforation caused by external trauma should be treated by thoracotomy, primary repair, and buttressing of the repair with a thick Grillo pleural flap.[88,90] Missed esophageal injuries result in an intense inflammatory reaction. Complex injuries or delayed

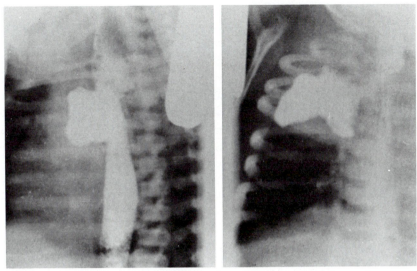

Figure 9–9. Iatrogenic perforation of the thoracic esophagus during endoscopy. Extravasation of dye on Gastrografin swallow. (From Van Der Zee DC, Festen C, van der Staak FH, Severijnen RS: *J Thorac Cardivasc Surg* 95:693, 1988.)

diagnosis of thoracic esophageal perforation may require esophageal exclusion and diversion, with cervical esophagostomy, thoracic drainage, gastrostomy, and jejunostomy.[88-90]

The presentation of iatrogenic esophageal perforation depends on the location of injury. Perforation occurs in 0.13% of all esophageal manipulations, especially following esophageal dilation.[91] Dilation is most often necessary in children for treatment of stenosis following repair of esophageal atresia or following corrosive pneumomediastinum. The patient may have pneumothorax, fever, leukocytosis, and shock. Unfortunately, up to half of iatrogenic injuries are not diagnosed until more than 24 hours after injury.[89] Diagnosis is confirmed and the location of injury ascertained in 93% of patients evaluated with a Gastrografin study (Fig. 9–9).[89,100] A negative study when clinical suspicion is high should prompt additional study with dilute barium. Treatment strategy includes nothing by mouth, resuscitation with intravenous fluids, and administration of antibiotics. The majority of older children require operative treatment.[88,89] Patients with an early diagnosis, in generally good health, and with no underlying esophageal disease may undergo a primary repair and drainage with good anticipated results. Patients with esophageal perforation and underlying esophageal disease with stricture may require esophagectomy. Patients with a late diagnosis and significant mediastinal and pleural inflammation may require esophageal exclusion and diversion and may expect a more dismal outcome. Nonoperative "curative" treatment is possible for select patients with minimal sepsis, a contained leak, and a cervical location of injury.[89] Treatment includes intravenous antibiotics and total parenteral nutrition. In one study of 13 children with iatrogenic esophageal perforation treated nonoperatively, 11 had a good outcome.[91]

Complications follow esophageal repair in 42% of patients and include anastomotic leaks, empyema, wound infection, pneumonia, sepsis, multiple organ failure, stricture, tracheoesophageal fistula, and hemorrhage.[89] Overall mortality is at least 10% to 36% depending on the length of delay in diagnosis and the location of injury.[88–90,100] Thoracic injuries are more lethal than cervical esophageal perforation.[88] Abdominal esophageal perforation is rare and may be manifest as an acute condition of the abdomen or free air. Abdominal esophageal perforation is repaired via laparotomy.

REFERENCES

1. Sinclair MC, Moore FC: Major surgery for abdominal and thoracic trauma in childhood and adolescence, *J Pediatr Surg* 9:155–162, 1974.
2. Eichelberger MR, Randolph JF: Progress in pediatric trauma, *World J Surg* 9:222–235, 1985.
3. Smyth BT: Chest trauma in children, *J Pediatr Surg* 14:41–47, 1979.
4. Peclet MH, Newman KD, Eichelberger MR, et al: Thoracic trauma in children: an indicator of increased mortality, *J Pediatr Surg* 25:961–966, 1990.
5. Eichelberger MR, Randolph JG: Thoracic trauma in children, *Surg Clin North Am* 61:1181–1197, 1981.
6. Eichelberger MR: Trauma of the airway and thorax, *Pediatr Ann* 16:307–316, 1987.
7. Nakayama DK, Romanofsky ML, Rowe MI: Chest injuries in children, *Ann Surg* 210:770–775, 1989.
8. Sivit CJ, Taylor GA, Eichelberger MR: Chest injury in children with blunt abdominal trauma evaluation with CT, *Radiology* 17:815–816, 1989.
9. Velcek FT, Weiss A, DiMaio D, et al: Traumatic death in urban children, *J Pediatr Surg* 12:375–384, 1977.
10. Haller JA: Thoracic injuries. In Welch KJ, ed: *Pediatric surgery,* Chicago, 1986, Year Book.
11. Meller JL, Little AG, Shermata DW: Thoracic trauma in children, *Pediatrics* 74:813–819, 1984.
12. May T, Matlak ME, Johnson DG, et al: The Modified Injury Severity Score in pediatric multiple trauma patients, *J Pediatr Surg* 15:719–726, 1980.
13. Haller JA: Major thoracic trauma in children, *Pediatr Clin North Am* 22:341–347, 1975.
14. Haller JA, Shermata DW: Acute thoracic injuries in children, *Pediatr Ann* 5:637–641, 1976.
15. McGuirt WF, Holmes KD, Feehs R, et al: Tracheobronchial foreign bodies, *Laryngoscope* 98:615–618, 1988.
16. Black RE, Choi KJ, Syme WR, et al: Bronchoscopic removal of aspirated foreign bodies in children, *Am J Surg* 148:778–781, 1984.

17. Musemeche CA, Kosloske AM: Normal radiographic findings after foreign body aspiration, *Clin Pediatr* 25:624–625, 1986.
18. Mantor RC, Tuggle DW, Tunell WP: An appropriate negative bronchoscopy rate in suspected foreign body aspiration, *Am J Surg* 158:622–624, 1989.
19. Cotton E, Yameda K: Foreign body aspiration, *Pediatr Clin North Am* 31:937–941, 1984.
20. Vane DW, Pritchard J, Colville CW, et al: Bronchoscopy for aspirated foreign bodies in children, *Arch Surg* 123:885–888, 1988.
21. Esclamado RM, Richardson MA: Laryngotracheal foreign bodies in children, *Am J Dis Child* 141:259–262, 1987.
22. Holinger L: Diagnostic endoscopy of the pediatric airway, *Laryngoscope* 99:346–348, 1989.
23. Swensson EE, Rah KH, Kim MC, et al: Extraction of large tracheal foreign bodies through a tracheostoma under bronchoscopic control, *Ann Thorac Surg* 39:251–253, 1985.
24. Wood RE, Gauderer MWL: Flexible fiberoptic bronchoscopy in the management of tracheobronchial foreign bodies in children, *J Pediatr Surg* 19:693–698, 1984.
25. Roxburgh JC: Rupture of the tracheobronchial tree, *Thorax* 42:681–688, 1987.
26. Hancock BJ, Wiseman NE: Tracheobronchial injuries in children, *J Pediatr Surg* 26:1316–1319, 1991.
27. Mahboubi S, O'Hara AE: Bronchial rupture in children following blunt chest trauma, *Pediatr Radiol* 10:133–138, 1981.
28. Amauchi W, Birolini D, Branco PD, et al: Injuries to the tracheobronchial tree in closed trauma, *Thorax* 38:923–928, 1983.
29. Shimazu T, Sugimoto H, Nishide K, et al: Tracheobronchial rupture caused by blunt chest trauma, *Am J Emerg Med* 6:427–434, 1988.
30. Ramzy AI, Rodriguez A, Turney SZ: Management of major tracheobronchial ruptures in patients with multiple system trauma, *J Trauma* 28:1353–1357, 1988.
31. Baumgartner F, Sheppard B, Virgilio C, et al: Tracheal and main bronchial disruptions after blunt chest trauma, *Ann Thorac Surg* 50:569–574, 1990.
32. Taskinen SO, Salo JA, Halttunen PEA, et al: Tracheobronchial rupture due to blunt chest trauma: a follow up study, *Ann Thorac Surg* 48:846–849, 1989.
33. Morgan AS, Flancbaum L, Esposito T, et al: Blunt injury to the diaphragm: an analysis of 44 patients, *J Trauma* 26:565–568, 1986.
34. Melzig EP, Swank M, Salzberg AM: Acute blunt traumatic rupture of the diaphragm in children, *Arch Surg* 111:1009–1011, 1976.
35. Weincek RG, Wilson RF, Steiger Z: Acute injuries of the diaphragm, *J Thorac Cardiovasc Surg* 92:989–993, 1986.
36. Beal SL, McKennan M: Blunt diaphragmatic rupture, *Arch Surg* 123:828–832, 1988.
37. Sharma OP: Traumatic diaphragmatic rupture: not an uncommon entity—personal experience and collective review of the 1980s, *J Trauma* 29:678–682, 1989.
38. Holm A, Bessey PQ, Aldrete JS: Diaphragmatic rupture due to blunt trauma: morbidity and mortality in 42 cases, *South Med J* 81:956–962, 1988.
39. Voeller GR, Reisser JR, Fabian TC, et al: Blunt diaphragm injuries, *Am Surg* 56:28–30, 1990.
40. Pipkin NL, Hamit HF: Traumatic perforation of the diaphragm, *South Med J* 81:1347–1350, 1988.

41. Estera AS, Landry MJ, McClelland RN: Blunt traumatic rupture of the right hemidiaphragm: experience in 12 patients, *Ann Thorac Surg* 39:525–530, 1985.

42. Flancbaum L, Morgan AS, Esposito T, et al: Non-left sided diaphragmatic rupture due to blunt trauma, *Surg Gynecol Obstet* 161:266–270, 1985.

43. Madden MR, Paull DE, Finkelstein JL, et al: Occult diaphragmatic injury from stab wounds to the lower chest and abdomen, *J Trauma* 29:292–298, 1989.

44. Stylianos G, King TC: Occult diaphragm injuries at celiotomy for left chest stab wounds, *Am Surg* 58:364–368, 1992.

45. Roux P, Fisher RM: Chest injuries in children: an analysis of 100 cases of blunt chest trauma from motor vehicle accidents, *J Pediatr Surg* 27:551–555, 1992.

46. Levy JL: Management of crushing chest injuries in children, *South Med J* 65:1040–1044, 1972.

47. Bonadio WA, Hellmich T: Post-traumatic pulmonary contusion in children, *Ann Emerg Med* 18:1050–1052, 1989.

48. Stellin G: Survival in trauma victims with pulmonary contusion, *Am Surg* 57:780–784, 1991.

49. Fredland M, Wilson RF, Bender JS, et al: The management of flail chest injury: factors affecting outcome, *J Trauma* 30:1460–1468, 1990.

50. Wagner RB, Sleviko B, Jamieson PM, et al: Effect of lung contusion on pulmonary hemodynamics, *Ann Thorac Surg* 52:51–58, 1991.

51. Frame SB, Marshall WJ, Clifford TG: Synchronized independent lung ventilation in the management of pediatric unilateral pulmonary contusion: case report, *J Trauma* 29:395–397, 1989.

52. Garcia VT, Gotschall CS, Eichelberger MR: Rib fractures in children: a marker of severe trauma, *J Trauma* 30:695–700, 1990.

53. Feldman KW, Brown DK: Child abuse, cardiopulmonary resuscitation, and rib fractures, *Pediatrics* 73:339–342, 1984.

54. Harris GJ, Soper RT: Pediatric first rib fractures, *J Trauma* 30:343–345, 1990.

55. Kleinman PK, Marks SC, Spevak MR, et al: Fractures of the rib head in abused infants, *Radiology* 185:119–123, 1992.

56. Eddy C, Rusch VW, Fligner CL, et al: The epidemiology of traumatic rupture of the thoracic aorta in children: a 13 year review, *J Trauma* 30:989–992, 1990.

57. Ali IS, Fitzgerald PG, Gillis DA, et al: Blunt traumatic disruption of the thoracic aorta: a rare injury in children, *J Pediatr Surg* 27:1281–1284, 1982.

58. Mure AJ, Unkle DW, Doolin E, et al: Blunt aortic trauma following deceleration in a seven year old, *Pediatr Emerg Care* 6:104–105, 1990.

59. Duhaylongsod FG, Glower DD, Wolfe WW: Acute traumatic aortic aneurysms: the Duke experience from 1970 to 1990, *J Vasc Surg* 15:331–343, 1992.

60. Schmidt CA, Wood MN, Razzouk AJ, et al: Primary repair of traumatic aorta rupture: a preferred approach, *J Trauma* 32:588–592, 1992.

61. Hilgenberg AD, Logan DL, Akins CW, et al: Blunt injuries of the thoracic aorta, *Ann Thorac Surg* 53:233–239, 1992.

62. Schmidt CA, Jacobson JG: Thoracic aortic injury, *Arch Surg* 119:1244–1246, 1984.

63. Mattox KL, Holzman M, Pickard LR, et al: Clamp/repair: a safe technique for treatment of blunt injury to the descending thoracic aorta, *Ann Thorac Surg* 40:456–463, 1985.

64. Olivier HF, Maher TD, Leibler GA, et al: Use of the Biomedicus centrifugal pump in traumatic tears of the aorta, *Ann Thorac Surg* 38:586–591, 1984.

65. Higgins RSD, Sanchez JA, DeGuidis L, et al: Mechanical circulatory support decreases

neurologic complications in the treatment of traumatic injuries of the thoracic aorta, *Arch Surg* 127:516–519, 1992.

66. Clark DE, Zeiger MA, Williams KL, et al: Blunt aortic trauma: signs of high risk, *J Trauma* 30:701–705, 1990.
67. Schmidt CA, Smith DE: Traumatic avulsion of arch vessels in a child: primary repair using hypothermic circulatory arrest, *J Trauma* 29:248–250, 1989.
68. Rosenberg JM, Bredenberg CE, Marvasti MA, et al: Blunt injuries to the aortic arch vessels, *Ann Thorac Surg* 48:508–513, 1989.
69. Langer JC, Winthrop AL, Wesson DE, et al: Diagnosis and incidence of cardiac injury in children with blunt thoracic trauma, *J Pediatr Surg* 24:1091–1094, 1989.
70. Eshel G, Gross B, Bar-Yochal A, et al: Cardiac injuries caused by blunt chest trauma in children, *Pediatr Emerg Care* 3:96–98, 1987.
71. Tellez DW, Hardin WD, Takahashi M, et al: Blunt cardiac injury in children, *J Pediatr Surg* 32:1123–1128, 1987.
72. Ildstad ST, Tollerud DJ, Weiss RG, et al: Cardiac contusion in pediatric patients with blunt thoracic trauma, *J Pediatr Surg* 25:287–289, 1990.
73. Hiatt JR, Yeatman LA, Child JS: The value of echocardiography in blunt chest trauma, *J Trauma* 28:914–922, 1988.
74. Wisner DH, Reed WH, Riddick RS: Suspected myocardial contusion, *Ann Surg* 212:82–86, 1990.
75. Rowland TW: Traumatic aortic insufficiency in children: case report and review of the literature, *Pediatrics* 60:893–895, 1977.
76. Abrunzo TJ: Commotio cordis, *Am J Dis Child* 145:1279–1282, 1991.
77. Mattox KL, Limacher MC, Feliciano DV, et al: Cardiac evaluation following heart injury, *J Trauma* 25:758–765, 1985.
78. Knott-Craig CJ, Dalton RP, Rossouw GJ, et al: Penetrating cardiac trauma: management strategy based on 129 surgical emergencies over 2 years, *Ann Thorac Surg* 53:1006–1009, 1992.
79. Golladay ES, Donahou JS, Haller JA: Special problem of cardiac injuries in infants and children, *J Trauma* 19:526–530, 1979.
80. Bar-Joseph G, Galvis AG: Perforation of the heart by central venous catheters in infants: guidelines to diagnosis and management, *J Pediatr Surg* 18:284–287, 1983.
81. Harris JP, Nanda NC, Moxley R, et al: Myocardial perforation due to temporary transvenous pacing catheters in pediatric patients, *Cath Cardiovasc Diagn* 10:329–333, 1984.
82. Haller JA, Donahoo JS: Traumatic asphyxia in children: pathophysiology and management, *J Trauma* 11:453–457, 1971.
83. Gorenstein L, Blair GK, Shandley B: The prognosis of traumatic asphyxia in childhood, *J Pediatr Surg* 9:753–756, 1986.
84. Lee M, Wong S, Chu J, et al: Traumatic asphyxia, *Ann Thorac Surg* 51:86–88, 1991.
85. Landercasper J, Cogbill TH: Long term followup after traumatic asphyxia, *J Trauma* 25:838–841, 1985.
86. Baldwin GA, Macnab AJ, McCormick AQ: Visual loss following traumatic asphyxia in children, *J Trauma* 28:557–558, 1988.
87. Rosato RM, Shapiro MJ, Keegan MJ, et al: Cardiac injury complicating traumatic asphyxia, *J Trauma* 31:1387–1389, 1991.
88. Attar S, Hankins JR, Suter CM, et al: Esophageal perforation: a therapeutic challenge, *Ann Thorac Surg* 50:45–51, 1990.

89. Flynn AE, Verrier ED, Way LW, et al: Esophageal perforation, *Arch Surg* 124:1211–1215, 1989.
90. Glutterer MS, Toon RS, Eldestad C, et al: Management of blunt and penetrating external esophageal trauma, *J Trauma* 25:784–792, 1985.
91. Van der Zee DC, Festen C, Severijnen RSVM, et al: Management of pediatric esophageal perforation, *J Thorac Cardiol Surg* 95:692–695, 1988.
92. Janik JS, Bailey WC, Burrington JD: Occult coin perforation of the esophagus, *J Pediatr Surg* 92:794–797, 1986.
93. Nachman BJ: Asymptomatic esophageal perforation by a coin in a child, *Ann Emerg Med* 13:627–629, 1984.
94. Krasna IH, Rosenfield D, Benjamin BG, et al: Esophageal perforation in the neonate: an emergency problem in the newborn nursery, *J Pediatr Surg* 22:784–790, 1987.
95. Vandenplas Y, Delree M, Bougatef A, et al: Cervical esophageal perforation diagnosed by endoscopy in a premature infant: review of recent literature, *J Pediatr Gastro Nutr* 8:390–393, 1989.
96. Whiteley S, Liu PH, Tellez DW, et al: Esophageal rupture in an infant secondary to esophageal placement of a Foley catheter gastrostomy tube, *Pediatr Emerg Care* 5:113–116, 1989.
97. Bar-Maor JA, Hayari L: Pneumatic perforation of the esophagus in children, *J Pediatr Surg* 27:1532–1533, 1992.
98. Curci MR, Dibbens AW, Grimes CK: Compressed air injury to the esophagus: case report, *J Trauma* 29:1713–1715, 1989.
99. Conlan AA, Wessels A, Hammond CA, et al: Pharyngoesophageal barotrauma in children: a report of six cases, *J Thorac Cardiovasc Surg* 88:452–456, 1984.
100. Yap RG, Yap AG, Obeid FN, et al: Traumatic esophageal injuries: 12 year experience at Henry Ford Hospital, *J Trauma* 24:623–625, 1984.
101. Feliciano DV, Bitondo CG, Mattox KL, et al: Combined tracheoesophageal injuries, *Am J Surg* 150:710–715, 1985.

INJURIES WITH SPECIAL CONSIDERATIONS

10

Alkali and Chemical Injuries of the Esophagus

Michael W. Paluzzi

Ingestion of caustic substances is one of the most common intoxications leading to hospitalization of children in Western countries.[1] In the United States, despite legislation in the Safety Packaging Act of 1970 mandating child-resistant containers for the most dangerous chemicals (potassium hydroxide, sodium hydroxide, and sulfuric acid), an estimated 26,000 caustic ingestions still occur each year in pediatric patients.[2] The majority of ingestions occur in children less than 5 years of age. A wide variety of agents are implicated; the most common cause is ingestion of foreign bodies (e.g., dry ice, Clinitest tablets, button batteries) by a curious infant or young child. Familiarity with the classes of chemicals involved, their spectrum of injury, clinical presentations, evaluation, management, and prognosis is important for clinicians caring for children. This chapter discusses the major management considerations for chemical injury to the upper aerodigestive tract with emphasis on strong alkali exposures, which account for the greatest morbidity and mortality (Fig. 10–1).

CLASSIFICATION OF AGENTS

Caustic ingestion is a disease of young children. After 6 years of age the magnitude of the problem becomes negligible. Most reports, including all those mentioned here, describe a patient population less than 6 years of age.

Cleaning substances comprise the largest group of chemical ingestions in children.[3] These agents rarely cause significant injuries.[4,5] Denture cleaners are an exception because they contain caustic alkaline salts and are capable of causing significant esophageal injury. If the child is known or thought to have ingested denture cleaners, endoscopy should be routinely performed.[3,5] If significant injury is confirmed, management follows the principles outlined below. Stricture formation after cleaning substance ingestion is rare.

Household bleach and related products account for approximately 15% of

279

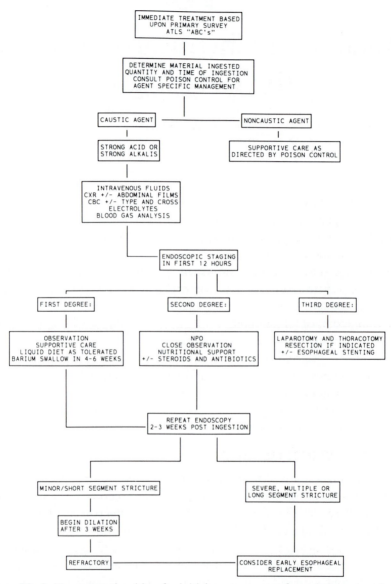

Figure 10–1. Treatment algorithm for initial management of caustic ingestions in children.

cleaning substances ingested by young children.[3] Sodium hypochlorite, the active ingredient in these products, is considered an esophageal irritant. It rarely causes significant injury beyond the mucosal level.[6–8] Patient management is geared to supportive care and is directed at the symptoms, which are usually minimal.[4,8,9]

Fifty-three percent of ammonia ingestions reported in 1990 occurred in children less than 6 years of age.[3] Ammonia solutions frequently result in esophageal burns, but these too are generally superficial and confined to the mucosa. Endoscopic evaluation is recommended.[9–11] Vigilant monitoring of respiratory status is important, since these solutions liberate ammonia vapors that may lead to pulmonary compromise.[9,12]

More than 1500 strong acid ingestions, usually of sulfuric, hydrochloric, or phosphoric acid, were reported in 1990 in children less than 6 years of age.[3] These products are mostly in the form of toilet bowl cleaners and disinfectants. Fortunately, these solutions cause clinically significant esophageal injury in less than 20% of patients.[12]

The most severe esophageal injuries are caused by lye ingestion (sodium or potassium hydroxide). In 1990 there were more than 13,000 reported pediatric ingestions of various forms of alkali, with 80% occurring in children under 6 years of age. Drain cleaners are the most common domestic source of strong alkalies, but these substances are also found in alkaline disk batteries and Clinitest tablets. Tablets and batteries tend to lodge at the level of the carina and cause thermal as well as caustic injury. Although deep, the burns are characteristically localized to a small area of the esophagus. Complications such as stricture formation can generally be managed nonoperatively or repaired by segmental resection with an esophageal end-to-end anastomosis.[1,3,14]

Of the more than 1900 button batteries reportedly ingested in 1990, most were hearing aid batteries, 40% of which came from the child's own hearing aid.[1,4] Corrosion of the battery results in leakage of its 45% solution of sodium or potassium hydroxide.[15,16] The vast majority of ingested batteries pass through the gastrointestinal tract harmlessly. If a battery becomes lodged in the esophagus, endoscopy should be performed to attempt removal and to evaluate concomitant injury. Subsequent management is based on the extent of the burn. Once the battery passes beyond the stomach, serial examinations, radiographs, close observation for signs of perforation, and monitoring of stool for passage of the battery are essential. Elimination generally occurs within a week but can be delayed up to 4 weeks.[16,17] Cathartics have been employed to shorten transit time.

MECHANISM OF INJURY

Acids cause a coagulation necrosis on contact with mucosal surfaces. The degree of injury is somewhat self-limited. The adherent coagulum that forms helps to protect unburned deeper tissues by preventing penetration of the caustic agent into deeper muscular layers. Strong acid products primarily damage the stomach, particularly the antrum and pylorus. The pylorus is extremely sensitive to caustic stimulation. Pylorospasm from contact with the ingested acid causes pooling of the agent in the antrum, resulting in concentration of the injury in this area. The degree of injury ranges from gastritis to full-thickness necrosis and perforation of the prepyloric antrum.[4,18-22] Strong acids are bitter to taste and result in immediate pain on contact with the oral mucosa. The child usually expectorates before much acid is actually swallowed. Because in most cases only a small quantity is ingested, the esophagogastric injury is usually limited in depth and extent.[4,5,18,22]

Conversely, ingested lye and other strong alkalies cause liquefaction necrosis.[5,10,11,22-24] The solvent action of alkali on contact with lipoprotein linings, such as the mucosa, results in denaturation of intracellular proteins, cell death, and acute necrosis.[5,10,22] After this initial phase the intense inflammatory reaction causes fat saponification and small vessel coagulation and thrombosis, resulting in necrosis of surrounding tissue.[24-26] Sloughing of the superficial necrotic layers occurs 2 to 4 days after the injury.[5,10] During the next week, fibroblasts infiltrate the wound and collagen deposition begins. The muscularis is replaced by fibrous tissue covered by a single layer of squamous epithelium devoid of glands.[11] Stricture formation results from scar contracture and is the most common delayed complication of esophageal burns. Strictures may be localized or involve the entire length of the esophagus. Evidence of stricture formation may be observed as early as 21 days after injury, but formation is usually not complete until 28 to 42 days and occasionally occurs as late as 9 to 12 months after injury.[10,23,27]

Ingestion of solid or crystalline lye-containing products results in significant esophageal burns in approximately 10% to 25% of cases. Approximately 30% of these burns cause some degree of stricture formation.[4,9-11,23] Solid products stick to the mucosa of the oropharynx and esophagus and rarely pass into the stomach in sufficient quantities to cause significant injury. The areas of the esophagus most susceptible to injury are regions of normal anatomic narrowing: the cricopharyngeus muscle, the aortic arch, the left mainstem bronchus, and the diaphragmatic hiatus or lower esophageal sphincter.[5,11]

In contrast, injury and stricture formation resulting from ingestion of liquid lye products are much more severe. An esophageal burn is diagnosed in 90% to 100% of patients with liquid lye ingestions, and 70% to 80% of those are second- or third-degree burns.[24,26-30] Animal studies have demonstrated that a 30-second exposure of the esophagus to 8.3% sodium hydroxide produces complete liquefaction of the mucosa and submucosa, with thrombosis of regional blood vessels.[31] When the agent reaches the pharynx, the cricopharyngeus muscle develops spasms and the esophagus propels the material into the stomach. The high viscosity of these liquids ensures that the ingested bolus will reach the stomach with full potency. Here it remains (because of a closed pyloric sphincter), churning between the esophagus and the pylorus and causing damage until it is neutralized.[32] Concomitant gastric injury is common. Its extent depends on a variety of factors, including the presence of residual food that can act as a buffer. The occurrence of necrosis is associated with a mortality rate approaching 100%. Death may occur from the development of severe mediastinitis with secondary sepsis, or as a result of various fistulas, such as tracheoesophageal, esophagoinnominate, or esophagoaortic. Fistula formation may occur within 72 hours or be delayed until 1 to 2 weeks after injury.[18,24]

The high mortality rate associated with transmural injury in liquid lye ingestion mandates an aggressive approach with rapid evaluation and early operative intervention to fully assess the extent of necrosis. Operative findings of full-thickness injury mandate radical resection such as esphagogastrectomy, which may be the only treatment method to prevent a fatal outcome.[27-30]

DIAGNOSIS AND MANAGEMENT

As with any traumatic injury, the patient is approached first with the intention of satisfying the ABCs of trauma care. Careful evaluation and meticulous attention to detail are essential. A careful, detailed history helps to determine the exact type and quantity of material ingested and the time of the incident. The composition (acid, alkali, liquid, solid) and the strength (percentage solution) of ingested material are the most important determinants of depth of injury.[33] Such information from the history of the event is particularly useful in directing diagnostic investigation and subsequent therapy.[5]

Several authors have suggested that the presence of symptoms is related to the extent of injury.[34,35] The absence of signs or symptoms in children with suspected chemical ingestions, particularly of caustic substances, does not rule out the presence or possibility of injury. Twelve percent of patients without symptoms after ingestion have second-degree burns at esophagoscopy.[36] Patients with second- or third-degree esophageal burns usually have at least two of three specific signs: drooling, spontaneous vomiting, or stridor. Presence of these symptoms may suggest a more selective approach toward invasive evaluation, but the classic approach is early and liberal endoscopic investigation.

Symptoms characteristic of strong alkali ingestion include vomiting (33%), dysphagia (25%), excessive salivation (24%), and epigastric pain (24%).[36] Respiratory distress, manifest as stridor or hemodynamic instability, is indicative of more severe injury. Again, absence of respiratory distress does not rule out laryngeal burns.[35]

Solid-state caustic substances stick to mucosal surfaces. Crystalline caustic materials characteristically cause oropharyngeal burns, whereas high-viscosity liquid caustic agents are easily swallowed and are more often associated with esophagogastric burns.[5,9,11,18] Approximately one in three children with oropharyngeal burns has esophageal burns. Oropharyngeal burns are absent in 2% to 15% of patients with clinically significant esophageal burns.[11,18,35,36]

Since all therapy is based on the presence and staging of esophageal burns, and since not all patients who have esophageal burns are symptomatic, timely and liberal use of esophagoscopy is recommended in evaluating this patient population.[9,11,36] Flexible endoscopy is most commonly performed, but rigid esophagoscopy is acceptable. The endoscopic modality employed depends on the skill and experience of the endoscopist. Endoscopy is performed within 24 to 48 hours of ingestion, and optimally within 12 to 24 hours.* Although several burn classification systems have been proposed, usually involving three degrees of injury, the most commonly used system is that first described by Hollinger. This system classifies the burn in a manner similar to burns of the skin[22,28,40]:

- First-degree burns exhibit mucosal hyperemia, edema, and superficial sloughing. This most superficial injury involves only the mucosa.
- Second-degree burns are characterized by patchy exudate, ulceration, blistering, and hyperemia.
- Third-degree injuries are full thickness and may be associated with erosion into the surrounding tissues.

Endoscopic identification of second- or third-degree burns is the most critical distinction, since it identifies the child at greatest risk.[4,5,9–11,27–30] Some practitioners advocate advancing a small endoscope beyond areas of circumferential injury. I believe the risk of further injury or perforation of devitalized tissue exceeds the theoretical benefits and does not improve the diagnostic yield or significantly alter management.†

If thorough esophagogastroduodenoscopy reveals no injury or only mild first-degree burns, management is simplified and supportive. The child is given a liquid diet and observed in the hospital overnight. It is important that these patients be reevaluated in 3 to 4 weeks. Cinefluoroscopy clearly identifies lesions if any symptoms suggestive of esophageal stricture develop.[5,9,11]

Early management of patients with severe second- or third-degree esophageal burns is mainly resuscitative. To prevent further injury, the patient is kept as quiet as possible. Emesis is discouraged to prevent reexposure of the esophagus to the burning agent, as well as to avoid placing the patient at risk for aspiration. Emetics and gastric lavage are contraindicated for the same reasons.

---

*References, 4, 6, 9–11, 18, 30, 37–39.
†References 4, 9–11, 22, 28, 30, 37, 40, 41.

Some clinicians encourage early oral intake for a diluent effect to neutralize the agent, but it is now generally accepted that heat produced in the neutralization reaction could exacerbate tissue damage. The child should have nothing by mouth.[4,12,28,37,40] A nasogastric tube may be placed at the time of endoscopy in children with second- or third-degree burns. The tube may then be used for gastric decompression and later for enteral nutrition. Blind nasogastric tube placement puts the patient at risk of perforation and should be avoided.[12] Chest roentgenography should be performed, intravenous fluids administered, and baseline electrolyte measurement and complete blood cell count performed.[5,11] Endoscopic evaluation is repeated in 2 to 3 weeks for all second- or third-degree burns.[5]

Following the initial stabilization and endoscopic staging, the patient remains in the hospital for close observation. Attention is turned to early recognition of acute complications such as perforation, and plans are initiated to address the most common long-term complication, stricture formation. Corrosive injury is the most common cause of pediatric esophageal strictures.[18,37] Methods used in an attempt to minimize stricture formation include pharmacologic, mechanical, and surgical regimens. The standard medical regimen includes steroid and antibiotic administration. Bougienage and surgical placement of esophageal stents are the mechanical and surgical modalities most often employed.

Intravenous steroid administration was first described as having a beneficial effect in preventing experimental esophageal strictures when applied in an animal model.[42] Since then, a wide variety of reports suggest a possible beneficial role in second-degree injuries in humans; however, the data are inconclusive.* Anderson, in a prospective randomized study of 60 children with esophageal burns, failed to prove a significant benefit from steroid treatment.[47] The risk of esophageal stricture was related only to the severity of injury. Hawkins found that in patients with second-degree burns, only one stricture occurred in seven patients treated with steroids versus four strictures in five patients treated without steroids.[9] Others report similar results in patients with second-degree burns treated with steroids and antibiotics.[11,12,23,25] Burn inflammatory changes occur early and are thought to contribute to stricture formation. To be effective, steroids must be administered immediately after confirmation of second-degree esophageal burns.

Most authors agree that steroid use has no value in preventing stricture formation in patients with third-degree injury and that in fact steroids may lead to a more complicated course. Steroids should not be routinely used in liquid alkali ingestions, since these burns are usually transmural.[28] Steroid use sup-

---

*References 4, 9–11, 19–23, 26–28, 33, 40, 43–47.

presses the normal inflammatory responses of injury, which may increase the risk of infection. Antibiotics are routinely used concurrently with steroid administration.[19,23] A common regimen consists of methylprednisolone (2 mg/kg in divided doses) or equivalent for a 3-week course and ampicillin (10 to 50 mg/kg every 6 hours) for 7 days or longer if the patient remains febrile.[5] Fever that persists for more than 2 weeks without an obvious source may be indicative of mediastinitis or peritonitis or may indicate a localized abscess in the mediastinum or abdomen.[28] Computed tomography and magnetic resonance imaging are useful for narrowing the differential diagnosis in these particularly complex patients.

Oral fluids are given as soon as the child is able to swallow his or her own saliva. The diet is cautiously advanced as tolerated. Histamine (H_2) antagonists or oral antacids are administered for 6 to 8 weeks after middle or distal esophageal injuries to prevent secondary injury from reflux. If the child cannot eat within 3 days, parenteral or enteral nutrition is initiated.[5,11,22,35]

Esophageal dilation with Malony mercury-filled dilators or Savory dilators threaded over a wire and passed under fluoroscopic guidance can be used to reduce the degree of stricture formation. Esophageal dilation as a management option was first shown effective in experimental injuries.[48] Both antegrade and retrograde methods have been employed at various times after injury in humans. The optimal time to begin dilation is 3 weeks after ingestion. Dilation is repeated every 7 to 10 days as needed to allow the child to tolerate a regular diet.[5,11] Dilation results in a prohibitively high perforation rate when attempted before 3 weeks after injury.[23,28,40,44-46] Once the esophagus is perforated, either iatrogenically or as a result of caustic erosion, esophageal replacement is the only viable option.[41] Dilation is most successful when employed in patients with short-segment strictures.

Principles of intraluminal splinting of full-thickness esophageal lye burns were developed and proved effective in experimental strictures in cats.[49,50] The technique was successfully applied in three children and one adult.[51] After endoscopic confirmation of third-degree burns, laparotomy is performed. A Silastic intraluminal esophageal stent is placed under direct endoscopic guidance. The proximal end of the stent is positioned 5 to 10 mm above the cricopharyngeus, and the distal end undergoes direct intragastric fixation. A nasogastric feeding tube may be passed through the stent and used for tube feedings. The stent remains in place for 3 weeks. During this time the patient is positioned with the head of the bed elevated 45 degrees to prevent aspiration. Chest roentgenograms are performed three times weekly to ensure correct stent placement. The child is restrained as necessary. The splint is removed under general anesthesia in 21 days, and esophagoscopy is performed. The first meal is thick barium, which is followed by cinefluoroscopy and plain films to define baseline anatomy.

A liquid diet is then given for 2 days with progression to regular diet by day 7.[51] Hill and associates[52] applied this technique and reported excellent results in two toddlers. In 1986 Estrera and co-workers[30] reported 62 caustic ingestions; 27 of these caused severe esophagogastric burns, which were treated with intraluminal splinting in 6 patients. Four patients healed without sequelae, and 2 required subsequent dilation for localized stricture.[30]

Some authors suggest a benefit from nasogastric tube placement alone as an effective esophageal stent.[9,21,53] Wijburg and co-workers[53] reported on 32 patients in whom "deep circular burns" were treated with a siliconized nasogastric tube. Strictures developed in only two patients, but the specific agents involved were not reported.[53]

PROGNOSIS

The severity of the esophageal burn injury is related to the strength and composition of the ingested material. The severity of the primary injury is the main determinant of development and degree of esophageal stricture formation.[46] Multiple areas of full-thickness injury have a high potential for stricture formation, regardless of the initial management.[32,33,44,54] Once strictures are formed, approximately one third respond to dilation.[33,46] Patients with multiple strictures or a single long stricture are less likely to respond to dilation and should be considered for early esophageal replacement. A colonic segment is the most commonly used conduit for reconstruction.[5,53] Expected complications of esophageal replacement include aspiration (25%), cervical restenosis (19%), cervical anastomotic leak (5%), and colonic necrosis (5%).[55]

Lye ingestion is implicated as a risk factor for esophageal carcinoma.[4,22] In one review of 2414 cases of esophageal carcinoma, 2.6% of patients had a history of lye ingestion in childhood. All these patients had squamous cell carcinoma; 84% of lesions were found at or just below the carina. The mean age at diagnosis of esophageal cancer is significantly lower (48 versus 70 years) than for those with no history of lye ingestion. Patients with history of lye ingestion may have a risk of esophageal carcinoma 1000 times greater than the general population.[56]

SUMMARY

Alkali and other chemical injuries to the esophagus in children result in a significant number of emergency department visits. The strong liquid alkalies cause the greatest injury and require vigilant monitoring and aggressive management. Early endoscopy is essential for diagnosis and is necessary to direct appropriate therapy. The use of parenteral antibiotics to reduce septic complications is important, but parenteral steroids are of questionable value. Expedient surgical intervention for significant or complicated injuries is essential and may be lifesaving. Currently available surgical procedures include intraesophageal stent placement and radical resection with subsequent colon interposition. Patients with esophageal burns require long-term follow-up, since late strictures develop in as many as 20%. These patients also have a 1000-fold increased risk of esophageal carcinoma compared with the general population.

REFERENCES

1. Cello JP, Fagel RP, Boland CR: Liquid caustic ingestion: spectrum of injury, *Arch Intern Med* 140:501–504, 1980.
2. Lovejoy FH: Corrosive injury of the esophagus in children, *N Engl J Med* 323:668–669, 1990.
3. Litovitz TL, Bailey KM, Schmitz BF, et al: 1990 annual report of the American Association of Poison Control Centers national data collection system, *J Emerg Med* 9:461–509, 1991.
4. Moore WH: Caustic ingestions, pathophysiology, diagnosis and treatment, *Clin Pediatr* 25:192, 1986.
5. Roghstein FC: Caustic injuries to the esophagus in children, *Pediatr Clin* 33:665, 1986.
6. Abramson AL: Corrosive injury to the esophagus, *Arch Otol* 104:514, 1978.
7. Weeks RS, Ravitch MN: Esophageal injury by liquid chlorine bleach: experimental study, *J Pediatr* 74:911, 1969.
8. Yarrington CT: The experimental causticity of sodium hypochlorite in the esophagus, *Ann Otol* 79:895, 1970.
9. Hawkins DB, Daxmeter MJ, Barnett TE: Caustic ingestion: controversies in management: a review of 214 cases, *Laryngoscope* 90:98, 1980.
10. Adam JS, Birch HG: Pediatric caustic ingestion, *Ann Otol Rhinol Laryngol* 91:656, 1982.
11. Haller JA Jr, Andrews HG, White JJ, et al: Pathophysiology and management of acute corrosive burns of the esophagus: results of treatment in 285 children, *J Pediatr Surg* 6:578, 1971.
12. Daly JF, Cardona JC: Acute corrosive esophagitis, *Arch Otol* 74:629, 1961.
13. Maull KI, Scher LA, Greenfield LJ: Surgical implications of acid ingestion, *Surg Gynecol Obstet* 148:895, 1979.
14. Burrington JD: Clinitest burns of the esophagus, *Ann Thorac Surg* 29:400, 1975.
15. Litovitz TL: Battery ingestions: product accessibility and clinical course, *Pediatrics* 75(16):349, 1985.
16. Litovitz TL: Button battery ingestions, *JAMA* 249(15):2495, 1983.
17. Votteler TP, Nash JC, Rutledge JC: The legend of ingested alkaline disk batteries in children, *JAMA* 249(14):2504, 1983.
18. Ashcraft KW, Holder TM, eds: *Pediatric esophageal surgery,* New York, 1986, Grune & Stratton, pp 73–88.
19. Steigman F, Dolehide RA: Corrosive (acid) gastritis: management of early and late cases, *N Engl J Med* 254:981, 1956.
20. Chong QC, Beahrs OH, Palyne WS: Management of corrosive gastritis due to ingested acid, *Mayo Clin Proc* 49:861, 1974.
21. Citron BP, Pincus IJ, Geokas MC, Huverback BJ: Chemical trauma of the esophagus and stomach, *Surg Clin North Am* 48:1303, 1968.

22. Goldman LP, Weigart JM: Corrosive substance ingestion: a review, *Am J Gastroenterol* 79:85, 1984.
23. Haller JA Jr, Bachman K: The comparative effect of current therapy on experimental caustic burns of the esophagus, *Pediatrics* 34:236–245, 1964.
24. Ray JF, Myers WO, Lawton BR: The natural history of liquid lye ingestion: rationale for aggressive surgical approach, *Arch Surg* 109:436, 1974.
25. Allen RE, Thoshinsky MJ, Stalone RJ: Corrosive injuries of the stomach, *Arch Surg* 100:409, 1970.
26. Leape LL, Ashcraft KW, Scarpell DG: Hazard to health—liquid lye, *N Engl J Med* 284:578, 1971.
27. Ritter FN, Gago O, Kirsh MM, et al: The rationale of emergency esophagogastrectomy in the treatment of liquid caustic burns of the esophagus and stomach, *Ann Otol Rhinol Laryngol* 80:513, 1971.
28. Kirsh MM, Peterson KA, Brown JW, et al: Treatment of caustic injuries of the esophagus: a ten year experience, *Ann Surg* 188:675, 1978.
29. Gago O, Ritler FN, Marte IW: Aggressive surgical treatment of caustic injury of the esophagus and stomach, *Ann Thorac Surg* 13:243, 1972.
30. Estera A, et al: Corrosive burns of the esophagus and stomach: a recommendation for an aggressive surgical approach, *Ann Thorac Surg* 41:276, 1986.
31. Ashcraft KW, Padula RT: The effect of dilute corrosives on the esophagus, *Pediatrics* 53:226–232, 1974.
32. Kirsh MM, Ritter F: Caustic ingestion and subsequent damage to the oropharyngeal and digestive passages, *Ann Thorac Surg* 21:74–82, 1986.
33. Moazam F, Talbert JL, Miller D, Mollett DL: Caustic ingestion and its sequelae in children, *South Med J* 80:187–190, 1987.
34. Crain EF, Gershel JC, Mezy AP: Caustic ingestions: symptoms as predictors of esophageal injury, *Am J Dis Child* 138:863, 1984.
35. Lovejoy FH: Corrosive injury of the esophagus in children, *N Engl J Med* 323:668–669, 1990.
36. Gaudrealeaut P, Parent M, McGuigan MA, et al: Predictability of esophageal injury from signs and symptoms: a study of caustic ingestion in 378 children, *Pediatrics* 71:767, 1983.
37. Cotton R, Fearon B: Esophageal strictures in infants and children, *Can J Otol* 1:224, 1972.
38. Sellars SL, Spence RAJ: Chemical burns of the oesophagus, *J Laryngol Otol* 101:1211, 1987.
39. Sugawa C, Mullins RJ, Lucas CE, Leibold WC: The value of early endoscopy following caustic ingestion, *Surg Gynecol Obstet* 153:553, 1981.
40. Hollinger PH: Management of esophageal lesions caused by chemical burn, *Ann Otol* 77:819, 1968.
41. Cardona JC, Daly JF: Current management of corrosive esophagitis—an evaluation of results in 239 cases, *Ann Otol* 80:521, 1971.
42. Rosenberg N, Kunderman DJ, Vroman L, Moolten SE: Prevention of experimental lye strictures of the esophagus by cortisone, *Arch Surg* 63, 1951.
43. Webb WR, Koutrus P, Ecker RR: An evaluation of steroids and antibiotics in caustic burns of the esophagus, *Ann Thorac Surg* 9:95, 1970.
44. Oakes DD, Shick JP, Mark JBD: Lye ingestion: clinical patterns and therapeutic implications, *J Thorac Cardiovasc Surg* 83:19, 1982.

45. Middlekamp MD, et al: The management and problems of caustic burns in children, *J Thorac Cardiovasc Surg* 57:341, 1969.

46. Ferguson MK, Migliore M, Stuszak VM, Little AG: Early evaluation and therapy for caustic esophageal injury, *Am J Surg* 157:116–120, 1989.

47. Anderson KD, et al: A controlled trial of corticosteroids in children with corrosive injury of the esophagus, *N Engl J Med* 323:637–640, 1990.

48. Knox WA, Scott JR, Zintel HA, et al: Bougienage and steroids used singularly or in combination in experimental corrosive esophagitis, *Ann Surg* 166:930, 1967.

49. Fell SC, Dinize A, Becker N, Hursitt ES: The effect of intraluminal splinting in the prevention of caustic stricture of the esophagus, *J Thorac Cardiovasc Surg* 52:675, 1986.

50. Reyes HM, Lin CY, Schluink FF, Reploge RL: Experimental treatment of corrosive esophageal burns, *J Pediatr Surg* 9:317, 1974.

51. Reyes HM, Hill JL: Modification of experimental stent technique for esophageal burns, *J Surg Res* 20:65, 1976.

52. Hill JL, Norberg HP, Smith MD, et al: Clinical technique and success of the esophageal stent to prevent esophageal stricture, *J Pediatr Surg* 11:443, 1976.

53. Wijgurg FA, Beakers MW, Hegmans HS, et al: Nasogastric intubation as sole treatment of caustic esophageal lesions, *Ann Otol Rhinol Laryngol* 94:337, 1985.

54. Belsey RHR: Corrosive strictures of the esophagus. In DeMeester T, Skinner DB, eds: *Esophageal disorders: pathophysiology and therapy,* New York, 1985, Raven Press, pp 261–269.

55. Berkowitz WP, Roger CL, Sessions DG, et al: Surgical management of severe lye burns of the esophagus by colon intraposition, *Ann Otol* 84:576, 1975.

56. Appleqvist P, Salmo M: Lye corrosion carcinoma of the esophagus, *Cancer* 45:2655, 1980.

11

Burn Injury

James E. Foster, II
Edward G. Ford

Human beings have had to deal with the consequences of burn injuries since their association with fire in prehistoric times. The treatment of burn wounds was directed for many generations by regional folklore or religious teachings rather than by principles based on the scientific method. The apparent earliest recorded treatment for burn wounds is found within the Papyrus Ebers dating from 1600 BC. The recipes found within this papyrus include various plants and animal parts that were cooked into a liniment and applied to the burn.[1] Chinese writings from the fifth and sixth centuries BC described similar remedies derived from teas. The Romans often debated the efficacy of emollients, astringents, and exposure therapy.

In the *Apologie Treatise Containing the Voyages Made into Divers Places with Many Writings upon Surgery,* Ambroise Pare described differences in physical injury with various types of traumatic wounds and commented on the identifying characteristics of partial- and full-thickness burns. Although his descriptions were quite detailed, his burn wound therapy still referred to mixtures first documented at the time of the Roman Empire:

> One of the Marshall of *Montejan* his Kitchin boyes, fell by chance into a Caldron of Oyle being even almost boyling hot; I being called to dresse him, went to the next Apothecaries to fetch refrigerating medicines commonly used in this case; there was present by chance a certaine old countrey woman, who hearing that I desired medicines for a burne, perswaded mee at the first dressing, that I should lay to raw Onions beaten with a little salt; for so I should hinder the breaking out of blisters or pustules, as shee had found by certaine and frequent experience. Wherefore I thought good to try the force of her Medicine upon this greasy scullion. I the next day found those places of his body whereto the Onions lay, to bee free from blisters, but the other parts which they had not touched, to be all blistered.[2]

During the 300 years following the observations of Pare, the study of burns remained primarily descriptive.

The first modern understanding of the pathophysiology and related treatment of burn wounds occurred between World Wars I and II. That was the time at which the physical and physiologic differences among environmental burns, flame burns, scald injuries, and phosphorous-type burns became apparent. The U.S. Army Surgical Research Unit at the Brooke Army Medical Center in San Antonio, Texas, provided a central focus for advances in burn wound treatment, grafting, treatment of associated complications, and nutritional support of burned patients. Care specifically directed to children with burn wound injuries began in Galveston, Texas, in 1962 with the establishment of the first Shriner's Hospital for Crippled Children Burn Institute. The Galveston Shriner's Hospital and subsequent Shriner's Burn Centers in Cincinnati and Boston have made major contributions to the understanding and specialized treatment of burn injuries in the pediatric population.[3]

Although our environmental association with fire has been modified somewhat since prehistoric times, thermal injury remains a significant cause of injury and death. Vectors of thermal injury include hot liquids and solids, flammable fabrics, volatile combustible liquids, and combustible portions of domestic dwellings. Common igniters include matches, poorly protected space heaters, kitchen ranges, and water heaters. Scalds are the leading cause of burn injury during the first 3 years of life (50% of all injuries), whereas flame burns are usually seen in older children.

Burn injuries are the second leading cause of nonvehicular accidental death in the United States. Acute medical care for burn injuries accounts for approximately 2 million emergency center patient visits a year in the United States. One hundred thousand patients a year require hospitalization, and approximately 7800 of those die as a direct result of their burn injuries. Thirty percent of burn-related deaths are of children less than 15 years of age, with most of those occurring in the home between 6 PM and midnight. Burns are the second leading cause of death in the home for children between 1 and 4 years of age and the third leading cause of accidental home death in children 5 to 14 years of age.[4-7]

Disability and rehabilitation from burn injury have significant long-term economic consequences for the child, the family, and the health care system. Any estimate of economic impact depends a great deal on assumptions made in determining indirect costs that may be generated from premature death or prolonged disability. The Consumer Product Safety Commission (CPSC) has developed an injury cost model that estimates the cost of burn injury to a child to range from $40,750 to $77,350, depending on the child's age. In 1985, 1461 children (up to 19 years of age) died as a result of burn injury in the United States. A total of 23,638 children were hospitalized out of 440,000 children who were treated for burns in emergency centers. Of those burns,

92.3% were considered unintentional. Considering the entire 1985 burned pediatric population, 101,000 life-years and 389 million dollars in productivity were lost as a direct result of fire and burn deaths. The cost of the nonfatal injuries included 383 million dollars for medical care, 221 million dollars for disability and rehabilitative services and 116 million dollars for "other" direct and indirect costs. "Pain and suffering" were valued by the CPSC model at 2.8 billion dollars. Therefore the total cost of pediatric burn injuries in 1985 was approximately 3.5 billion dollars.[8] Clearly, prevention of burn injuries is the best treatment strategy. Fire prevention, education, improved product safety, reduced flammability of common igniters, and an organized approach to education of the public must be supported to spare children the effects of a major burn injury.

DEFINITIONS

Proper assessment and classification of burn wounds aid in treatment planning, communication between providers at different levels of care, evaluation of outcomes, and determination of the effectiveness of various therapeutic interventions. The following definitions are standard. A classification of the severity of burn injury is presented in Table 11–1.

Assessment of Burn Depth[9,10]

First-degree burns. A first-degree burn involves the epidermis (Fig. 11–1) and is characterized by erythema and mild discomfort. Tissue damage is minimal, and skin integrity is maintained. Pain is the primary symptom and

Table 11–1. Severity of Burn Injury

Classification	Criteria
Critical	Second degree involving >30% TBSA
	Third degree involving >10% TBSA
	Any burn with respiratory tract injury or fracture or in critical area (face, hands, feet, perineum)
	High-voltage electrical burn
	Burn associated with significant preexisting disease
Moderate	Second degree involving 15%-20% TBSA
	Third degree involving 2%–10% TBSA
	(Above not to include critical areas)
Minor	Second degree involving <15% TBSA
	Third degree involving <2% TBSA
	(Above not to include critical areas)

Data from Demling RH: Burns. In Greenfield LJ, ed: *Surgery: scientific principles and practice*, Philadelphia, 1990, WB Saunders, pp 1–11.
TBSA, Total body surface area.

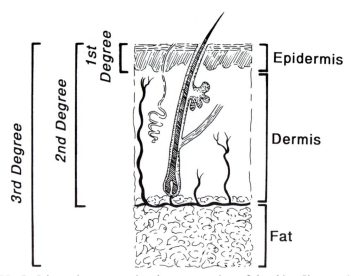

Figure 11–1. Schematic cross-sectional representation of the skin. Characteristic areas of injury are identified for first-degree, second-degree (superficial and deep), and full-thickness (third-degree) burns.

generally resolves within 72 hours. Damaged epithelium peels off in 5 to 7 days with no residual scarring. Sunburn and brief scalding episodes are the most common examples (Fig. 11–2).

Second-degree burns. A second-degree burn involves the entire epidermis layer and various amounts of underlying dermis. These are often referred to as

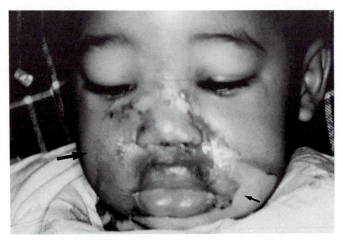

Figure 11–2. First-degree *(large arrow)* and second-degree *(small arrow)* burns of the face following scalding with hot water.

partial-thickness burns and are subclassified as superficial or deep (Fig. 11–3).

Superficial second-degree burns. Injury involves the outer one third of the dermis (see Fig. 11–1). Capillaries are damaged, and increased local vascular permeability leads to leakage of plasma into the interstitial space with subsequent blister formation. Wounds heal in 7 to 14 days by rapid reepithelialization from deep dermal skin appendages. Scarring is minimal.

Deep second-degree burns. Injury extends deep into the dermis (see Fig. 11–1), with a significant reduction in the number of viable deep dermal epithelial cells. Reepithelization is extremely slow. Pain is present but at a lesser degree than in superficial injuries. Blister formation is unusual, although fluid loss from damaged vessels is significant. Fluid losses and metabolic effects are similar to those of third-degree burns (see the following discussion). Dense scarring results if the wounds are not grafted.

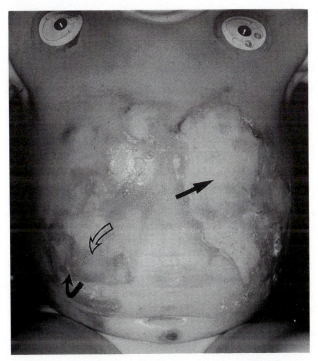

Figure 11–3. A 3-year-old who was burned by pulling hot coffee from a tabletop. The chest wounds show characteristic changes of second-degree (partial-thickness) burns. These burns are characterized by blister formation *(curved solid arrow)*. Areas of more superficial burn are characterized by slight erythema with punctate areas of epithelialization *(open arrow)*. Deep, second-degree burns are whiter in color, with fewer of the epidermal appendages evident around hair follicles *(solid straight arrow)*. These burns are painful when touched.

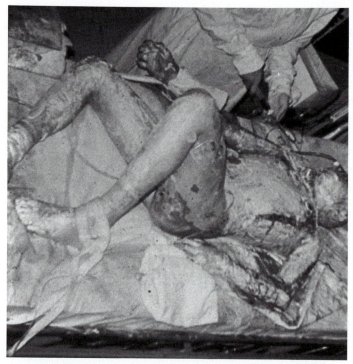

Figure 11–4. A child with third-degree burns. The skin has an opalescent, waxy appearance. Dermal blood vessels have thrombosed, and all dermal neural elements have been destroyed. The skin has a leathery texture and may cause extremity constriction as edema increases in tissues beneath the burn wound.

Third-degree burns. Injury is full thickness, with the entire epidermis and dermis destroyed (see Fig. 11–1). The skin has a waxy, avascular appearance (Fig. 11–4). Pain is absent because of destruction of dermal nerve endings. Painlessness differentiates full-thickness from partial-thickness burns. The most common cause of third-degree burns is a short exposure to a very high temperature, such as a flame burn or prolonged contact with a hot liquid.

IMMEDIATE MANAGEMENT

The immediate management of a burn injury usually comes under the purview of the family or local emergency services. The first consideration is to stop the burning process. Clothing that has been exposed to flames or hot water may retain heat for long periods. Synthetic fibers may melt when exposed to high temperatures, then stick to a patient's skin and concentrate heat exposure to localized areas. Chemicals and solvents may be absorbed by clothing fabric and held next to the skin for long periods. The degree of burn injury (heat, chemical, or scald) is related to the degree of heat or concentration of chemicals and the length of time the burning agent is applied to the skin. All clothing should be immediately removed from the patient.

The patient suffering chemical burns should have the exposed skin irrigated with large quantities of water to dilute the chemical agent. Attempts to use specific neutralizing agents may result in unexpected chemical reactions and heat generation and should be avoided. In the hemodynamically stable patient, prolonged irrigation (30 to 60 minutes) may be particularly beneficial in alkali burns. Prompt irrigation of chemical burns also decreases the potential for absorption of toxic elements. Since exposing the patient's skin by clothing removal and irrigation of chemical burns may predispose the patient to hypothermia, the patient should be covered with clean, dry sheets or dressings as soon as possible.[4,9,10]

Airway

Neutralization of the burning source does not take precedence over rapid assessment of the patient's airway. Early death in burn victims is often due to inhalation of smoke toxins or carbon monoxide poisoning. Airway injury may also occur as a result of thermal effects.

Inhalation injuries are commonly present in patients who are burned in a closed space such as a small building, basement, or mobile home. These patients often have burns of the face, singed nasal hairs, hoarseness or wheezing, or carbonaceous sputum. The upper airway (oropharynx, larynx, and upper trachea) absorbs most of the thermal energy, so heat injuries are usually confined to the upper aerodigestive tract. An important exception is the patient who is exposed to activated steam. Steam carries thermal energy to even the smallest airways and causes distal bronchial injury. No test reliably predicts the degree of airway injury. Fiberoptic laryngoscopy and bronchoscopy are sensitive and specific both for identifying injury on admission and for follow-up examinations. The most important management concerns for upper airway injuries are recognition and a realization that inhalational injuries are progressive. Laryngeal edema increases during the first 18 to 24 hours; airway injury mandates early intubation for airway control.[9,11]

Endotracheal intubation is indicated in patients with deep facial burns, inhalation injury demonstrated by laryngoscopy or bronchoscopy, and massive burns of the upper torso where ventilation compromise caused by decreased chest wall compliance may be anticipated. Tube size should be appropriate for the child's age, with the understanding that a larger endotracheal tube permits better tracheobronchial toilet if progressive lung injury develops. Tracheostomy in the early period after the burn should be avoided. Ventilatory support is instituted with administration of humidified oxygen. Inspired oxygen concentrations of 90% to 100% are indicated for the treatment of carbon monoxide toxicity. Continuous positive airway pressure or positive end-expiratory pressure is indicated to maintain an adequate functional residual capacity in the presence of progressive airway edema. Full-thickness burns to the upper torso may lead to severe impairment of ventilation from impaired chest wall compliance as edema develops deep to the inelastic burn eschar. Significant chest wall restriction must be relieved by chest wall escharotomy. Anesthesia is not necessary for escharotomy. The full thickness of eschar is sharply incised to the subcutaneous tissues. Bilateral incisions are made in the anterior axillary lines and connected across the anterior surface by a subcostal incision (Fig. 11–5). This technique is also applicable to circumferential extremity burns when neurovascular compromise develops from progressive tissue edema. Escharotomy wounds are dressed with topical antimicrobial preparations, as discussed later in the chapter.[11]

Humidified oxygen, chest physiotherapy, aerosol bronchodilators, and frequent repositioning assist in maintaining adequate small airway patency. The risk of pulmonary infections in burned patients is greatest from the seventh to fourteenth day after injury. Although prophylactic systemic antibiotics are not indicated for either pulmonary infection or the burn wound, diligent surveillance of the bronchial secretions assists in detecting bacterial bronchitis before the development of pneumonia. Pathogen-specific therapy should be instituted as soon as culture results indicate a proliferating pathogen. The length of time to maintain artificial airway control and ventilation depends on the patient's management course. Tissue edema may begin to resolve in 48 to 72 hours. A

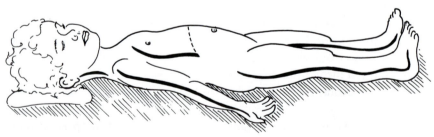

Figure 11–5. Third-degree burn wounds that gird an extremity or the torso may restrict normal physiologic functions. In the chest, ventilation may become difficult as compliance is restricted. In the extremity, progressive tissue edema may lead to neurovascular compromise. Incision through the burn wound (burn wound escharotomy) relieves such pressure and allows increased compliance of the chest cavity and return of perfusion to the distal extremities. Escharotomy incisions are placed laterally on the torso and medially and laterally on the extremities. The lateral chest wounds are connected via incision over the anterior portion of the chest.

predictable decrease in pulmonary function occurs after each debridement or excision of inflamed or infected eschar. Early burn wound excision and grafting may require prolonged intubation because of repeated operations and the use of significant quantities of narcotic analgesics. Metabolic demands can also be reduced by decreasing the work of breathing and maintaining mechanical support. The decision to extubate the burned patient is based on the following[12,13]:

- General condition of the patient
- Return of adequate respiratory mechanics
- Subsidence of edema
- Development of an air leak, indicating lessening of airway edema
- Character of secretions; sooty secretions or evidence of pulmonary infection should militate against extubation
- Clearing of pulmonary infiltrates
- Successful pattern of weaning from assisted ventilation
- Timing; extubation should occur at a time that the patient can be carefully observed for recurrent obstruction or respiratory insufficiency
- Planning; the patient should not be extubated if surgery is planned for the following day

Carbon monoxide is a product of incomplete combustion and binds to hemoglobin approximately 200 times more readily than does oxygen. Carbon monoxide toxicity should be suspected in patients with ruby red lips or mucosal surfaces and in patients with a persistent and profound metabolic acidosis despite restoration of adequate tissue perfusion. The diagnosis is confirmed by elevated carboxyhemoglobin levels. Treatment for carbon monoxide poisoning is the early administration of high concentrations of inhaled oxygen. Since all trauma protocols for field management of injured patients include the use of high-flow oxygen, most patients with carbon monoxide poisoning will have already received treatment before arrival in the emergency center. The half-life of carboxyhemoglobin is approximately 30 minutes when the patient is treated with 90% to 100% oxygen. Thus it is not uncommon to find normal carboxyhemoglobin levels even in patients with severe torso and facial burns or those who may have been injured in closed spaces. For patients with persistently elevated carboxyhemoglobin levels, hyperbaric oxygen therapy may return the oxygen levels to normal more expeditiously. These patients are extremely rare.[9,11]

Fluid Management

Airway and ventilation management is followed by determination of the patient's burn size and estimation of fluid requirements. Children have a larger body surface/weight ratio than adults. The larger surface area leads to relatively larger evaporative fluid losses, which must be considered during fluid resuscitation and temperature regulation.

Burn size in children over 10 years of age may be accurately estimated with the Rule of Nines (Table 11–2).[10] Estimation of burn size in younger children should be guided by the use of a Lund-Browder burn chart (Fig. 11–6).[14] Reasonable estimates of the burn surface area may also be based on the observation that the area of the *patient's* palm is approximately 1% of his or her total body surface area (TBSA). The presence of soot, burned clothing, and singed hair may lead to an initial overestimation of burn size. Calculation of the TBSA burned should be made after the wounds are cleaned and debrided. The original estimate of TBSA must be accurate because it is the basis for initial fluid management.

Calculated fluid requirements for the first 24 hours are usually supplied as crystalloid. One half of the estimated requirements is provided in the first 8 hours, and the second half is provided over the subsequent 16 hours. These estimates are from the time of burn injury, not from the time of arrival in the emergency center. If a patient arrives in the emergency center 4 hours after the time of burn injury, half of the fluid requirement would be administered during the first 4 hours in the hospital, that is, within 8 hours from the burn. Several formulas are available, each using a different calculation schema (weight in kilograms, percent body surface area burned, square meter of surface area) and each varying slightly on the type of fluid administered (Table 11–3).[15] We consider each of the formulas to be appropriate and suggest the emergency center provider choose the formula he or she prefers. Fluids should be administered by peripheral venous catheters preferentially placed through nonburned skin. Peripheral venous catheters placed through the burn wound and central venous catheters should be avoided until all other peripheral sites have been exhausted. Vascular access through areas of burned tissue is associated with a higher rate of septic complication and should be used only if access through nonburned tissue cannot be obtained. Reliable access may be established in

Table 11–2. Rule of Nines for Estimating Percentage of Body Surface Involved in Burns

Anatomic Area	Percent of Body Surface
Head	9
Right upper extremity	9
Left upper extremity	9
Right lower extremity	18
Left lower extremity	18
Anterior trunk	18
Posterior trunk	18
Neck	1

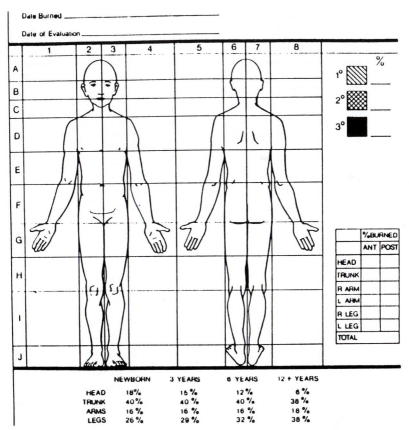

Figure 11-6. Lund-Browder burn chart for estimation of burn wound size. The percentage a given body part contributes to total surface area is age dependent and indicated in the lower portion of the chart.

pediatric patients by performing a cut-down over the long saphenous vein at the ankle. This vessel is reliably found 1 cm anterior and 1 cm superior to the medial malleolus. The surgeon exposes the vein by making a 1 cm transverse incision through the skin and gently spreading the subcutaneous tissues. The vein should be immediately apparent. Central venous catheters are much less efficient in delivering the large fluid volumes required in burn resuscitation, so they should be reserved primarily for monitoring.

Fluid resuscitation is begun with the objective of maintaining adequate tissue perfusion. See Table 11-4 for a sample administration plan. Adequate tissue perfusion correlates with a urine output of 1 to 1.5 ml/kg/hr. Overresuscitation in infants and children may rapidly lead to pulmonary edema. The initial fluid estimates by the standard formulas are simply *estimates* of fluid

Table 11-3. Standard Formulas for Estimating Fluid Requirements for Burned Children for the First 24 Hours of Therapy

Formula	Fluid Type	First 24 Hours
Parkland	Colloid	None
	Electrolyte	4 ml/kg/% burn
	Glucose in water	None
Brooke	Colloid*	1.5 ml/kg/% burn
	Electrolyte†	0.5 ml/kg/% burn
	Glucose in water	2000 ml
Evans	Colloid	1 ml/kg/% burn
	Electrolyte	1 ml/kg/% burn
	Glucose in water	2000 ml
Carvajal (1975)	Electrolyte with 12.5 g human serum albumin per liter	5000 ml/m² body surface area burned + 2000 ml/sq total body surface area

*Colloid = plasmanate, plasma, dextran.
†Electrolyte = Ringer's lactate.

requirements. Approximately 50% of patients require adjustment of the fluid rate to maintain the desired urine output.[16] The main total fluid replacement may be as high as 6.3 ± 2.2 ml/kg/percent TBSA in children.[17]

Maintenance of adequate hemodynamic stability in the early period after the burn includes ensuring adequate oxygen-carrying capacity with attention to plasma volume and red blood cell mass. Cardiac output and oxygen consumption increase by two to three times immediately after injury. Intravascular volume decreases as tissue edema "leaks" into the interstitial space. This process is

Table 11-4. Administration of Fluids Calculated with the Parkland Formula

First 24 Hours

Electrolyte solution (lactated Ringer's): 4 ml/kg body wt/percent of second- and third-degree burn
Administration rate: one half in first 8 hours, one fourth in second 8 hours, one fourth in third 8 hours
Urine output: 30 to 70 ml/hr

Second 24 Hours

Glucose in water (D_5W): To replace evaporative water loss, maintaining serum sodium concentration of 140 mEq/L
Colloid solution (plasma): To maintain plasma volume in patients with more than 40% second- and third-degree burns
Urine output: 30 to 100 ml/hr

accentuated in burn patients with concomitant inhalation injury.[13] Hypovolemia is corrected with crystalloid fluids as discussed previously. Hypoproteinemia should be corrected to normal serum protein levels with fresh-frozen plasma. The half-life of red blood cells is reduced both by direct erythrocyte damage from the burn injury and by increased fragility from released inflammatory mediators of the acute injury response. Red blood cell production is also impaired during the early period after the burn by direct bone marrow suppression. Anemia should be aggressively corrected with red blood cell transfusions to maximize tissue oxygen delivery.

Fluid and protein losses into the interstitium are diminished after the second day after the burn. Evaporative losses from the disrupted skin barrier continue until the burned portion of the integument is closed by skin grafting. Evaporative losses may be estimated by use of the following formula:

$$\text{Evaporative loss (ml of water per hour)} = (25 + \% \text{ TBSA}) \times \text{TBSA (m}^2)$$

Evaporative losses are primarily free water and must be replaced as such. On about the third or fourth day the patient's capillary leak seals and edema fluid moves from the interstitium to the vascular space. The mobilization of edema fluid, combined with continued aggressive volume support, may predispose a child to hypervolemia and congestive cardiovascular changes. Administration of small amounts of diuretics may assist in excreting the excess salt and water load. Salt loading during this period should specifically be avoided.[9]

Burn Wound Sepsis

Once the patient has an adequately controlled airway and reliable venous access and the burn resuscitation has begun, attention is turned to prevention of the next most important complication in burn patients, burn wound sepsis. Sepsis is most effectively prevented by early and aggressive burn wound debridement, frequent daily dressing changes, and early excision with grafting.

Burn wound sepsis is a major cause of morbidity and mortality in burn victims but is a relatively minor concern in the acute emergency center management. Immediately following the burn, burn surfaces are sterile or have low populations of normal skin microflora. Rapid colonization takes place during the first 72 hours after injury. Sources of bacterial colonization include the patient's own skin, hair follicles, and sweat glands and the environment in which the patient is maintained. The emergency center rarely is colonized with other than community-type organisms. The modern intensive care or burn unit may be a source of virulent nosocomial organisms.

Burned skin loses its barrier function, and the dead tissue with its markedly impaired blood supply encourages rapid proliferation of bacteria. Bacterial invasion of a partial-thickness burn can, in fact, convert the injury to a deeper or full-thickness burn in a matter of hours. Topical antibiotic preparations have been developed to assist in preventing bacterial colonization of the wounds. *After* the patient has been hemodynamically stabilized, topical preparations are applied directly to the eschar and covered with clean dressings. If the emergency center patient is to be moved quickly to an intensive care unit or burn center, application of topical antibacterials can wait until the transfer has been completed. If the patient is to be maintained in the emergency center for over an hour, or if several hours have passed since the burn injury, topical antibiotics should be applied as soon as possible. Silver sulfadiazine, mafenide acetate, bacitracin ointment, and silver nitrate solution are the standard topical antibiotics currently used in most emergency and burn centers.

Silver sulfadiazine (1%). Silver sulfadiazine (Silvadene cream) is the most widely used topical burn agent in the United States. Primary antibacterial properties are directed at gram-negative organisms with some gram-positive coverage. Gram-negative resistance has been documented to *Enterobacter, Escherichia coli,* and *Candida.* Silvadene does not penetrate the burn eschar and therefore is an excellent first-line preventive agent rather than a therapy for deeper established infections. The most prevalent complication resulting from the use of Silvadene is a mild transient leukopenia that follows reversible bone marrow suppression. Silvadene is thinly applied to the burn eschar, covered with fine mesh gauze, and wrapped with a bulky Kerlex dressing. Silvadene should be applied twice daily.

Mafenide acetate (10%). Mafenide acetate (Sulfamylon) has strong gram-negative and gram-positive coverage. This antibiotic is especially effective against *Pseudomonas,* but it has no efficacy against *Providencia stuartii* and no antifungal activity. Sulfamylon can penetrate the eschar and is used as a second-line topical agent for the treatment of deep or subeschar infections. Sulfamylon has significant side effects, which limit its use in the emergency center. It is a potent carbonic anhydrase inhibitor, and application is painful.

Neosporin and bacitracin. Neosporin and bacitracin are transparent and not toxic to the eyes, so they are safe and cosmetically appealing for use on burns to the face. Toxic effects may occur if they are used on very large burns. The ointment is applied as needed through the day and night.

Silver nitrate (0.5%). Silver nitrate is applied as a solution that tends to react with the skin, producing a blackish discoloration. The antibacterial spectrum includes gram-positive organisms and fungi, with some resistance in the gram-negative group. The metabolic complications include hyponatremia, hypokalemia, and methemoglobinemia. The rapid absorption limits the use of this antibiotic to burns under 50% TBSA. The solution must be applied in bulky wet dressings every 2 hours and is extremely messy.

Dressing Changes

Burn dressing changes are tedious and painful, involve large numbers of support personnel, and produce a great deal of anxiety in younger children. Children must be approached with an understanding of the cause of their anxiety. The degree of anxiety may be minimized by including the child in his or her interventional procedures. The optimal approach includes the following[9]:

- Before the burn dressing change, the child is told what to expect and then is kept informed as the burn dressing change progresses.
- Emphasis is placed on the need for the child's help with the burn dressing change.
- The choices offered to the child are appropriate and reasonable.
- The nurse maintains control by setting reasonable time limits for the child's help with procedures.
- The child's attention is focused on the task by encouragement to watch, help, and look at the burned area being treated.
- Generous praise is given for the child's help.
- Predictability is increased by telling the child when to expect the next burn dressing change.
- Most importantly, no child of any age is ever forced to do anything that he or she clearly does not want to do or is not ready to do.

Patients with burns should undergo tetanus prophylaxis and treatment if needed according to the recommendations of the American College of Surgeons (Table 11–5).

Definitive Burn Care

Once the patient is hemodynamically stable, the circulating blood volume has been augmented to normal hemoglobin concentrations, and burn wound colonization has been attended to, the next major issue is the main goal of burn therapy, wound closure. Management from this point is outside the purview of the emergency center and is usually accomplished at a burn center or by surgeons experienced in burn wound excision and grafting. The operative procedures are relatively straightforward, but the support services and cost in resources (e.g., blood banking, nursing services, operating room specialty services, pediatric intensivists, nutritional support) may be substantial. For these reasons it is recommended that the pediatric burn victim be transferred to a center experienced specifically in the management of *pediatric* burns.

A significant move has been made in the adult literature suggesting treatment of burn wounds by immediate complete total excision and skin grafting with homograft or xenograft. The complication rate and cost of such therapy are similar to those of serial excisions and graftings, but the hospital stay is significantly less. For large wounds (greater than 20% TBSA) such an approach

Table 11–5. Recommendations of the Committee on Trauma of the American College of Surgeons: Specific Measures for Patients with Wounds: Tetanus Prophylaxis and Treatment

I. Previously immunized individuals
  A. When the attending physician has determined that the patient has previously been fully immunized and the last dose of toxoid was given within 10 years:
    1. For non-tetanus-prone wounds, no booster of toxoids is indicated.
    2. For tetanus-prone wounds and if more than 5 years has elapsed since the last dose, 0.5 ml absorbed toxoid should be given. If excessive prior toxoid injections have been given, this booster may be omitted.
  B. When the patient has had two or more prior injections of toxoid and received the last dose more than 10 years previously, 0.5 ml absorbed toxoid for both tetanus-prone and non-tetanus-prone wounds should be given. Passive immunization is not considered necessary.
II. Individuals not adequately immunized, i.e., the patient has received only one or no prior injection of toxoid or the immunization history is unknown
  A. For non-tetanus-prone wounds, 0.5 ml absorbed toxoids should be given.
  B. For tetanus-prone wounds:
    1. A dose of 0.5 ml absorbed toxoid and 250 units (or more) of human tetanus immune globulin (using different syringes, needles, and sites of injection) should be given.
    2. Administration of antibiotics should be considered, although the effectiveness of antibiotics for prophylaxis of tetanus remains unproved.

in very young children produces enormous surgical and physiologic stress. We recommend serial excision and grafting for young children. Among the major expected complications of excision and grafting are major hemorrhage, pulmonary dysfunction, sepsis, malnutrition, myocardial dysfunction, and loss of grafts. The following treatment philosophies may be used to minimize the complication rate in small children[9]:

- Limiting operative time to less than 2 hours
- Excision and grafting of not more than 20% TBSA at a time
- Limiting the operative interventions when the blood loss exceeds half the patient's circulating blood volume
- Maintaining the operating room ambient temperature above 30° centigrade
- An aggressive approach to nutritional support

Which burns to graft? Any third-degree (full-thickness) burn has lost all its epithelial elements and requires grafting. First-degree burns and superficial second-degree burns have retained varying but substantial amounts of epithelium and if treated in a timely fashion usually do not require skin grafting. There is some debate as to the best management for deep second-degree burns.[19,20]

The epithelial elements of these burns are somewhat limited, but reepithelialization will eventually occur. Epithelial growth may require many weeks, and the patient may suffer substantial hypertrophic scar formation with the possibility of requisite follow-up operative interventions for contracture release. Because of the thickness of the injury and the relatively few epithelial elements, deep partial-thickness wounds are at a substantial risk of conversion to full-thickness injuries if an infection develops. That infection need not be one of the burn itself; conversion to full-thickness injury may occur with remote infections such as sinusitis, pneumonitis, or decubitus ulcers. We recommend early excision and grafting of deep second-degree burns, especially when those wounds are associated with larger full-thickness injuries.

During the time the patient is undergoing serial excision and grafting, portions of the burn wound that have not yet been excised are at risk for progressive infection. Invasive infection, or subeschar collections, may be clinically subtle but easily lead to overwhelming burn sepsis. Burn wound infection may be suggested by erythema around the wound edges, progressive patient agitation, increased ventilator requirements, increasing oxygen use, progressive anemia, or premature separation of the burn wound eschar with subeschar purulent collections. Periodic wound surveillance biopsy and quantitative cultures of the eschar should be performed to detect the development of invasive infections. Biopsy requires 1 cm^3 of tissue, which includes a portion of the viable tissue deep to the eschar. The specimen is obtained after the surface of the wound has been cleansed of all exudate and dried. The biopsy specimen is transported to the laboratory in a moist gauze. Quantitative cultures with greater than 10^5 organisms per gram of eschar indicate burn wound sepsis, necessitating treatment with systemic antibiotics and consideration of aggressive eschar excision. Histologic examination of the biopsy specimen may also show bacterial invasion of the tissue.

Associated injuries must be identified and managed along with the burn injury. In children burned in vehicular accidents or blast accidents or those who may have been injured trying to escape from a fire, associated injuries are often overlooked. Traumatic blunt or penetrating injuries should be managed as described elsewhere in this book.

The American Burn Association identifies the following as burn injuries requiring referral:

- Partial- and full-thickness burns involving greater than 10% TBSA in patients under 10 years of age
- Partial- and full-thickness burns involving greater than 20% TBSA in older patients
- Partial- and full-thickness burns involving the face, eyes, ears, hands, feet, genitalia, perineum, and major joints

- Third-degree burns greater than 5% TBSA in any age group
- Electrical burns
- Chemical burns
- Burns associated with significant fracture or other major injury in which the burn poses the most significant morbidity
- Burn injury with associated inhalation injury
- Lesser burns in patients with other significant preexisting disease

Several factors are critical for safe and appropriate transfer. The most significant factor is direct communication between the referring and receiving physicians. The referring physician is responsible for identifying injuries, initiating resuscitative efforts, and stabilizing the patient. A careful documentation of injuries, an explanation of initial therapy, and a record of the patient's responses to that therapy must accompany the patient. The receiving physician recommends procedures or interventions that may be beneficial to the patient during transfer. Both should ensure that the patient's airway is secured and that oxygen and ventilatory support are available during transfer. A urinary catheter is placed for monitoring, and a nasogastric tube is placed for decompression. Personnel who accompany the patient should be briefed on possible problems during transfer and should be trained to provide the level of support that may be necessary. The development of standard transfer protocols assists all parties in arranging safe transfers.

NUTRITIONAL SUPPORT

Burn injury induces a catabolic response that makes burns the most physiologically stressful of all disease processes. Nutritional support must be instituted early, be aggressively monitored, and employ the enteral route whenever possible. Chapter 15 details nutritional support of burned children.

REFERENCES

1. Breasted JH: Edwin Smith surgical papyrus. In *Surgical treatise, translation and commentary,* vol 1, Chicago, 1930, University of Chicago Oriental Institute Publications, p 83.
2. Keynes AG, ed: *The apologie and treatise: the first discourse wherein wounds made by gunshot are freed from being burnt or cauterized according to* Vigoes *methode,* London, 1951, Falcon Educational Books, p 140.
3. Artz CP: History of burns. In Artz CP, Moncrief JA, Pruitt BA Jr, eds: *Burns: a team approach,* Philadelphia, 1979, WB Saunders, pp 3–16.
4. Carvajal HF: Burn injuries. In Behrman RE, Kliegman RM, Nelson WE, Vaughan VC III, eds: *Nelson textbook of pediatrics,* ed 14, Philadelphia, 1992, WB Saunders, p 233.
5. East MK, Jones CA, Feller IL, et al: Epidemiology of burns in children. In Carvajal HF, Parks DH, eds: *Burns in children,* Chicago, 1988, Year Book.
6. Robinson MD, Seward PN: Thermal injury in children, *Pediatr Emerg Care* 3(4):266–270, 1987.

7. Lenoski EF, Hunter KA: Specific patterns of inflicted burn injuries, *J Trauma* 17:11, 1977.
8. McLoughlin E, McGuire A: The causes, cost, and prevention of childhood burn injuries, *Am J Dis Child* 144:677–683, 1990.
9. Demling RH: *Care of the surgical patient,* New York, 1988, Scientific American Medicine, pp 8–10.
10. Briggs SE: First aid, transportation, and immediate care of thermal injuries. In Martyn JAJ, ed: *Acute management of the burned patient,* Philadelphia, 1990, WB Saunders, pp 1–11.
11. Strongin J, Hales C: Pulmonary disorders in the burn patient. In Martyn JAJ, ed: *Acute management of the burned patient,* Philadelphia, 1990, WB Saunders, pp 25–45.
12. Goudsouzian N, Szyfelbein SK: Management of upper airway following burns. In Martyn JAJ, ed: *Acute management of the burned patient,* Philadelphia, 1990, WB Saunders, pp 45–56.
13. Lalonde C, Knox J, Youn Y, Demling R: Burn edema is accentuated by a moderate smoke inhalation injury in sheep, *Surgery* 112(5):908–917, 1992.
14. Lund CC, Browder NC: Estimation of areas of burns, *Surg Gynecol Obstet* 79:352–358, 1944.
15. Pruitt BA Jr, Goodwin CW Jr, Pruitt SK: Burns. In Sabiston DC Jr, ed: *Textbook of surgery,* ed 14, Philadelphia, 1991, WB Saunders, p 185.
16. Carvajal HF: Resuscitation of the burned child. In Carvajal HF, Parks DH, eds: *Pediatric burn management,* Chicago, 1988, Year Book, pp 78–98.
17. Graves TA, Cioffi WG, McManus WF, et al: Fluid resuscitation of infants and children with massive thermal injury, *J Trauma* 28(12):1656–1659, 1988.
18. Sharp RJ: Burns. In Ashcraft KW, Holder TM, eds: *Pediatric surgery,* ed 2, Philadelphia, 1992, WB Saunders, pp 89–102.
19. Gore D, Desai M, Herndon DN, et al: Comparison of complications during rehabilitation between conservative and early surgical management in thermal burns involving the feet of children and adolescents, *J Burn Care Rehab* 9(1):92–95, 1988.
20. Briggs SE: Rationale for acute surgical approach. In Martyn JAJ, ed: *Acute management of the burned patient,* Philadelphia, 1990, WB Saunders, pp 118–127.

Head and Neck Trauma

Daniel A. Beals

Facial and neck injuries, unlike head injuries, are much less common in children than adults. Patients less than 6 years of age rarely sustain facial fractures because of characteristic differences in the pediatric craniofacial skeleton.[1,2] By the age of puberty the child's craniofacial anatomy and the associated frequency and pattern of traumatic injuries begin to parallel those of the adult. Although the initial treatment of facial injuries is basically the same in children and adults, the management of injuries is different because of the unique ability of the growing child to remodel the facial skeleton.

Automobile-related accidents account for a large number of severe injuries and related facial trauma in children.[3,4] Other causes of facial injuries include falls, thermal injuries, and animal bites; athletic injuries may be a source of facial fractures in older children. Unfortunately, gunshot wounds and injuries related to violence are becoming more common even in the very young age groups.

Several aspects of pediatric facial trauma management require special attention. Therapy may be difficult simply because patients are often unable to cooperate in rehabilitation. Injuries in children also have the potential for late complications from altered continued growth of the facial skeleton. A posttraumatic facial deformity in a child may be a result not only of the displacement of the bony structures because of fracture, but also of faulty or arrested growth.[5] Developmental malformations in teenagers and young adults are often caused by early childhood injuries. Growth-related abnormalities are particularly common in relation to injuries involving the nasomaxillary complex and the condylar region of the mandible. The parents of a child with maxillofacial trauma should be informed that, despite timely and adequate reduction and treatment, maldevelopment in growth may occur.

CLINICAL EXAMINATION

Assessment and care of the airway are of paramount importance in the initial management of the injured child. Trauma to the head and neck may

310

directly influence the ability to provide and maintain a patent airway. The team leader in a trauma resuscitation should be positioned at the patient's head. Rapid assessment of the head, neck, and chest is performed to ensure an adequate airway. Although this assessment may not be difficult in a crying, awake child, the presence of an adequate airway can seldom be determined by simple observation of the more severely injured patient. There is no substitute for a methodical, unhurried examination.

Initial assessment of the airway should always include attention to cervical spine immobilization, regardless of dramatic injuries that may be obvious at presentation. For example, the physician must not assume that penetrating trauma to the lower extremity cannot be associated with cervical spine injury. The patient may have suffered an unwitnessed fall resulting from the lower extremity trauma. Primary emergency responders now carry and freely use cervical spine immobilization collars. Occasionally a child arrives in the emergency department with no spinal immobilization or improper immobilization. These patients should receive manual in-line traction and immobilization while the initial assessment is performed.

When the trauma patient arrives in the emergency room, the most rapid way to assess the airway is simply by asking a question, for example, "What is your name?" or "How are you?"[6] Appropriate verbal response indicates the level of consciousness, airway, ventilation, and perfusion. In infants and younger children the appropriate response to trauma is crying. These children may not be capable of conversation, so the quality and strength of the cry become important factors in airway assessment. The Advanced Trauma Life Support course defines the procedure for recognizing airway problems: *look, listen, and feel*. The examiner should look at the patient. Is the patient lying quietly or combative? Is there obvious facial or neck trauma? Does the chest rise and fall with respiration? The examiner should then listen to respiration and auscultate breath sounds. Are there upper airway secretions? Are the breath sounds bilaterally equal? Is the voice hoarse, suggesting laryngeal trauma? The examiner should feel for air movement at the mouth. Is there crepitus? Is the trachea midline? These same maneuvers usually give immediate clinical indicators of facial trauma.

The child with traumatic injury responds much differently to the emergency treatment environment than does the adult. Young patients are sometimes unable or unwilling to provide a history of their injury. Emergency medical and paramedical personnel who were at the scene of the accident can sometimes provide insight into the type, cause, and mechanism of the accident and what other injuries may have been incurred. Parents may not be available when the injured child arrives in the emergency room, and sometimes parents who are present are either injured or overly apprehensive about their child's injuries, which may only add to the confusion and the patient's anxiety. Extra time should be taken to gain the child's confidence, especially if he or she has maxillofacial trauma.

The maxillofacial area of a patient with traumatic injuries should be examined completely and methodically. First the contour of the face is observed for obvious defects in symmetry. Areas of laceration or bruising should be carefully inspected because they frequently signify underlying fracture (Fig. 12–1). The mouth is inspected, and any loose or missing teeth are noted. In the childhood population missing teeth may be a normal finding unrelated to the trauma. The parents if present can usually give a reliable dental history.

The stability of the mandible and maxilla are determined by direct intraoral palpation. Bimanual examination exerting lateral external pressure is useful in diagnosing fractures of both the mandible and the maxilla (Fig. 12–2). Malocclusion may be an important sign of maxillofacial fracture but is often difficult to assess in an uncooperative or severely injured child (Fig. 12–3).

After inspection of the midface the remainder of the face and scalp are examined. The scalp, orbital rims, zygomatic arches, and temporal areas are palpated for signs of fracture: pain, "step-off," discontinuity, or crepitus. Func-

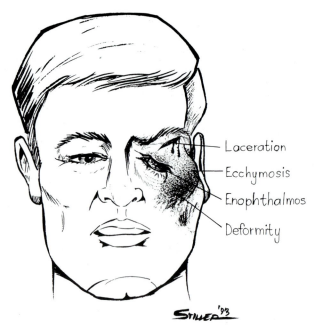

Figure 12–1. Signs of maxillofacial fracture.

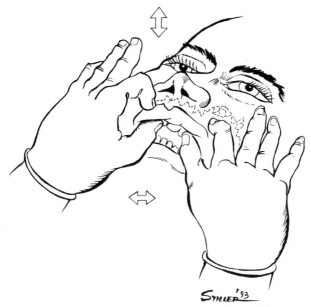

Figure 12–2. Bimanual examination for facial fractures.

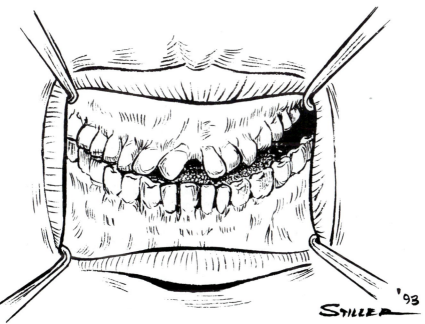

Figure 12–3. Malocclusion after maxillofacial fracture.

tional use is also evaluated. Limitation of jaw movement, malocclusion, or double vision may be signs of injury or fracture.

The examination of the neck warrants special consideration in the trauma patient. Initially the neck is immobilized until potential neurologic injury is evaluated. Direct injury to the neck may cause hemorrhage or airway compromise, necessitating early intervention. In these patients care must still be taken to maintain in-line traction and avoid flexion, extension, or rotation. Direct injury to the neck may result from penetrating or blunt trauma. Penetrating injuries, such as gunshot or knife wounds, are examined with attention to trajectory of the missile or stab; type, size, or caliber of the wounding agent; and the victim's position at the time of trauma. The location and size of entrance and exit wounds are also noted. The presence of hematoma or subcutaneous emphysema may indicate major vascular or airway injury. Air bubbling from a laceration or gunshot wound with respiration is evidence of a major airway injury. Abnormalities of laryngeal contour associated with hoarseness may signify a laryngeal fracture (Fig. 12–4).

Careful palpation and auscultation of the neck may add further information to the evaluation for significant traumatic injuries. Pulsatile, expanding masses are usually due to major vascular trauma when they are associated with penetrating injuries. The presence of vascular bruit in a child's neck is distinctly

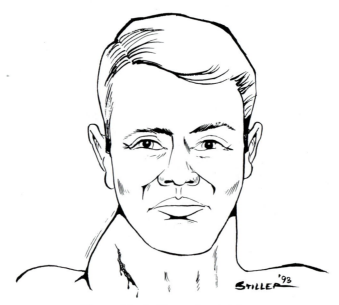

Figure 12–4. Signs of neck injury.

abnormal and may be due to traumatic arteriovenous fistula formation or arterial intimal disruption from either blunt or penetrating trauma. Crepitus may be due to airway or esophageal injury.

RADIOGRAPHIC EXAMINATION

The injured child may be unable to cooperate with positioning for radiographic examination.[7] In the initial radiographic evaluation of a child with head and neck trauma, the cervical spine series is the first priority. Evaluation of films may prove difficult because the child's spine commonly has incomplete vertebral ossification, epiphyseal variation, and greater mobility than an adult's. The examiner must always be aware that an unstable fracture, with or without spinal injury, may occur without obvious evidence of bony disruption because of the incomplete ossification in children less than 10 years of age.[8] Therefore a single cross-table lateral cervical radiograph is not sufficient for evaluating a multiply injured child. Radiographs of the entire spinal column, as well as cervical anteroposterior, lateral, and odontoid views, are necessary to assess the possibility of an injury to the spine. These radiographs should be obtained regardless of anticipated computed tomography (CT) scans, since CT is inadequate for complete evaluation of the spine. In some patients flexion-extension views are helpful in the evaluation of spinal stability.

After the cervical spine has been completely evaluated, radiographic examination of maxillofacial injuries may proceed. Several plain radiographic views are traditionally used in evaluation of the maxillofacial region. The Waters view is useful in evaluating the midface, zygoma, maxilla, orbital floors, and nasal pyramid.[9] In children fracture lines may be difficult to visualize because of slight patient movements or because of the higher ratio of cancellous to cortical bone. CT scanning has become the diagnostic tool of choice for the complete evaluation of extent and degree of pediatric facial fractures.[10] CT also offers the opportunity to evaluate head-injured patients for concomitant intracranial injury. Axial orientation of the CT scan is preferred initially to examine both the face and the skull. Facial fractures should additionally be evaluated with coronal imaging. The combination of axial and coronal views may be further supplemented with three-dimensional reconstructions (Fig. 12–5). This modality offers a major advance in the evaluation and operative planning for reconstruction of complex maxillofacial fractures.

Penetrating injuries to the neck are becoming commonplace in children. These injuries may require angiographic documentation before operative intervention. A complete discussion of cervical vascular injuries, their evaluation, and treatment is found in Chapter 13.

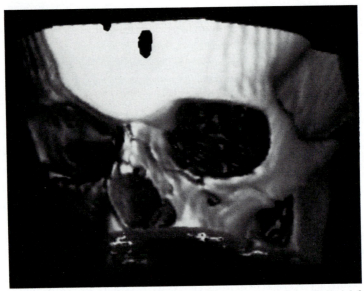

Figure 12–5. Three-dimensional reconstruction tomograms of maxillofacial fractures.

EMERGENCY MANAGEMENT

In a patient with maxillofacial injury, securing the airway may be intimidating. The American College of Surgeons manual used in the Advanced Trauma Life Support course provides an excellent outline of assessment and management of the airway in both an adult and a child.[11] Once the airway has been assessed by the look, listen, and feel method as previously discussed, initial management is begun with the delivery of supplemental oxygen via an oxygen rebreather mask at an FIO_2 of 100%. In patients with upper airway obstruction resulting from altered sensorium, the chin lift or jaw thrust method is useful to provide adequate ventilation (Fig. 12–6). A disadvantage of the jaw thrust method is that two people are needed to ventilate the patient, one to lift up the mandible and secure the face mask and the other to ventilate. Although oropharyngeal and nasopharyngeal airways are useful in adult trauma patients, these devices have little use in children, especially those with maxillofacial injury and respiratory distress.

Instruments to create a surgical airway should be readied before any airway intervention. Having to find and open the proper instruments after intubation has failed is an invitation to disaster.

Oral endotracheal intubation is the primary means of securing the airway in pediatric patients with respiratory distress. Contraindications to orotracheal

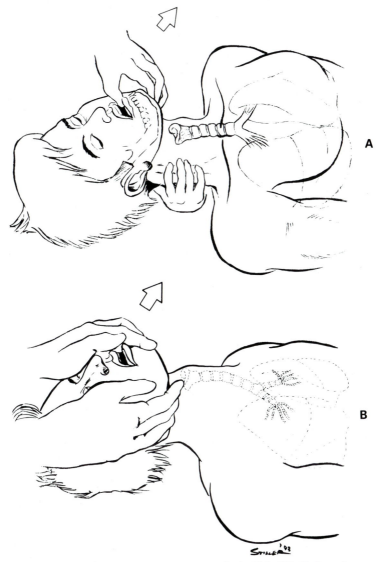

Figure 12–6. Methods of initial airway control. **A,** Chin lift. **B,** Jaw thrust.

intubation include massive maxillofacial trauma with inability to visualize the upper airway, unstable cervical spine injury with inability to visualize the glottis without neck extension, and foreign body aspiration to the glottis with respiratory arrest. After three unsuccessful attempts at orotracheal intubation, a surgical airway should be created.

In noncombative, obtunded, or very young patients, oral intubation is usually accomplished without premedication or topical anesthetic agents. The avoidance of narcotic and paralytic agents offers several advantages. The patient is able to continue respiratory efforts and to help protect the airway in case of regurgitation. The patient's neurologic status may continue to be monitored for localizing signs or signs of deterioration. Older patients who are conscious or combative usually cannot tolerate awake orotracheal intubation. These patients are treated with a rapid induction anesthetic to obtain an airway in the shortest possible time and to return the patient's reflexes to a preintubation state as quickly as possible (so neurologic evaluation can continue). A recommended approach is pretreatment during the initial oxygenation with atropine at 0.02 mg/kg, followed by succinylcholine 2 mg/kg and fentanyl 2 µg/kg. Although longer acting agents such as vecuronium and the diazepams are useful for maintaining sedation, these agents have a significantly longer onset of action. Whenever sedation must be used in airway control, preparations for surgical airway intervention should be made beforehand.

If an airway cannot be secured after usual methods of bag-mask ventilation or orotracheal intubation, surgical cricothyrotomy should be performed. Although cricothyrotomy may lead to complications, it should be used without hesitation if reasonable attempts at intubation have failed. In cases of foreign body aspiration or massive maxillofacial trauma with respiratory arrest, little time should be spent on less secure methods of airway control.

Cricothyrotomy is performed by either of two techniques, depending on the patient's age. In children less than 12 years of age, needle cricothyrotomy is preferred (Fig. 12–7). The child's head and neck are held in midline traction by an assistant. The neck is prepped with betadine, and a 16- or 14-gauge Angiocath catheter is advanced through the cricothyroid membrane. A syringe attached to the Angiocath with 2 to 3 cc of air demonstrates a sudden decrease in resistance to pressure on the plunger as the trachea is entered. Likewise, air should be easily aspirated from within the trachea. The catheter is then advanced over the needle and secured in place with suture. Insufflation of the trachea with high-flow oxygen (15 L/min) for 1 second with an exhalation phase of 3 to 4 seconds provides adequate short-term ventilation. Insufflation may be facilitated by use of a Y-type connector (Fig. 12–8). After initial ventilation is established by needle cricothyroidotomy, a definitive airway may be placed in the operating room within 30 to 40 minutes.

In patients over 12 years of age, or when needle cricothyrotomy has failed, open cricothyrotomy is indicated (Fig. 12–9). As with the needle technique, the head is held in midline traction by an assistant and the neck prepped. A vertical incision is made in the skin just above the cricoid cartilage. The cricothyroid membrane is incised transversely, and an endotracheal tube is inserted and secured with umbilical tape. Care must be taken not to insert the tube too

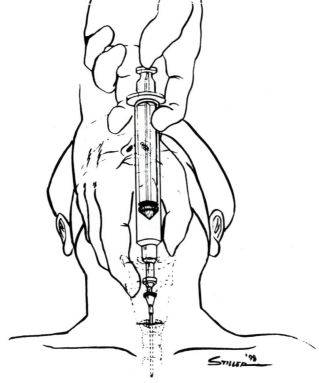

Figure 12–7. Technique of needle cricothyrotomy.

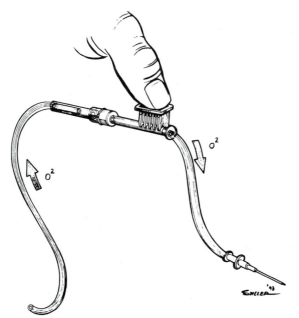

Figure 12–8. Equipment for insufflation with needle cricothyrotomy.

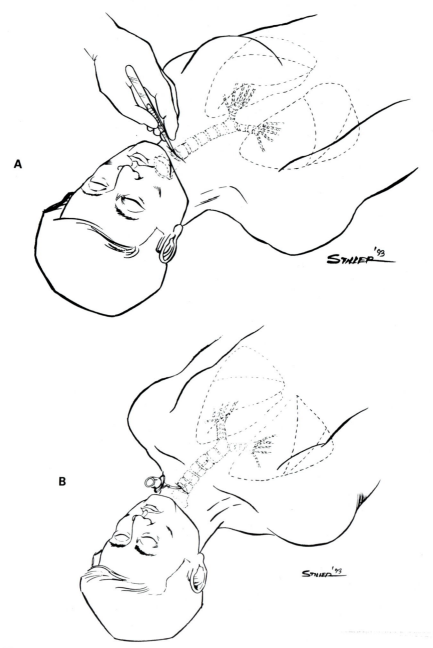

Figure 12–9. Technique of open cricothyrotomy. **A,** Incision in cricothyroid membrane. **B,** Placement of endotracheal tube.

far into the mainstem bronchus or to attempt placement of too large a tube that would fail to pass the cricoid cartilage. All patients who undergo cricothyrotomy should have an alternative airway placed electively within 12 hours of insertion. This may be done by conversion to a formal tracheotomy or by orotracheal intubation with fiberoptic guidance.

Both needle cricothyrotomy and open cricothyrotomy are subject to complications. Inadvertent damage to the larynx or posterior tracheal perforation with tracheoesophageal fistula formation may be avoided by not performing overvigorous attempts at airway placement. Hemorrhage from the great vessels of the neck may be avoided by careful attention to midline placement of the needle or incision. Pneumothorax may follow energetic ventilation through a small-bore tube or misplacement of the endotracheal tube with forced ventilation outside the trachea.

Bleeding associated with maxillofacial trauma is usually not life threatening. However, careful evaluation is necessary to ensure that significant bleeding is recognized. Nasomaxillary bleeding is especially insidious because patients may swallow large amounts of blood before external signs of bleeding are evident. In the majority of cases of scalp or facial bleeding, direct pressure is the most effective and efficient method of hemorrhage control. Hemostats or other instruments should not be blindly applied without formal exploration of the wound. After a careful evaluation of the entire patient, bleeding wounds may be readdressed. To prevent ongoing blood loss, scalp wounds may be closed with a simple running suture before CT scanning and diagnostic tests. Facial lacerations usually stop bleeding spontaneously within 15 minutes with constant direct pressure. Wounds that continue to bleed after this time may require formal exploration in the operating room.

Maxillofacial fractures rarely cause a life-threatening source of bleeding. A significant amount of blood may be rapidly lost with some complex fractures, and the patient may be at risk for aspiration of blood into the tracheobronchial tree. In these instances rapid control of bleeding is necessary until the remainder of the patient can be evaluated and proper fixation of the fractures undertaken in the operating room. Anteroposterior nasal packing may be accomplished either with a cloth (Nugauze) bolster or by using a Foley balloon for posterior packing and gauze for anterior packing. Before either method, displaced fractures may be approximated to their normal position to lessen bleeding. Nasal packing is not without complications. The Foley catheter may inadvertently enter the orbit or anterior cranial fossa in the patient with severely comminuted fractures. Necrosis of the columella may occur if packing is maintained for more than 6 hours. In patients with cerebrospinal fluid leak, nasal packing should be avoided or packs should be removed early to prevent ascending meningeal infections.

In a very few patients bleeding cannot be stopped by packing or operative reduction. These patients may benefit from selective arterial ligation or angiographic embolization. Usually this requires embolization of the internal maxillary ethmoidal arteries. At times, ligation or embolization of the external carotid and temporal arteries may be required. These modalities are reserved for the most severe cases in which all other therapy has failed.

SPECIFIC INJURIES
Soft Tissue

Facial lacerations and abrasions commonly require at least some care in the emergency room. All injuries should be carefully examined, foreign bodies removed, and the wound edges conservatively debrided. Clean lacerations of the face may be closed for up to 8 hours after the injury. The operator should allow 15 minutes for every centimeter of laceration to be repaired. Lacerations that require longer than 1 hour to repair are probably best repaired in the operating room. If the patient requires surgical intervention for other injuries, the facial lacerations may be repaired in the operating room.

Several special problems in facial lacerations should be kept in mind during evaluation and repair. A "trapdoor deformity" may result from underlying subcutaneous tissue loss. The facial nerve is prone to injury and must be evaluated before injection of local anesthetics. Nerve injuries lateral to the lateral canthus of the eye require repair; such repairs are best accomplished in the operating room (Fig. 12–10).

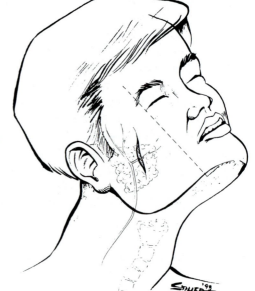

Figure 12–10. Facial nerve injuries in facial lacerations.

The parotid duct may be injured in lacerations of the buccal area contiguous to the parotid gland. The location of the wound or saliva issuing from the wound should alert the physician to parotid duct injury (Fig. 12–11). Injury can be documented by careful exploration in the emergency room, but repair should be performed in the operating room.

Lacerations to the medial canthus of the orbit or medial portions of the eyelid sometimes injure the lacrimal apparatus (Fig. 12–12). The lower lacrimal duct is most important in the prevention of epiphora, but injuries of either the superior or inferior duct should also be recognized and repaired.

The nose, eyelids, and lips can be difficult to repair. The free margins of these organs require precise approximation to prevent an unacceptable cosmetic outcome. The underlying muscle must also be correctly approximated if proper function is to be ensured. If the laceration is complex or the operator is unfamiliar with plastic technique, appropriate consultation and repair in the operating room may be indicated.

Scalp laceration may be responsible for significant blood loss, especially in the very young patient. Before repair the underlying skull should be palpated to evaluate for fracture. Depressed skull fractures or open skull fractures require neurosurgical consultation. Simple lacerations may be sutured to prevent additional bleeding while other tests are being performed. Unless the patient has an extensive stellate type of laceration, only minimum amounts of hair need to be removed to suture the wound.

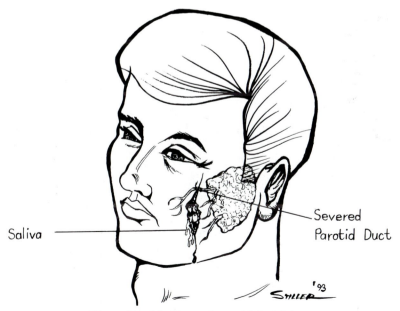

Saliva

Severed Parotid Duct

Figure 12–11. Signs of parotid duct injury.

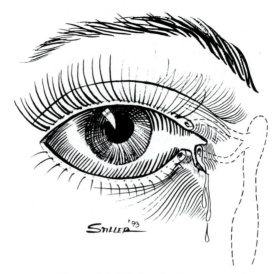

Figure 12–12. Lacrimal injuries.

Ear

The ear consists of an external appendage and the neurosensory components of the middle and inner ear. The external ear is injured much more often than the middle or inner portions. Repairing the external ear requires precise approximation of the free margin. All portions of cartilage should be salvaged and covered. Ragged lacerations may be excised in a V fashion and closed primarily (Fig. 12–13).

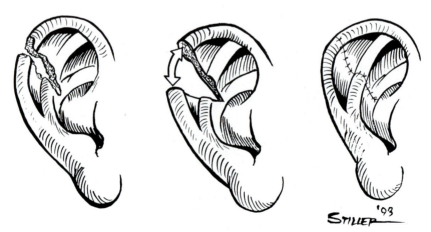

Figure 12–13. Excisional repair of the ear.

Middle and inner ear injuries consist of penetrating injuries (cotton-tipped applicators, pencils), concussive injuries (blast, blow to ear), temporal bone fractures extending into the middle ear, deceleration injuries with skull trauma, barotrauma (diving or airplane accidents), or lightning injuries. In an evaluation for possible middle ear injuries, it is important to determine whether the cochlea or vestibular structures have been damaged. Perception of the spoken word gives an estimate of hearing level. Clear repetition of spoken words militates against severe inner ear damage. Vestibular injury is characterized by vertigo and nystagmus, usually accompanied by nausea and vomiting. Immediately after injury the fast component of nystagmus is toward the involved ear. However, after several hours the findings are reversed, with the fast component being away from the affected ear. Suspicion of middle or inner ear injury should prompt an immediate consultation with an otolaryngologist, since emergency repair often restores hearing.

Neck

The neck is a compact area full of vital structures. Soft tissue injuries should be evaluated after cervical spine injury has been excluded. Shallow wounds that do not penetrate the platysma muscle may be cleaned and closed primarily in the emergency room. Punctate or deep wounds are more worrisome because the airway or major vascular structures may be injured. These injuries require operative exploration. In stable patients specific injuries are best evaluated before surgical exploration. The investigative tools include arteriography, laryngoscopy, bronchoscopy, esophagoscopy, and CT scanning. The neck is divided into three anatomic areas: zone I, clavicle to cricoid cartilage; zone II, cricoid cartilage to the angle of the mandible; and zone III, angle of the mandible to the base of the skull (Fig. 12–14).[12] Trauma with suspected vascular injury in zones I and III should be evaluated with arteriography. Proper planning for vascular control, evaluation of cerebral cross-over flow, and documentation of the extent of injury are all ascertained by arteriography. Patients with injuries to zone II also benefit from arteriography if it can be performed safely and expeditiously, but operative exploration of zone II rarely misses a carotid artery injury. Therefore in zone II injuries arteriography may be reserved for patients who are stable but have clinical features suggestive of carotid arterial injury.

Arterial injuries in the neck are usually amenable to primary repair.[13-15] Ligation should be used only when repair is impossible or the patient is dying from other injuries. Even patients with neurologic deficits or in a coma should undergo primary repair if possible. Concern about hemorrhagic infarction with revascularization in these patients seems unwarranted.[16] In cases of loss of the arterial wall, autologous grafting with saphenous vein provides acceptable reconstruction. Prosthetic material such as Gore-tex is acceptable in older patients

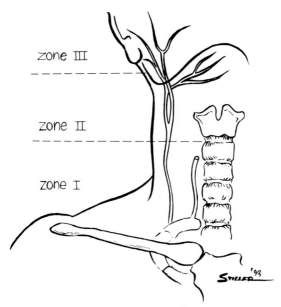

zone III

zone II

zone I

Figure 12—14. Anatomic zones of the neck.

but should not be used in patients who will continue to grow significantly after the injury.

Vertebral artery injuries are rare and usually caused by penetrating trauma. Surgical ligation is the mainstay of treatment.[17,18] Arteriographic embolization has been reported in adults.[19] In the pediatric population, surgical ligation and neck exploration are advisable because the incidence of concomitant injury is high.

Esophageal injuries are notoriously difficult to diagnose preoperatively. Most injuries are confined to the cervical area and are manifest as dysphasia, hematemesis, and odynophagia. Some patients may have no preoperative signs of injury. Simple physical examination is usually not sufficient to rule out esophageal injury in penetrating neck trauma. The combination of water-soluble contrast esophagography and rigid esophagoscopy (if the contrast study is equivocal or suggestive of an injury) leads to the correct diagnosis in more than 90% of patients with esophageal trauma. Primary esophageal repair should be accomplished if possible; otherwise, cervical esophagostomy is employed. The interposition of muscle such as the sternocleidomastoid between the damaged esophagus, trachea, and great vessels, is important to prevent fistula formation.

Injuries to the laryngotrachea are characterized by hoarseness, hemoptysis, crepitation, and dysphonia. When acute airway obstruction is the initial symptom, creation of a surgical airway is necessary. Proper diagnosis can be established with direct laryngoscopy and bronchoscopy. Primary repair is usually possible. The use of a protective tracheotomy with primary repair is controversial. CT can be used for further delineation of laryngeal fractures.

Face

Facial fractures occur less frequently in children than in adults because of the relative small proportions of the face compared with the skull of the child and because the developing bones in childhood are more resilient.

ASPECTS OF FACIAL DEVELOPMENT

Early growth of the face is rapid. At 3 months of age a child's face is less than half the size of an adult's. Approximately 70% of adult facial size is attained by 2 years of age, and by 5½ years the face grows to approximately 80% of adult size.[20] The relative craniofacial proportions also change remarkably with age. Although the majority of cranial growth is completed by 3 years of age, facial growth occurs in several stages. Generalized rapid growth takes place during the first 6 months of life, followed by a slower, more gradual increase in size between 4 and 7 years of age. After puberty a second period of rapid growth occurs between the fifteenth and nineteenth years, mainly in the naso-maxillary complex. This final portion of growth is most important in differentiation of male and female facial features. At birth the relative ratio of cranium to facial area is 8:1, at 5 years of age 4:1, and in adulthood 2:1. These changes are due to actual growth of the face and to modifications in facial proportions with characteristic remodeling into male and female features.

The mandible is the facial bone most frequently involved in long-term, posttraumatic malformations. The mandible grows in two ways: (1) bone growth and (2) development of the alveolar process accompanying development of the teeth. The child has both deciduous and permanent teeth within the mandible, which results in a higher tooth to bone ratio than in the adult. This higher density affords the mandible a greater resilience to trauma. The condylar neck is also shorter and thicker in the child, which gives additional protection from fracture and displacement. However, the growing condylar articular cartilage is susceptible to traumatic damage. Injury to the articular cartilage, especially before 5 years of age, may result in mandibular hypoplasia.

The skeleton of the midface, with the exception of the nasal cartilaginous capsule, is formed from membranous bone. The role of the nasal septum in growth of the midface is unclear. Some believe that the septum actually controls midface growth, whereas others consider the nasal septum to be less important. Just as the facial skeleton is relatively smaller in neonates than in adults, the nasal cavity and paranasal sinuses are also relatively small. The nasal cavities are as wide as they are high in the newborn. At this age the maxillary sinuses are narrow and not sufficiently developed to reach laterally beyond the infraorbital foramen. At birth the nasal septum is continuous with the cartilage of the cranial base. The floor of the maxillary sinus remains above the level of the floor of the nose up to the age of 8 years.[21] At approximately 1 year of age the perpendicular plate of the ethmoid begins ossification from the nasoethmoidal center. By 3 years of age bony union occurs between the ethmoid and vomer bones. Growth of the face then occurs in three main steps: (1) displacement away from the cranial base, (2) posterior enlargement of the nasomaxillary complex, and (3) anterior resorption, which forms the normal nasomaxillary contour of the face.

The effects of traumatic injury on the midface and nasomaxillary complex of children are difficult to determine. Most children recover from major maxillofacial trauma with good anatomic reduction and uninhibited posttraumatic growth, but in a few patients significant growth retardation occurs.

Dentoalveolar injuries are relatively common in children. Dental trauma in toddlers usually injures the anterior maxillary teeth. Intraoral inspection should include an evaluation of occlusion and the mobility of teeth. However, primary teeth undergoing resorption of newly erupted permanent teeth may be somewhat mobile in the absence of trauma. If several teeth together are mobile, an alveolar process fracture is suspected. Luxation injuries and fractures not involving the root canal can usually be reduced and immobilized with intradental wire splinting, but heroic attempts to maintain injured deciduous teeth are contraindicated. Root fractures of deciduous teeth require extraction. Permanent teeth with immature root formation may be reimplanted after complete avulsion if this can be accomplished within a few minutes of injury.[22] Alveolar fractures are treated with arch bar fixation or application of an acrylic splint (Fig. 12–15).

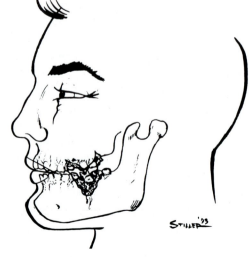

Figure 12–15. Alveolar fracture.

Mandibular fractures are common in children (Fig. 12–16). Treatment of these fractures is a challenge in the pediatric age group because of the rapidly changing growth and dentition. Older patients with permanent teeth in place can usually be treated with intermaxillary fixation. Younger children with mixed dentition or unerupted teeth require acrylic splint fixation or open interosseous fixation. In the latter technique, great care must be maintained to avoid injury to the underlying tooth bud follicles.

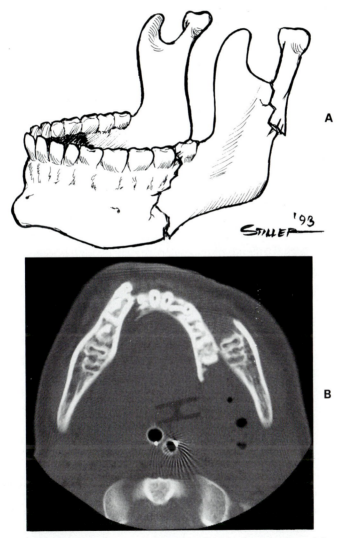

Figure 12–16. Mandibular fractures. **A,** Fracture of the body and subcondylar mandible. **B,** Computed tomographic scan of severe mandibular fracture.

Subcondylar fractures of the mandible have the greatest potential for growth disturbance. Most injuries may be treated nonoperatively. Severe fracture-dislocations may require intermaxillary fixation for immobilization. These fractures occasionally produce ankylosis of the temporomandibular joint with growth retardation and limitation of movement.

Midface fractures are uncommon in children under 12 years of age. When these fractures are seen in a child, a tremendously high-energy impact has occurred. The typical LeFort fractures (Fig. 12–17) are usually not seen in children. The LeFort classification does provide a good academic framework for categorizing midface fractures.

The low maxillary, LeFort type I fracture is rare in children because of the relative underdevelopment of the midface. Pyramidal or LeFort II fractures are more common and frequently unilateral (hemi-LeFort). LeFort III, or panfacial, fractures occur in severe trauma such as automobile accidents involving unrestrained passengers.

In cases of facial fracture, accurate alignment within 1 to 2 days of the injury is preferred. Wire interfragmentary fixation is sometimes unsatisfactory because the soft bone is cut through when placed under tension. Wire fixation to the piriform aperture or microplate fixation is preferred.

Zygomatic fractures are more common in adolescents than in younger children. Considerable force is required to fracture the zygoma, and the injury usually results in a fracture-dislocation. Treatment of these fractures is similar to that of adult zygomatic fractures. The presence of palpable step-off deformity or asymmetry with flattening of the malar eminence requires operative reduction and wire or microplate fixation. Unlike in an adult, accurate reduction in a child must be accomplished within 5 to 7 days of the injury to prevent later dysfunction and deformity.

Orbital "blow-out" fractures are usually the result of a blow to the orbit with a ball, fist, or deceleration injury. Diplopia, enophthalmos, and entrapment of the inferior rectus muscle are usually seen on presentation (Figs. 12–18 and 12–19). Treatment is restoration of the continuity of the orbital floor. Small alloplastic implants or bone grafts may be used to cover the orbital floor defect. Early repair prevents adhesions between the globe, the periorbital fat, the inferior rectus and inferior oblique muscles, and the orbital floor.[22]

Nasal fractures are common in children. In early childhood the nasal skeleton is relatively more cartilaginous than bony, which makes the diagnosis of nasal fractures more difficult. As with other types of childhood facial fractures, postinjury growth and development may be affected even after accurate diagnosis and reduction. Hematoma may form in any area between the lateral cartilages and the undersurface of the nasal bones. A child who cannot breathe through the nose after trauma should be evaluated for septal hematoma and concomitant

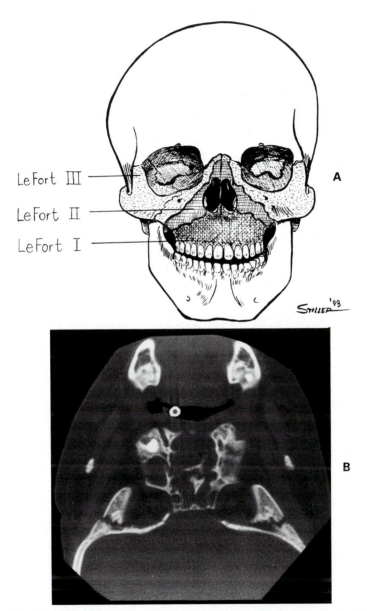

Figure 12–17. LeFort fractures. **A,** Classification of LeFort fractures. **B,** Computed tomographic scan of LeFort III fracture.

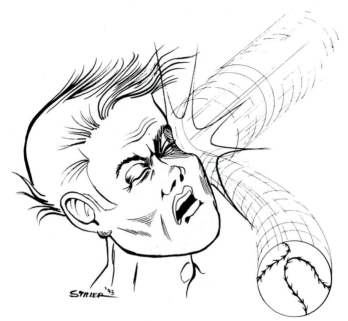

Figure 12–18. Mechanism of injury in orbital fracture.

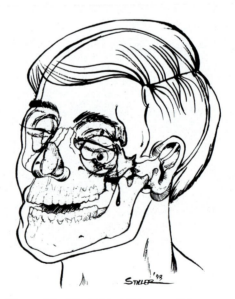

Figure 12–19. Orbital "blow-out" fracture.

nasal fracture. Often general anesthesia is necessary for adequate examination. Hematomas should be drained with an L-shaped incision extending through the mucoperichondrium from the vomer to the septal cartilages. Reduction of septal fractures and realignment of the lateral cartilages are splinted with an external splint and nasal packing. Parents should be warned that despite accurate reduction, hypertrophic callus often develops, resulting in widening of the nasal bridge years after the injury.

Compound, multiple, and comminuted fractures offer a special challenge to the surgeon (Fig. 12–20). Proper primary treatment prevents severe facial disfigurement. Partially avulsed flaps of soft tissue and bone fragments should be preserved and replaced, since the blood supply of the face in children ensures survival. In severe midface fractures the first goal should be proper occlusion, followed by fixation of the upper facial bones. Suspension wires are rarely useful in complex midface fractures, the preferred method being interfragmentary microplate and screw fixation.

SUMMARY

Severe maxillofacial injuries are uncommon in children and are usually seen in conjunction with severe head trauma or multiple injuries. Control of the airway may be difficult in a child with head and neck trauma, but an orderly,

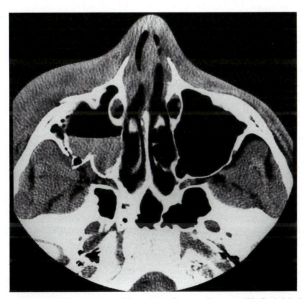

Figure 12–20. Computed tomographic scan of complex maxillofacial injury with multiple fractures and extensive soft tissue damage.

methodical evaluation and treatment plan will help prevent problems. Once an airway has been ensured and ventilation is adequate, a more thorough examination of the head and neck can be performed. Special aspects of facial injury include facial nerve laceration, parotid or lacrimal duct injury, and maxillofacial fractures. Penetrating injury to the neck is unfortunately becoming more common in the pediatric population. Appropriate evaluation and treatment are necessary to determine whether a vital structure has been injured and to deal properly with that injury.

REFERENCES

1. Rowe NL: Fractures of the facial skeleton in children, *J Oral Surg* 26:505–515, 1968.
2. Morgan BDG, Madan DK, Bergerot JPC: Fractures of the middle third of the face: a review of 300 cases, *Br J Plast Surg* 25:147–151, 1972.
3. Agran A, Dunkle DE: Motor vehicle occupant injuries to children in crash and noncrash events, *Pediatrics* 70:993–996, 1982.
4. Agran PF, Dunkle DE, Winn DG: Motor vehicle childhood injuries caused by noncrash falls and ejections, *JAMA* 253:2530–2533, 1985.
5. Duresne CR, Manson PN: Pediatric facial trauma. In McCarty J, ed: *Plastic surgery,* Vol 2. *The face,* Philadelphia, 1990, WB Saunders, pp 1142–1187.
6. Ramenofsky ML et al: Advanced trauma life support, Chicago, 1990, American College of Surgeons, p 34.
7. Spine injury in the multiply injured child. In Kling TF Jr: *Trauma in children,* 1986, Aspen, pp 175–197.
8. Aufdemaur M: Spinal injuries in juveniles: necropsy findings in twelve cases, *J Bone Joint Surg* 56B:513–519, 1974.
9. Pollack RA, Rohrich RJ, Sheffield RW: Facial fractures II: upper and middle face (overview), *Selected Readings Plast Surg* 4:2, 1987.
10. Children's fractures. In Rowe NL, Williams JC: *Maxillofacial injuries,* New York, 1985, Churchill Livingstone.
11. Committee on Trauma, American College of Surgeons: *Advanced trauma life support manual,* Chicago, 1990, The College.
12. Roon AJ, Christianson N: Evaluation and treatment of penetrating surgical injuries, *J Trauma* 19:391, 1979.
13. Bradley EL III: Management of penetrating neck injuries: an alternative approach, *J Trauma* 13:248, 1973.
14. Brown MF, Graham JM, Feliciano DV, et al: Carotid injuries, *Am J Surg* 144:748, 1982.
15. Richardson JD, Simpson C, Miller FB: Management of carotid artery trauma, *Surgery* 104:673, 1988.
16. Ledgerwood AM, Mullins RJ, Lucas CE: Primary repair vs ligation for carotid artery injuries, *Arch Surg* 115:488, 1980.
17. Reid JD, Weigelt JA: Forty-three cases of vertebral artery trauma, *J Trauma* 28:1007, 1988.

18. Meier DE, Brink BE, Fry WJ: Vertebral artery trauma, *Arch Surg* 16:2361, 1981.
19. Golueke P, Sclafani SJA, Phillips T, et al: Vertebral artery injury: diagnosis and management, *J Trauma* 27:856, 1987.
20. Enlow DH: Handbook of facial growth, ed 2, Philadelphia, 1982, WB Saunders.
21. Bernstein L: Pediatric sinus problems, *Otol Clin North Am* 4:126, 1971.
22. Berkowitz R, Ludwig S, Johnson R: Dental trauma in children with adolescents, *Clin Pediatr* 19:166, 1980.
23. Manson PN, Clifford CM, Su CT, et al: Mechanisms of globe support and posttraumatic enophthalmos. I. The anatomy of the ligament sling and its relation to intramuscular cone orbital fat, *Plast Reconstr Surg* 77:193, 1986.

13

Vascular Trauma

Chris Cribari
Jay S. Miller
Matthew L. Lukens

Vascular trauma has challenged surgeons caring for the injured as far back as records exist. Over 230 years have passed since Hallowell[1] performed the first crude arteriorrhaphy of a brachial artery injury. He placed a pin through the arterial walls and held them in apposition with a figure-of-8 suture wrapped around the pin. The first successful end-to-end arterial anastomosis was performed by J.B. Murphy[2] in 1896. In 1902 Carrel[3] conceived the technique of triangulation, a simple concept that proved to be a monumental advance in vascular surgery. That technique was modified to a quadrangulation technique by Frouin[4] in 1908. In 1906 Goyanes[5] successfully bridged an arterial defect with a vein graft using the triangulation technique developed by Carrel and Guthrie.

Over the next 50 years numerous valuable lessons were learned as thousands of vascular injuries were treated during World Wars I and II. Although the Germans attempted repair of arterial injuries during World War I, infection plagued virtually all of the wounded and thereafter any serious consideration to attempting repair was considered time consuming and foolhardy.[6] DeBakey and Simeone[7] analyzed 2471 arterial injuries treated during World War II. Only 81 repairs were attempted, with a 35% eventual amputation rate. Ligation, with an accompanying 49% amputation rate, remained the wartime procedure of necessity, despite agreement that the techniques of repair were available. Not until the Korean conflict was routine successful vascular repair accomplished. Hughes[8] reported 304 arterial injuries (269 repaired, 35 ligated) in which the overall amputation rate dropped to 13%. In addition to the availability of vascular clamps and improved suture material of smaller size, factors contributing to this dramatic decrease in amputations included the rapid evacuation of casualties, improvements in anesthetic management, and the availability of antibiotics and blood transfusions.

336

With the lessons learned from the Korean conflict and the widespread teaching of vascular surgical techniques in surgical residencies, arterial repair became the highly successful standard of care for arterial injuries beginning in the late 1950s. One of the first large series of civilian arterial injuries was reported by Morris, Creech, and DeBakey[9] in 1957. Over a 7-year period, 136 acute arterial injuries were treated at Baylor-affiliated hospitals in Houston. Upper extremity arterial injuries accounted for 50% of the reported injuries. Four years later, in 1961, Ferguson, Byrd, and McAfee[10] reported 200 arterial injuries treated at Grady Memorial Hospital over a 10-year period; the superficial femoral artery was most frequently injured. Acts of violence accounted for the majority of the injuries in both these early civilian series.

The Vietnam conflict contributed a wealth of experience and knowledge about management of military casualties and vascular trauma. The Vietnam Vascular Registry, established in 1966 at Walter Reed General Hospital, allowed the documentation and analysis of all vascular injuries treated in U.S. Army hospitals in Vietnam. In 1970 Rich, Baugh, and Hughes[11] reported their analysis of 1000 cases. Vascular injuries in the extremities accounted for 91% of the cases, with 56.8% involving the lower extremity and 34.2% involving the upper extremity. Despite implementation of all the valuable lessons learned in the previous 25 years, the amputation rate remained at 13%. The stable amputation rate reflected the magnitude of wartime injuries, many of which have no adequate reconstructive option. Over the past 23 years experience in civilian trauma centers has continued to refine the vast amount of information accumulated in wartime. The magnitude of the civilian experience is exemplified by the report of Mattox and associates[12] on 5760 cardiovascular injuries treated at a single institution over a 30-year period. Although the knowledge base for diagnosing and treating vascular injuries in adults is enormous, data specific to the management of pediatric vascular injuries have lagged. The first report of a case series of peripheral arterial injuries in infants and children did not appear until 1968. In this report from Johns Hopkins Hospital, White, Talbert, and Haller[13] showed that pediatric peripheral arterial injuries occurred more frequently than was generally recognized. They grouped their cases by etiology to illustrate a pattern of injuries peculiar to this age group. The first group included arterial injuries associated with trauma to an extremity. In this group were injuries resulting from penetrating wounds and fractures. Specific emphasis was placed on injuries resulting from falls through glass storm doors and vascular injuries associated with supracondylar humoral fractures. The second etiologic group encompassed iatrogenic injuries resulting from retrograde arterial catheterization. The authors stressed concern about impairment of limb growth if thrombosis went unrecognized and if blood flow was left dependent on collateral flow. The final etiologic group was cases of iatrogenic injuries occurring from "other" procedures such as "needling an extremity." The insight and conclusions contained in this landmark article have withstood the test of time. Subsequent reports on pediatric vascular injuries have confirmed many of the early findings and therapeutic concerns. This chapter presents a summation of the literature in English and discusses current concepts in the management of pediatric vascular injuries.

SPECIAL CONSIDERATIONS

Advances achieved in the treatment of adult trauma victims have gradually been applied to children. As experience in managing pediatric vascular injuries has accumulated, important differences and special considerations have been elucidated. Many of these special considerations center on patient size and concerns for growth. First is the recognition that a child's smaller blood volume allows a relatively smaller margin of safety from exsanguination. Also related to size is the character of the vessel itself. The vessel's smaller size adds to the technical challenge of repair and increases the propensity for thrombosis. These considerations are further complicated by the marked arterial vasospasm that is noted to occur in the younger age groups. Vasospasm may not only promote the likelihood of thrombosis, but also make the diagnosis of occlusion extremely difficult.[14] Infants and small children are also characteristically more prone to thrombosis because of polycythemia, dehydration, hyperviscosity, or congenital hypercoagulable states.[15-24] The issue of future growth is of paramount importance. Any treatment plan or technique of repair must take into consideration the effect it may have on the later growth of the vessel and extremity.

ETIOLOGY

Blunt vascular trauma related to high-speed motor vehicle accidents and falls has become a well-recognized mechanism of vascular injury. As in the early literature concerning adults, the majority of pediatric vascular injuries involve the extremities and are related to acts of violence (i.e., gunshot wounds, stab wounds). Most children are injured in accidents involving motor vehicles. The introduction of invasive monitoring techniques and techniques for pediatric cardiac catheterization has produced a group of patients at risk for iatrogenic vascular trauma that may require operative repair. Pediatric patients with iatrogenic vascular injuries became particularly evident in the landmark article from Johns Hopkins.[13,25] The classification of vascular injuries is commonly based on the mechanism of injury. The three broad categories of injury are blunt, penetrating, and iatrogenic. Each of these may be subdivided based on the specific mechanism (Table 13–1).

The potential mechanisms of injury must be recognized and understood to allow a high index of suspicion during patient evaluation. The prevalence of

Table 13–1. Classification of Vascular Injuries by Cause

Blunt Trauma (falls, motor vehicle accidents, crush injury)

Fractures (supracondylar humeral fractures, tibial plateau fractures, knee dislocations)
Neck hyperextension/rotational injury
Deceleration injury
Direct contusion

Penetrating Injuries

Lacerations (e.g., falls through plate glass)
Projectiles from lawnmowers, air rifles, handguns, rifles, and shotguns
Stab wounds from knives, pencils, sticks, glass shards, and other sharp objects

Iatrogenic

Vascular procedures
   Cardiac catheterization
   Arteriography
   Umbilical artery catheters
   Central venous access
   Radial artery catheters
Other nonvascular invasive procedures
   Operative misadventure
   Kyphectomy for lumbar kyphosis

the different mechanisms varies based on the age of the pediatric patient. O'Neil,[26] in his treatise on traumatic vascular lesions in infants and children, divided the children into three age groups: less than 2 years of age, 2 to 6 years of age, and older than 6 years of age. In the youngest age group, iatrogenic injuries accounted for 81% of the vascular injuries. In the 2- to 6-year age group the incidence of noniatrogenic injuries approximated that of iatrogenic injury. This increase in noniatrogenic mechanisms corresponds to the toddler's increasing independent ambulation and accompanying falls. In the oldest age group, noniatrogenic injuries prevailed. The group has a greater proportion of penetrating injuries as children become exposed to the violence in our society. There remains controversy as to the upper age cutoff for inclusion in a pediatric series. In some series the limit is 14 years of age, but others include patients up to 18 or 19 years of age. Regardless, the distribution of the mechanisms of injury during the teenage years appears to be no different from that of adults. Extremity vascular injuries following violence predominate.

We have reviewed, compiled, and tabulated all series reported in peer review journals from the literature in English to characterize the pediatric population at risk for vascular injury (Table 13–2). Altogether, 1049 cases were tabulated; 381 (36.3%) resulted from iatrogenic injuries and 668 (63.7%) from non-

Table 13−2. Compilation of the Literature

Author	Iatrogenic	Noniatrogenic (Blunt/Penetrating)	Age Range
White[13]	7	3 (1/2)	3 mo—8 yr
Cahill[25]	6		
Mansfield[27]	29		4 mo—25 yr
Stanford[28]	1	42 (10/32)	14 mo—18 yr
Bloom[29]	3		
Whitehouse[30]	11	9 (9/10)	1 mo—16 yr
Shaker[31]	41	30 (8/22)	All <15 yr
Meagher[32]	3	50 (14/36)	24 days—14 yr
Smith[33]	5		All <2 yr
O'Neil[26]	54	53 *3 spontaneous	All <16 yr
Richardson[34]	4	24 (11/13)	8 mo—13 yr
Navarre[35]		59	10 mo—19 yr
Klein[36]	32		1 day—16 yr
Perry[37]	4		All <1 yr
Flanigan[38]	45		1 day—13 yr
LeBlanc[39]	40	8 (3/5)	5 days—17 yr
Villavicencio[40]	59	36 (11/25)	
Evans[41]	92	(28/64)	14 mo—18 yr
Solak[42]		83 (23/60)	5 yr—20 yr
Myers[43]		20 (7/13)	7 yr—18 yr
Wolf[44]		30 (4/26)	4 yr—14 yr
Mills[45]		40 (29/11)	5 mo—12 yr
Eren[46]	2	89 (21/68)	3 yr—14 yr
LaQuaglia[47]	9		All <2 yr
TOTAL CASES: 1049	381 (36.3%)	668 (63.7%)	

iatrogenic mechanisms. We recognize that this tabulation does not include individual case reports, nor does it include vascular injuries reported in reviews of thoracic, abdominal, or orthopedic injuries. Our review may include some overlap of cases because of institutions reporting their earlier cases in later series. Despite these flaws we believe that one third to one half of vascular injuries in children are due to iatrogenic mechanisms, with most of these occurring before 6 years of age.

Specific mechanisms of vascular injury in the pediatric population have repeatedly appeared in the literature. Supracondylar fractures of the humerus in children are associated with injury to the brachial artery in 12% of patients.[48] Fractures in other sites may also result in vascular injury, including fractures of the femur, tibia, fibula, radius, ulna, and clavicle. Significant vascular injury is, however, far less common than in those with supracondylar fractures.[49] Other orthopedic injuries that may be associated with vascular injury include dislocations of the knee, elbow, and shoulder.[50,51] Green[51] reported a 32% overall incidence of popliteal artery injury with dislocation of the knee.

Blunt trauma causing vascular injury that is not related to orthopedic injuries may occur with stretching, shearing, or crushing of the vessel. Deceleration injury to the aorta results from shearing forces generated at sites where the aorta is relatively well fixed (e.g., the proximal descending thoracic aorta at the level of the ligamentum arteriosum). These injuries cause partial or complete transection of the aortic wall. The occurrence of traumatic aortic rupture in the pediatric population may be more common than was previously recognized, although less prevalent than in adults. Eddy and co-workers[52] reported 13 children who sustained traumatic rupture of the thoracic aorta; in 6 the injury occurred in automobile versus pedestrian accidents, in 5 as a result of high-speed motor vehicle accidents, and in 2 as the result of off-road motorcycle accidents.[52] Blunt abdominal aortic and iliac artery injuries are also reported in association with lap belt trauma in motor vehicle accidents, direct blows to the abdomen, and crush injuries.[53,54] Hyperextension and rotational injuries of the neck, which may occur with relatively minor trauma, have resulted in dissections of the carotid and vertebral arteries.[55-57] Manifestations of carotid and vertebral artery injuries may first appear days after the traumatic event and may include headache, intermittent neurologic signs, or frank stroke. Another unusual mechanism of injury leading to internal carotid artery thrombosis is associated with intraoral trauma to the soft palate. The typical example is a running toddler who trips and falls with an object in the mouth. The carotid arteries are relatively superficial behind the tonsils and easily approachable via intraoral routes. These injuries may be blunt or penetrating. Pearl[58] in his review of the literature found 20 cases of childhood stroke resulting from intraoral trauma to the carotid artery.

The mechanisms of most noniatrogenic penetrating vascular injuries are obvious (e.g., gunshot wounds, stab wounds, and lacerations).[32,43] More subtle mechanisms requiring a high index of suspicion during evaluation include puncture wounds from glass shards,[13,28] dog bites,[59] airgun pellets,[60] and projectiles from lawnmowers.[28] Any patient with a penetrating wound near a vascular structure must be considered to have a potential vascular injury until that injury is ruled out by further diagnostic studies or surgical exploration.

Iatrogenic vascular injuries are subdivided into two categories. The first category includes vascular complications associated with procedures that directly involve the vascular system (i.e., any procedure involving arterial or venous access). This group represents the majority of iatrogenic vascular injuries. A vascular complication or injury may occur during almost any procedure that involves entering a vessel, but the majority of iatrogenic pediatric vascular injuries reported have been associated with cardiac catheterization, arteriography, the use of umbilical artery catheters, central venous catheterization, and radial artery catheterization. The potential complications of intravascular instrumentation include perforation or rupture of the vessel with hemorrhage and hematoma formation, thrombosis of the vessel, embolization, pseudoaneurysm or mycotic aneurysm formation, arteriovenous fistula, and late stenosis.[61] Local complications, such as hematoma formation at the site of puncture, are the most common. They rarely require intervention other than close follow-up to rule out the development of a pseudoaneurysm or an arteriovenous fistula.

Thrombosis is the most common complication that requires intervention. Thrombosis occurred in up to 30% of patients undergoing arteriotomy for cardiac catheterization as reported in the early literature.[13,25] Numerous improvements in technique, including a percutaneous approach and the use of intravenous heparin, have reduced the incidence of thrombosis to 2% to 3%.[62] Similar improvements have reduced the incidence of thrombosis associated with arteriography. Thrombosis of the radial artery following removal of intraarterial monitoring catheters occurs in 63% to 80% of neonates, but blood flow almost always reappears in 1 to 29 days.[63] The evaluation and management of iatrogenic thrombosis are discussed later in the chapter.

The use of umbilical artery catheters in the management of critically ill newborns is also associated with thrombosis and a variety of vascular complications. Perforation of the artery during placement of the catheter is rare but carries the potential for fatal hemorrhage. Thrombosis of the aorta and iliac arteries associated with umbilical artery catheters may require a much more aggressive approach than thrombosis resulting from cardiac catheterization or arteriography because the more proximal thrombus may occlude the visceral or renal vessels.[64-66] Ischemia distal to the area of thrombosis may also lead to gluteal necrosis, lower extremity gangrene, paraplegia, and visceral infarction.[65-67] The level of the tip of the catheter usually determines the potential proximal extent of thrombosis. This has led some authors to recommend low placement of the catheter just above the bifurcation of the aorta.[67] Another rare but often disastrous complication is the formation of mycotic aneurysms of the aorta and iliac arteries. These aneurysms are typically reported in neonates with umbilical artery catheters who have staphylococcal sepsis.[68] A consistent relationship has been shown between the duration of catheterization and the risk of both increased intimal damage and incidence of infection.[67-69] Most aneurysms occur adjacent to the catheter tip, yet another reason for recommending more caudad placement of the catheter.[68]

As the pathogenesis of vascular complications during medical procedures becomes clear and new techniques are introduced, the incidence of many of these iatrogenic vascular injuries will probably decrease. On the other hand, as newer procedures are introduced, so will the potential for other types of iatrogenic injury.

The second category of iatrogenic injury encompasses a variety of vascular complications that occur during procedures not directly involving the vascular system (e.g., aortic occlusion following kyphectomy for congenital kyphosis[61] or any vascular injury occurring during nonvascular surgical procedures).

Although prevention plays the most important role in the management of any injury, whether noniatrogenic or iatrogenic, once the injury occurs an efficient, accurate, cost-effective approach to diagnosis and treatment is essential.

DIAGNOSIS

The prompt, accurate detection of vascular injuries is critical in the management of pediatric trauma. Delays in diagnosis of vascular trauma are associated with poor outcomes.[41] Physicians evaluating trauma patients must be able to generate a high index of suspicion based on the mechanism of injury alone. The recognition of specific mechanisms associated with different vascular injuries may be the first clue leading to detection of an occult injury. (An example of this is the association of carotid and vertebral artery dissections with relatively minor hyperextension and rotational neck trauma.[33-35]) The history and physical examination provide sufficient information for the diagnosis of arterial insufficiency in 75% of cases of vascular injury.[70] The hard signs of arterial injury are absent distal pulse, active bleeding, expanding or pulsatile hematoma, and evidence of distal ischemia (pain, pallor, paresthesias, and paralysis). The presence of any of these hard signs in the nonneonate has such a high predictive value for a major vascular injury that immediate surgical exploration without further evaluation is indicated.

Pediatric trauma patients have a number of characteristics that make evaluation more challenging. The signs and symptoms of distal ischemia may be more difficult to evaluate in children. Infants and small children may be unable to describe their symptoms. Pain and paresthesias are often obscured by related injuries. Paralysis may not be readily evident in an uncooperative infant or child. Vasospasm may masquerade as arterial occlusion, further complicating the diagnostic dilemma. In children who have a cold, pulseless extremity after noniatrogenic trauma or who have an obvious vascular injury, *no further evaluation is necessary before surgical intervention.* Likewise, for an expanding hematoma, active bleeding from a penetrating injury, or a palpable thrill overlying an injury, operative intervention is mandatory. However, if the patient is stable and has softer signs of arterial injury (diminished pulse, nonexpanding hematoma, or proximity of the artery to a wound), or if the signs and symptoms are thought to be secondary to intense vasospasm, the possibility of a vascular injury must be ruled out with modalities short of surgical exploration.

In adults, policies of mandatory exploration of all potential vascular injuries were instituted to prevent missed injuries. This resulted in a high negative exploration rate. Subsequently, liberal use of arteriography to exclude vascular injury decreased the negative exploration rate from 58% to 35%.[71] Arteriography has been shown to have a sensitivity of 97% to 100% and a specificity of 90% to 98% and remains the "gold standard" to which newer techniques are compared.[71,72]

The increased incidence of iatrogenic arterial trauma and the characteristically severe vasospasm associated with arterial catheterization in infants and smaller children have limited routine use of arteriography in pediatric patients. In pediatric series reported the use of arteriography has ranged from none to 65% of the patients.[28-47] This wide variance is related not only to the different types of patients included in the different series (with the greater use of arteriography in series of older children with penetrating injuries), but also to the availability of experienced interventional radiologists and to the confidence the surgeons have in their abilities. Apprehension about further injury, vasospasm, and other complications associated with arteriography has led to the use of other diagnostic modalities in children.

DIAGNOSTIC TESTS

The avoidance of arteriography in pediatric patients has been recommended by numerous authors,[47,73] and selective arteriography has been proposed by most others.* The obvious concern is that arteriography is an invasive procedure carrying a definite risk of arterial injury and thrombosis. The risk of arterial thrombosis is greatest in the smallest patients and is negligible after 10 years of age.[62,76] Digital venous subtraction angiography (DSA) has been used to evaluate pediatric vessels in elective circumstances,[33] to rule out spasm in emergency situations,[45] and to follow up vascular repairs.[76] DSA offers the advantage of being a venous technique that avoids the risks of arterial puncture. DSA is subject to motion artifact and is of limited use in small patients.

Doppler pressure measurements have been helpful in evaluating pediatric trauma patients (Fig. 13–1). Normal Doppler pressures nearly rule out the existence of mechanical vascular obstruction.[74] Doppler studies also provide objective measurement of peripheral perfusion that may be used later in follow-up. Duplex imaging has been useful in evaluating arterial injuries in patients with viable extremities, with and without normal Doppler measurements.[38] Duplex scanning has the added ability of graphically identifying small arterial injuries such as arteriovenous fistulas, pseudoaneurysms, intimal flaps, and venous injuries that might otherwise be missed with physical examination or Doppler pressure measurements.[38,76]

Isotope arteriography has been used in infants to avoid routine arteriog-

---

*References 30, 39, 43–45, 74, 75.

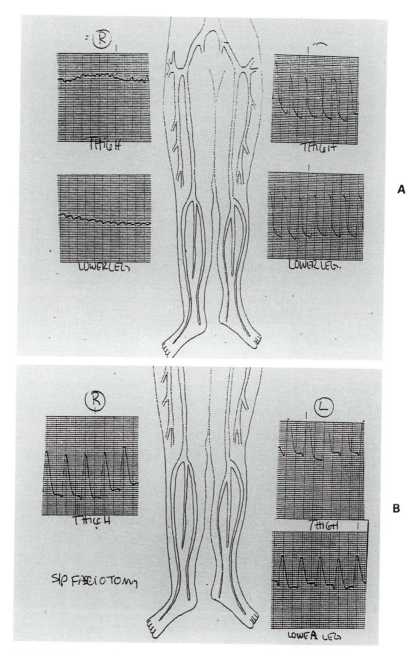

Figure 13–1. A, Preoperative arterial Doppler wave forms showing complete occlusion of the right superficial femoral artery following heart catheterization in a 2-year-old child. **B,** First postoperative day follow-up from thrombectomy and repair of the right superficial femoral artery. The Doppler wave forms show a brisk and normal arterial tracing on the right.

Illustration continued on following page

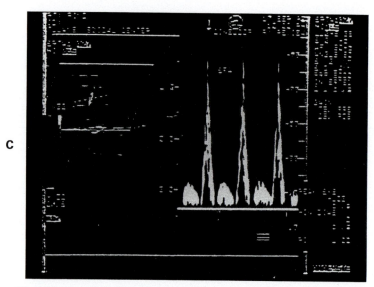

Figure 13–1 *Continued* **C,** The three-month follow-up study shows brisk arterial Doppler flows at the site of arterial repair.

raphy for the evaluation of aortoiliac occlusion.[25,73] Because of the poor resolution of detail in very small vascular structures, these nuclear medicine studies have a limited role in defining vascular injury.

The diagnostic approach of choice to pediatric vascular injury depends on the patient's age. Algorithms for the evaluation of pediatric patients under and over 6 years of age are shown in Figures 13–2 and 13–3, respectively.

MANAGEMENT

The management of arterial and venous injuries in infants and children has paralleled developments in vascular surgery on adults. As a result, a majority of surgeons now recommend prompt exploration and reconstruction of vascular injuries in children. Before definitive procedures the patient must be resuscitated like any other trauma victim. This includes securing an airway if one is lacking, initiating ventilation if the patient is not breathing, and achieving hemodynamic stability. To maintain hemodynamic stability, external hemorrhage is controlled with direct pressure, "large-bore" intravenous access is established, and crystalloid fluids and blood products are administered as required. All of these measures are performed to maintain a stable cardiac output. Arterial and venous reconstruction performed in patients with decreased cardiac output clearly increases the risk of postoperative thrombosis.[46] All life-threatening injuries (persistent bleeding, hypotension, and cardiopulmonary instability) must be addressed be-

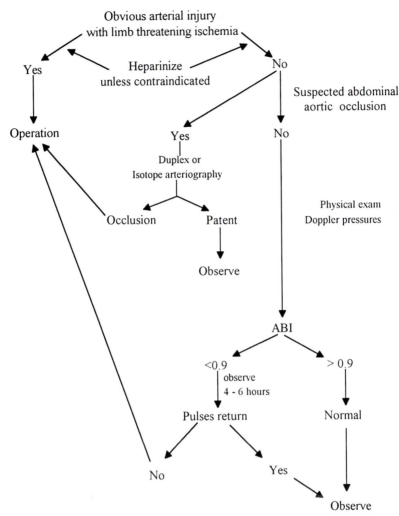

Figure 13–2. Algorithm for management of penetrating vascular injuries in children under 6 years of age.

fore definitive repair of an extremity vascular injury. During the hectic period of evaluation and resuscitation, tetanus prophylaxis for penetrating injuries and antibiotic prophylaxis for all operative candidates must not be neglected.

Following stabilization and diagnosis of a vascular injury, the decision is made as to whether operative treatment is required or whether a course of nonoperative observation may be pursued. Nonoperative management is considered only for selected patients, such as those with an intimal flap and preservation of distal flow or infants with an iatrogenic catheter-related loss of distal

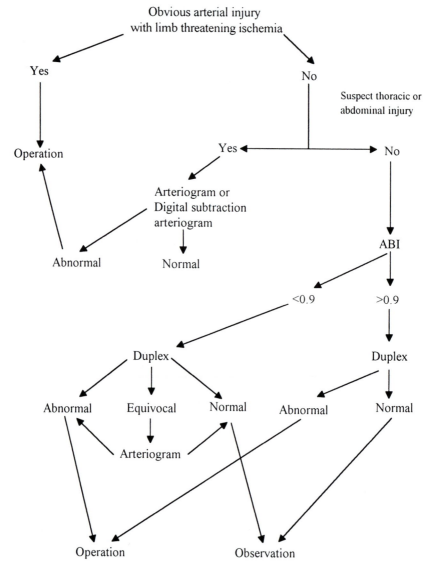

Figure 13–3. Algorithm for management of patients over 6 years of age.

pulses that may be secondary to vasospasm. In most other instances operative repair of vascular injuries is indicated and should be performed as expeditiously as possible.

All of the sequelae (e.g. arteriovenous fistulas, pseudoaneurysms, and thrombosis) reported following missed, or nonoperatively managed, adult vascular injuries may also occur in children. In addition, the possibility of growth impairment in the affected limb is a unique and important complication in the pediatric population. Currarino and Engle[77] first presented clinical evidence of limb growth retardation in patients who underwent a Blalock-Taussig shunt procedure. They found a significant reduction in length of the radius and a decrease in muscle mass in the affected limb. Several authors then looked for clinical evidence of limb length disparity in the lower extremities of children following cardiac catheterization and found growth disturbances in 0.8% to 85% of patients.[78–81] The wide variability among reports was believed to correlate with the variable frequency of arterial injury. Smith and Green[33] evaluated children with proven thrombosis after catheterization and reported decreased limb growth in all affected extremities, as well as claudication in more than half the affected limbs.[33] The limb growth disparity appears to be due to decreased blood flow both to the muscles in the affected extremity and to the epiphyseal region of the long bones.[29] Even though children usually have sufficient collateral vessels to maintain a viable extremity, the potential for limb growth disparity and significant morbidity strongly supports revascularization whenever possible.

Infants less than 1 year of age are considered separately because of their profound propensity for vascular spasm after injury (Fig. 13–4). Mortensson[82] demonstrated arterial occlusion caused by vasospasm around arterial catheters used for cardiac arteriography. Franken and associates[83] showed arterial spasm in 62% of 100 consecutive infants undergoing angiography of the left side of the heart via the femoral approach. Infants less than 1 year of age who have a catheter-induced pulseless extremity should be initially treated with anticoagulant therapy. Most authors recommend removal of the catheter and initiation of heparin (100 units/kg) for a 4- to 6-hour period.[32,37,84] Many infants are not thought to be suitable candidates for heparinization because of the potential for bleeding complications.[38,40] If the infant has contraindications to heparin use (e.g., intraventricular hemorrhage), low-molecular-weight dextran may be substituted. During the period of anticoagulation the patient is observed for bleeding and for worsening of the limb ischemia. If only a proximal pulse appears during the observation period, a duplex study should be performed to look for proximal artery thrombosis. If no thrombus is identified and the patient is a neonate, heparin therapy should be continued for up to 48 hours with continued observation. A local operative procedure is not possible in the neonate because the smallest balloon embolectomy catheter (2F) is too large to pass the superficial femoral, deep femoral, axillary, or brachial arteries.[38] However, if thrombus is documented in the common femoral artery or no femoral pulse is noted, operative intervention is warranted.

Case reports of thrombolytic therapy in the infant population have indicated varying results.[85] Further study regarding the use of thrombolysis in this patient population is under way.

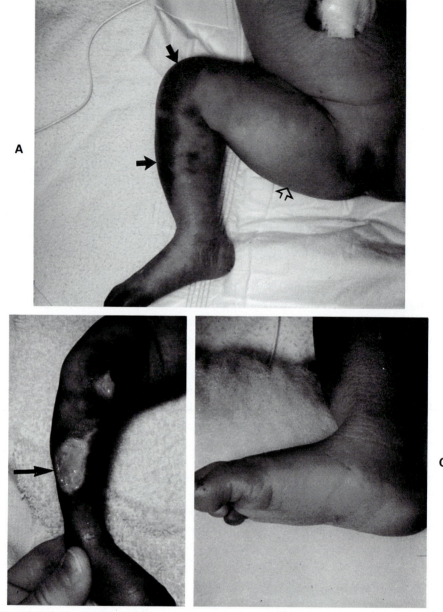

Figure 13–4. A, This patient is a neonate who suffered complete occlusion of the superficial femoral artery (SFA) following heart catheterization. The watershed vascular supply is clearly demonstrated. Tissues in the gluteal distribution are well-perfused (*open arrow*). Tissues in the SFA distribution are completely compromised (*closed arrows*). The tissue between the two is partially perfused. This patient was treated with thrombolytic therapy and heparin. **B,** Over the course of 48 hours the patient regained vascular supply to most of the extremity. The skin with only SFA supply sloughed (*arrow*). **C,** Tissues at the distal most distribution of the toes never re-perfused. These areas were allowed to mummify and slough.

350

Several differences between pediatric and adult patients in the management of and technical approach to treating vascular injuries must be emphasized. Infants and children have smaller vessels that require meticulous dissection and repair, necessitating the use of at least 2.5 × magnification. Any repair of the vessel must anticipate future growth of the patient. Interrupted suture techniques should be used to decrease the likelihood of a subsequent stenosis. A variety of treatment regimens may be necessary to reduce associated intense arterial vasospasm. Recommended therapy for spasm includes adequate volume resuscitation and topical or direct adventitial administration or intraarterial infusion of 1% lidocaine or 2% to 3% papaverine or both.[37,38,45]

All pediatric patients should have operative procedures performed under general anesthesia. Neonates with thrombosis resulting in an ischemic lower extremity should initially undergo exploration of the common femoral artery (CFA). Vascular control can be attained with small Silastic loops that cause less endothelial trauma than vascular clamps. A transverse arteriotomy is made in the CFA, and a 2F or 3F Fogarty embolectomy catheter is used to remove the thrombus from the vessel. Some authors have reported the use of small catheters to aspirate and remove thrombus from very small vessels.[25] This technique may have a higher failure rate because up to 60% of distal thrombus may not be continuous.[31] After excellent inflow and outflow are achieved, the arteriotomy is closed with meticulously placed, interrupted, very fine, monofilament suture (6-0 to 8-0). If this initial arterial repair fails, reoperation should be performed only for severe arterial ischemia. In a limb that is ischemic but viable, further surgery should be deferred because of the disappointing results with reoperation in neonates.[40]

The timing of revascularization to cause the least limb length disparity remains controversial. Bloom and co-workers[29] demonstrated a reduction of limb length disparity with delayed revascularization. However, in a later study by Whitehouse and associates,[30] delayed revascularization did not prevent or reverse limb length disparity. We believe that the best way to prevent limb length disparity is to achieve revascularization as soon as possible following diagnosis.

A special situation is acute aortic occlusion that occurs in neonates following umbilical artery catheter placement. If evaluation by ultrasonography, arteriography, or radionuclide scanning reveals thrombotic aortic occlusion associated with severe lower extremity ischemia, congestive heart failure, renal failure, or signs of multisystem organ failure, operative treatment is necessary. Delay in therapy may jeopardize patient survival. Systemic anticoagulation (unless contraindicated) is initiated, and the aorta is approached through a transverse mid-abdominal incision. A transverse aortotomy is performed in the infrarenal aorta. A longitudinal aortotomy is preferred in patients with renal artery thrombosis.

Thrombus is extracted from all vessels through 2F and 3F Fogarty catheters. The aortotomy is repaired with interrupted monofilament suture (6-0). Heparin therapy is then discontinued.[26,64]

Vascular surgical techniques in the remainder of the pediatric population are designed to ensure optimal growth of the artery. Unless anticoagulants are contraindicated, all patients receive heparin (100 units/kg) preoperatively. If systemic heparin is contraindicated, local heparin administration into the proximal and distal arterial segments is used. The simplest technique that provides a tension-free repair is often the best. For a longitudinal laceration involving greater than 50% of the circumference of an artery, we recommend a patch angioplasty with saphenous vein using an interrupted suture technique. A primary repair in this injury may constrict the vessel. If the injury has resulted in a severely traumatized artery, resection of nonviable arterial wall is performed. The proximal and distal segments of the artery are mobilized without sacrificing collateral vessels. A tension-free, generously spatulated, end-to-end anastomosis is constructed with interrupted suture. If a tension-free primary anastomosis cannot be created or if an extensive portion of artery is traumatized, a bypass procedure is performed with reverse saphenous vein graft harvested from the noninjured leg. Vein grafts provide durable bypass conduits in the pediatric population with the exception of bypass or replacement of major intraabdominal visceral arteries.[86,87] Aneurysmal degeneration of the vein graft with attendant embolization and thrombosis tends to occur in these larger central vessels. Aneurysmal dilation of saphenous vein aortorenal grafts occurs in 20% to 40% of cases.[87] The conduit of choice for repair of aorta or intraabdominal visceral vessels is autogenous hypogastric artery.[88,89] Whenever a graft is required, autologous sources should be considered first.* The successful use of PTFE and Dacron grafts has been reported in children.[32-34,39]

Many arterial injuries are accompanied by an associated venous injury. Venous injuries, especially those involving the femoral, popliteal, and brachial veins, should be repaired if technically feasible. Venous repair leads to a marked reduction in postoperative edema, a lower incidence of amputation, and a lower incidence of severe postphlebitic sequelae.[46,92,93] Acceptable options for repair include lateral venorrhaphy, patch venoplasty, or insertion of a saphenous vein interposition graft.[46,92,93]

After surgical therapy to relieve acute arterial ischemia, especially involving the lower extremity, many pediatric patients still face potential limb loss from compartment syndrome. Early recognition and proper treatment of compartment syndrome may prevent permanent neuromuscular disability, enhance limb salvage, and avoid myonecrosis with subsequent renal failure or death. Indi-

---

*References 30, 38, 43, 46, 47, 84, 90, 91.

cations for fasciotomy include limb ischemia for more than 6 hours, combined arterial and venous injuries, crush injuries, and massive tissue swelling. Fasciotomy is performed, if indicated, at the time of initial operation. A four-compartment lower extremity fasciotomy, as described by Mubarak and Owen,[94] is performed through a primary incision over the anterolateral aspect and a counterincision on the posteromedial aspect of the limb. Opening the fascia the full length of the lower leg is important to prevent subsequent tissue compromise.[95,96]

Another uncommon but interesting type of arterial injury is carotid and vertebral artery dissections. These injuries usually occur when forcible extension of the head stretches the internal carotid artery over the transverse process of the third cervical vertebra and the body of the second cervical vertebra, disrupting the intima and media. Dissection of these vessels has long been recognized in adults following blunt trauma with subsequent severe neurologic morbidity. This entity is now being identified more often in the pediatric population. Children and small infants may be more prone than adults to this injury because of the relatively larger size of the head in relation to the remainder of the body. There has been an evolution in the literature regarding the role of surgical versus medical management of these lesions. Currently medical management (volume resuscitation, blood pressure control, and anticoagulation) is the preferred initial therapy in light of the overall prognosis and limitations of surgical intervention. The role of anticoagulation in small children with this lesion has not been defined, and its use must be individualized. Medical therapy is based on the tenet that the majority of the neurologic deficits are embolic or thrombotic and may be preventable with anticoagulation. Surgical intervention is reserved for patients with progressive neurologic deficits secondary to hypoperfusion or embolic phenomena associated with a favorable anatomic lesion. Surgical options include thrombectomy, with or without intimal tacking, endarterectomy or intimectomy, embolectomy, and dilation. For lesions not amenable to surgical repair, ligation therapy, either operative or through endovascular occlusion techniques (balloon or coils), is used. In adult patients an internal carotid artery stump pressure greater than 60 mm Hg as determined by oculoplethysmography provides adequate circulation. If adequate collaterals are not present, an extracranial-intracranial byass can be employed. No experience with this technique exists in the pediatric population.[97-99]

Popliteal artery injury in the pediatric population is a difficult problem with potential for catastrophic consequences.[100,101] This specific injury deserves special emphasis because of the high amputation rate from acute ligation and thrombosis of this artery following trauma. In the literature concerning adults, acute ligation of the popliteal artery carries an amputation rate of 72.5%.[7] This injury is unusual in infants but is seen in adolescents. Infrequently, primary repair of the artery may be accomplished. Most often the artery is severely damaged and repair is accomplished with a saphenous vein bypass from the suprageniculate popliteal artery to the infrageniculate popliteal artery.

Although the results of the different pediatric vascular surgery series are difficult to compare, it is clear that prevention is the best means of approaching any traumatic problem. However, once an injury has occurred, an aggressive approach of diagnosis and management as outlined previously reduces morbidity. Promised advances in diagnosis and management include high-resolution duplex imaging, magnetic resonance angiography, and newer pharmacologic agents affecting vasospasm, platelet aggregation, coagulation cascade, and the fibrinolytic system. These advances may further reduce mortality and long-term disability.

SUMMARY

Vascular trauma remains a challenge to surgeons treating pediatric patients. A high index of suspicion and a thorough evaluation are indicated. A wait and see attitude is no longer acceptable because it may result in avoidable morbidity. We recommend an aggressive noninvasive evaluation and invasive diagnostic procedures when indicated. Factors that make pediatric patients with vascular trauma different from adult patients include propensity for intense vasospasm, anatomically small vessels, and the requirement for future growth. When an injury is identified, it should be immediately repaired in a fashion that allows normal development and minimizes long-term sequelae.

REFERENCES

1. Hallowell (1759): Cited by Lambert: Extract of a letter for Mr. Lambert, Surgeon at Newcastle upon a Tyne, to Dr. Hunter, *Med Observ Inq (London)*, Ch 30, p 360, 1762.
2. Murphy JB: Resection of arteries and veins injured in continuity—end to end suture—experimental and clinical research, *Med Rec* 51:73, 1897.
3. Carrel A: La technique ope'ratoire des anastomoses vasculaires et la transplantation des visce'res, *Lyone Med* 98:859, 1902.
4. Frouin A: Sur la sutre des vaisseaux, *Presse Med* 16:233, 1908.
5. Goyanes J: Neuvos trabajos de chirurgia vascular: substitucion plastica de las arterias por las venas, o arterio-plastia venosa, aplicado, como neuvo metodo, al traitamiento de las aneurismas, *El Siglo Med* 53:561, 1906.
6. Nolan B: Vascular injuries, *J R Coll Surg* 13:72, 1968.
7. DeBakey ME, Simeone FA: Battle injuries of arteries in World War II: an analysis of 2,471 cases, *Ann Surg* 123:534, 1946.
8. Hughes CW: Arterial repair during the Korean War, *Ann Surg* 147:555, 1958.
9. Morris GC Jr, Creech O Jr, DeBakey ME: Acute arterial injuries in civilian practice, *Am J Surg* 93:565, 1957.
10. Ferguson IA Sr, Byrd WM, McAfee DK: Experiences in the management of arterial injuries, *Ann Surg* 153:980, 1961.

11. Rich NM, Baugh JH, Hughes CW: Acute arterial injuries in Vietnam: 1,000 cases, *J Trauma* 10:359, 1970.
12. Mattox KL, Feliciano DV, Burch JM, et al: Five thousand seven hundred sixty cardiovascular injuries in 4459 patients, *Ann Surg* 209:698, 1989.
13. White JJ, Talbert JL, Haller JA: Peripheral arterial injuries in infants and children, *Ann Surg* 167:757, 1968.
14. Edwards WS, Lyons C: Traumatic arterial spasm and thrombosis, *Ann Surg* 140:318, 1954.
15. Raffensperger JG, D'Cruz IA, Hastreiter AR: Thrombotic occlusion of the bifurcation of the aorta in infancy: a case with successful surgical therapy, *Pediatrics* 34:550, 1964.
16. Moberg A, Reinand T: Aortic thrombosis in infancy: two cases of different etiology, *Acta Pathol Microbiol Scand* 39:161, 1956.
17. Salerno F, Collins DD, Redmond DC: External iliac artery occlusion in a newborn infant, *Surgery* 67:863, 1970.
18. Henry W, Johnson BB, Peterson AL: Left common iliac arterial embolectomy in the newborn, *West J Surg Obstet Gynecol* 68:352, 1960.
19. Bjarke B, Herin P, Blomback M: Neonatal aortic thrombosis: a possible clinical manifestation of congenital antithrombin III deficiency, *Acta Paediatr Scand* 63:297, 1974.
20. Stout C, Koehl G: Aortic embolism in a newborn infant, *Am J Dis Child* 120:74, 1970.
21. Gross RE: Arterial embolism and thrombosis in infancy, *Am J Dis Child* 70:61, 1945.
22. Rothstein JL: Progress in pediatrics: embolism and thrombosis of the abdominal aorta in infancy and in childhood, *Am J Dis Child* 49:1578, 1935.
23. Alstrup P, Anderson HJ, Schmidt KG: Neonatal aortic thromboembolism: surgical treatment and coagulation studies, *Dan Med J* 25:261, 1978.
24. Braly BD: Neonatal arterial thrombosis and embolism, *Pediatr Surg* 58:869, 1965.
25. Cahill JL, Talbert JL, Otteson OE, et al: Arterial complications following cardiac catheterization in infants and children, *J Pediatr Surg* 2:134, 1967.
26. Traumatic vascular lesions in infants and children. In O'Neil JA Jr: *Vascular disorders of children*, Philadelphia, 1983, Lea & Febiger, pp 181–192.
27. Mansfield PB, Gazzaniga AB, Litwin SB: Management of arterial injuries related to cardiac catheterization in children and young adults, *Circulation* 42:501, 1970.
28. Stanford JR, Evans WE, Morse TS: Pediatric arterial injuries, *Angiology* 27:1, 1976.
29. Bloom JD, Mozersky DJ, Buckley CJ, et al: Defective limb growth as a complication of catheterization of the femoral artery, *Surg Gynecol Obstet* 138:524, 1974.
30. Whitehouse WM, Coran AG, Stanley JC, et al: Pediatric vascular trauma, *Arch Surg* 111:1269, 1976.
31. Shaker HJ, White JJ, Signer RD, et al: Special problems of vascular injuries in children, *J Trauma* 16:863, 1976.
32. Meagher DP, Defore WW, Mattox KL, et al: Vascular trauma in infants and children, *J Trauma* 19:532, 1979.
33. Smith C, Green RM: Pediatric vascular injuries, *Surgery* 90:20, 1981.
34. Richardson JD, Fallat M, Nagaraj HS, et al: Arterial injuries in children, *Arch Surg* 116:685, 1981.
35. Navarre JR, Cardillo PJ, Gorman JF, et al: Vascular trauma in children and adolescents, *Am J Surg* 143:229, 1982.
36. Klein MD, Coran AG, Whitehouse WM, et al: Management of iatrogenic arterial injuries in infants and children, *J Pediatr Surg* 17:933, 1982.
37. Perry MO: Iatrogenic injuries of arteries in infants, *Surg Gynecol Obstet* 157:415, 1983.

38. Flanigan DP, Keifer TJ, Schuler JJ, et al: Experience with iatrogenic pediatric vascular injuries, *Ann Surg* 198:430, 1983.
39. Leblanc J, Wood A, O'Shea, et al: Peripheral arterial trauma in children, *J Cardiovasc Surg* 26:325, 1985.
40. Villavicencio JL, Gonzalez-Cerna JJ: Acute vascular problems in children, *Curr Probl Surg* 22:64, 1985.
41. Evans WE, King Dr, Hayes JP: Arterial trauma in children: diagnosis and management, *Ann Vasc Surg* 2:268, 1988.
42. Solak H, Yeniterzi M, Yuksek T, et al: Injuries of the peripheral arteries and their surgical treatment, *Thorac Cardiovasc Surg* 38:96, 1990.
43. Myers SI, Reed MK, Black CT, et al: Noniatrogenic pediatric vascular trauma, *J Vasc Surg* 10:258, 1989.
44. Wolf YG, Reyna T, Schropp KP, Harmel RP: Arterial trauma of the upper extremity in children, *J Trauma* 30:903, 1990.
45. Mills RP, Robbs JV: Paediatric arterial injury: management options at the time of injury, *J R Coll Surg Edinb* 36:13, 1991.
46. Eren N, Ozgen G, Ener BK, et al: Peripheral vascular injuries in children, *J Pediatr Surg* 26:1164, 1991.
47. LaQuaglia MP, Upton J, May JW: Microvascular reconstruction of major arteries in neonates and small children, *J Pediatr Surg* 26:1136, 1991.
48. Shaw BA, Kasser JR, Emans JB, Rand FF: Management of vascular injuries in displaced supracondylar humerus franctures without arteriography, *J Orthop Trauma* 4:25, 1990.
49. Eren N, Ozgen G, Gurel A, et al: Vascular injuries and amputation following limb fractures, *Thorac Cardiovasc Surg* 38:48, 1990.
50. Hofammann KE, Moneim MS, et al: Brachial artery disruption following closed posterior elbow dislocation in a child—assessment with intravenous digital angiography, *Clin Orthop Rel Res* 184:145, 1984.
51. Green A: Vascular injuries associated with dislocation of the knee, *J Bone Joint Surg* 59:236, 1977.
52. Eddy AC, Rusch VW, Fligner CL, et al: The epidemiology of traumatic rupture of the thoracic aorta in children: a 13 year review, *J Trauma* 30:989, 1990.
53. Lock JS, Huffman AD, Johnson RC: Blunt trauma to the abdominal aorta, *J Trauma* 27:674, 1987.
54. Stylianos S, O'Donnell TF, Harris BH: Femorofemoral artery bypass for blunt iliac artery occlusion in a child, *J Pediatr Surg* 26:1425, 1991.
55. Ueda T, Kikuchi H, Karasawa J, et al: Traumatic stenosis of the internal carotid artery in children, *Surg Neurol* 26:368, 1986.
56. Lewis DW, Berman PH: Vertebral artery dissection and alternating hemiparesis in an adolescent, *Pediatrics* 78:610, 1986.
57. Ko GD, Berbrayer D: Childhood stroke after minor neck trauma—case report, *Arch Phys Med Rehabil* 71:923, 1990.
58. Pearl PL: Childhood stroke following intraoral trauma, *J Pediatr* 110:574, 1987.
59. Rothrock SG, Howard RM: Delayed brachial artery occlusion owing to a dog bite of the upper extremity, *Pediatr Emerg Care* 6:293, 1990.
60. Psaila JV, Lakshman D, Knox R, Charlesworth D: Common carotid injury from an airgun pellet, *Injury* 20:173, 1989.
61. Loder RT, Shapiro P, Towbin R, Aronson DD: Aortic anatomy in children with myelomeningocele and congenital lumbar kyphosis, *J Pediatr Orthop* 11:31, 1991.

62. Freed MD, Keane JF, et al: Use of heparinization to prevent arterial thrombosis after percutaneous cardiac catheterization in children, *Circulation* 50:565, 1975.

63. Hack WWM, Vos A, Van der Lie J, Okken A: Incidence and duration of total occlusion of the radial artery in newborn infants after catheter removal, *Eur J Pediatr* 149:275, 1990.

64. Himmel PD, Sumner DS, Mongkolsmai GR, et al: Neonatal thoracoabdominal aortic thrombosis associated with the umbilical artery catheter: successful management by transaortic thrombectomy, *J Vasc Surg* 4:119, 1986.

65. Marsh JL, King W, Barret C, Fonkasrud EW: Serious complications after UAC for neonatal monitoring, *Arch Surg* 100:1203, 1975.

66. O'Neil JA Jr, Neblett WW, Born ML: Management of major thromboembolic complications of umbilical artery catheterization, *J Pediatr Surg* 16:972, 1981.

67. Symansky MR, Fox HA: Umbilical vessel catheterization: indications, management, and evaluation of technique, *J Pediatr* 80:820, 1972.

68. Cribari C, Meadors FA, Crawford ES, et al: Thoracoabdominal aortic aneurysm associated with umbilical artery catheterization: case report and review of the literature, *J Vasc Surg* 16:75, 1992.

69. Kristt DA, Rosenberg KA, Engel BT: Effect of prolonged intra-arterial catheterization on arterial wall, *Johns Hopkins Med J* 135:1, 1974.

70. Spencer AD: The reliability of signs of peripheral vascular injury, *Surg Gynecol Obstet* 114:490, 1962.

71. Snyder, WH, Thal ER, Bridges RA, et al: The validity of normal arteriography in penetrating trauma, *Arch Surg* 113:424, 1978.

72. Reid JD, Weigelt JA, Thal ER, Francis H: Assessment of proximity of a wound to major vascular structures as an indication for arteriography, *Arch Surg* 123:942, 1988.

73. Wagner ML, Singleton EB, Egan ME: Digital subtraction angiography in children, *Am J Radial* 140:127, 1983.

74. Meissner M, Paun M, Johansen K: Duplex scanning for arterial trauma, *Am J Surg* 161:552, 1991.

75. Friedman RJ, Jupiter JB: Vascular injuries and closed extremity fractures in children, *Clin Orthop Rel Res* 188:112, 1984.

76. Lynch K, Johansen K: Can Doppler pressure measurement replace "exclusion" arteriography in the diagnosis of occult extremity arterial trauma? *Ann Surg* 214:737, 1991.

77. Currarino G, Engle MA: The effects of ligation of the subclavian artery on the bones and soft tissues of the arms, *J Pediatr* 67:808, 1965.

78. Bassett FH, Lincoln CR, King TD, et al: Inequality in the size of the lower extremity following cardiac catheterization, *South Med J* 61:1013, 1968.

79. Hawker RE, Palmer J, Bury RG, et al: Results of percutaneous retrograde femoral arterial catheterization of the leg, *Br Heart J* 35:447, 1973.

80. Jacobsson B, Carlgren LE, Hedvall G, et al: Review of children after arterial catheterization of the leg, *Pediatr Radiol* 1:96, 1973.

81. Rosenthal A, Anderson M, Thompson S, et al: Superficial femoral artery catheterization: effect on extremity length, *Am J Dis Child* 124:240, 1972.

82. Mortensson W: Angiography of the femoral artery following percutaneous catheterization in infants and children, *Acta Radiol* 17:581, 1976.

83. Franken EA, Girud D, Sequeira FW, et al: Femoral artery spasm in children: catheter size is the principal cause, *Am J Radiol* 138:295, 1982.

84. Cikrit DF, Hekikson MA, Nichols WK, et al: Complete external iliac disruption after

percutaneous aortic valvuloplasty in two young children: successful repair with hypogastric artery transposition, *Surgery* 109:623, 1991.

85. Schmidt B, Wais U, Furste O, et al: Arterial occlusion in a preterm infant, successful nonsurgical treatment with urokinase and low dose heparin, *Helv Paediatr Acta* 37:438, 1982.

86. Ramirez A, Stallworth JM: Long-term behavior of vein grafts as replacements for arterial segments within the peritoneal cavity, *Surgery* 69:832, 1971.

87. Stanley JC, Ernst CB, Fry WJ: Fate of 100 aortorenal vein grafts: characteristics of late graft expansion, aneurysmal dilatation, and stenosis, *Surgery* 74:931, 1973.

88. Wylie EJ: Vascular replacement with arterial autografts, *Surgery* 57:14, 1965.

89. Stoney RJ, DeLuccia N, Ehrenfeld WK, et al: Aortorenal arterial autografts: long-term assessment, *Arch Surg* 116:1416, 1981.

90. Bergdahl L, Ljungqvist A: Long-term results after repair of coarctation of the aorta by patch grafting, *J Thorac Cardiovasc Surg* 80:177, 1980.

91. Reul GJ, Kabbani SS, Sandiford FM, et al: Repair of coarctation of the thoracic aorta by patch graft aortoplasty, *J Thorac Cardiovasc Surg* 65:696, 1974.

92. Rich NM, Hughes CW, Baugh JH: Management of venous injuries, *Ann Surg* 171:724, 1970.

93. Rich NM: Repair of lower extremity venous trauma: a more aggressive approach required, *J Trauma* 14:639, 1974.

94. Mubarek SJ, Owen CA: Double-incision fasciotomy of the leg for decompression in compartment syndromes, *J Bone Joint Surg* 59:184, 1977.

95. Garrett RC, Kerstein MD: Compartment syndrome in the newborn, *South Med J* 80:533, 1987.

96. Patman RD: Compartmental syndromes in peripheral vascular surgery, *Clin Orthop* 113:103, 1975.

97. Mokri B, Piepgras DG, Houser OW: Traumatic dissections of the extracranial internal carotid artery, *J Neurosurg* 68:189, 1988.

98. Zelenock GB, Kazmers A, Whitehouse WM, et al: Extracranial internal carotid artery dissection, *Arch Surg* 117:425, 1982.

99. Gee W, Kaupp HA, McDonald KM, et al: Spontaneous dissection of the internal carotid artery, *Arch Surg* 115:944, 1980.

100. Reed MK, Lowry PA, Myers SI: Successful repair of pediatric popliteal artery trauma, *Am J Surg* 160:287, 1990.

101. Holcomb GW, Meacham PW, Dean RH: Penetrating popliteal artery injuries in children, *J Pediatr Surg* 23:859, 1988.

CHRONIC SUPPORT OF THE INJURED CHILD

14

Metabolic Responses to Injury

Harry C. Sax

The focus of this chapter is the specialized nutritional needs of children. The modern era of pediatric nutritional support began in the laboratories of Dudrick, Wilmore, and Vars in the mid 1960s. They first described normal growth and development of beagle puppies and then of a child with a congenital short gut syndrome who received nutrients solely by vein.[1,2] The development of total parenteral nutrition (TPN) and of nutritional support teams, in addition to the emergence of the specialty of pediatric surgery, has allowed focus on the appropriate metabolic support of the injured child. Trauma remains one of the leading causes of death and disability in the pediatric age group.[3,4] Although the recognition of the importance of nutritional support has increased, many injured children still die of multiple inflammatory sepsis syndrome (MISS), which may be triggered at the level of the gut.[5] Furthermore, it is important to understand alterations in the metabolism associated with injury and how they affect nutrient needs. Among those changes are alterations in serum levels of catecholamines and increased secretion of cortisol and of the mediators of the inflammatory response such as the interleukins and prostaglandins.

METABOLIC RESPONSE TO INJURY

The response to injury is variable, with multiple factors determining its intensity. This has been extensively studied in adults but is not well understood in children.[6] Because of the disproportionate weight to surface area of a child as compared with an adult, children have a heightened metabolic response to injury. Regardless of the age of the injured person, however, for a response to occur the stimulus must be perceived at the central nervous system; this information is then integrated, output is determined, and changes ensue at the cellular level.

The input can take several routes. Primary afferent neurologic routes must be intact for injury to be perceived. The use of epidural anesthesia blocks the expected vasopressin release in response to surgical injury, whereas general anesthesia does not. Injury inflicted below a sensory level in spinal cord injury does not elicit the increase in adrenocorticosteroid secretion that occurs when the injury is inflicted above the lesion.[7,8] Further, injury is often associated with loss of effective circulating volume. This is detected at the baroreceptor level, and afferent signals are then transmitted to the brain. This results in release of the chronic down-regulation of the pituitary hypothalamic axis. Cortisol secretion in response to adrenocorticotropic hormone (ACTH) is elevated, as is conversion of angiotensinogen to angiotensin. During these events the patient may be in the "ebb" or "shock" phase of injury. Blood pressure and cardiac output are initially reduced until effective resuscitation takes place. This is associated with retention of large amounts of sodium and water at the level of the kidney.[9]

The body also responds to perceived decreases in oxygen delivery with increases in fractional extraction of oxygen at the tissue level. This leads to a widened arteriovenous oxygen difference perceived at chemoreceptors.

Pain and emotional arousal associated with the injury further yield increases in vasopressin, ACTH, and the endogenous opiates.[10] Elevation of catecholamine levels leads to the classic "fight or flight" phenomenon. This not only causes an initial vasoconstriction, but also supports a heightened catabolic response over time. Liver effects include glycogenolysis for the first 24 hours until glycogen stores are depleted, followed by fat mobilization and gluconeogenesis.

Neural responses are integrated in the brain through multiple pathways.[11] Initial evaluation takes place within the dorsal pons, with output mediated primarily through the hypothalamus and pituitary gland.[12] The output from the central nervous system and pituitary hypothalamic axis works in concert with local inflammatory responses, especially at a site of injury. These responses involve the arachidonic acid pathways, including the prostaglandins and leukotrienes, as well as specific factors, such as the interleukins released locally from wound macrophages in response to stimulation.

SPECIFIC METABOLIC AND HORMONAL CHANGES IN RESPONSE TO INJURY

Elevation in cortisol concentration has numerous effects at the cellular level.[13–15] After initial binding with a receptor, cortisol stimulates synthesis of cyclic adenosine monophosphate, which then migrates to the nucleus to alter protein synthesis. Cortisol moves amino acids out of the muscle to provide skeletons to the liver for gluconeogenesis as well as protein synthesis. Cortisol's central role is emphasized when acute adrenal crisis develops. The patient may not be able to mount an appropriate response because of previous suppression or injury to the adrenal glands. As a result, hypoglycemia, hyponatremia, hyperkalemia, shock, and hyperpyrexia develop. In these specific cases the use of steroids is lifesaving. The routine use of steroids in patients with sepsis has not led to increases in survival and may increase morbidity.

Contrary to what one might expect, the hypermetabolic state is not associated with elevation in thyroid hormone levels. Cortisol inhibits the conversion of T_4 to T_3, and therefore excessive amounts of T_4 are converted to the inactive reversed T_3.[16,17]

A potent stimulus to the retention of salt and water at the kidney level is provided by both aldosterone and the renin-angiotensin system. The baroreceptors at the kidney respond not only to decreases in effective circulating volume, but also to beta-adrenergic stimulation by catecholamines. This leads to secretion of renin with eventual conversion of angiotensin I to angiotensin II. Aldosterone is also stimulated, leading to fluid and sodium retention. These levels gradually fall as the patient moves into the flow phase after injury with diuresis of resuscitation fluids. If kidney function is maintained, the injured child initially concentrates urine to 1 to 2 ml of water per milliosmole of solid excreted, with an osmolarity corresponding to 1000 mOsm/L. In the patient below 2 years of age, this response may not be fully matured and the ability to excrete a water load after injury is reduced.[18]

NUTRITIONAL CONSIDERATIONS

During the "flow phase," energy expenditure is increased. This is most markedly seen in patients with burn injury. Although initially the increase in metabolic expenditure was thought to be related to the hyperdynamic state with increased cardiac output, studies of patients with unilateral extremity burn or injury show no correlation between oxygen consumption and blood flow.[19] Even though blood flow to the injured extremity is increased, oxygen consumption is not. The reason for this is vasodilation of the wound bed itself. The wound also is a mediating factor in the response. Increased blood flow supports the regenerative process by delivering additional oxygen to the underlying tissues. During injury, efflux of amino acids from the skeletal muscle to the liver provides substrate for gluconeogenesis and protein synthesis. In a study measuring substrate exchange across burned and unburned extremities, net glucose uptake across the uninjured extremity was low, suggesting that fat was a primary fuel in resting skeletal muscle. Glucose uptake was increased in the burned extremity. The injured extremity also released large quantities of lactate consistent with anaerobic metabolism of the glucose consumed. The lactate was metabolized through the Krebs cycle in the liver. These changes are consistent with differential nutrient requirements of inflammatory tissue such as fibroblasts, macrophages, and leukocytes.

NUTRITIONAL INTERVENTION

In addition to preserving lean body mass by meeting energy needs, nutritional support can alter the response to injury. This is of greatest importance during the ebb stage immediately after injury. At this time, blood flow to the splanchnic circulation is decreased, starving the mucosa and allowing the barrier function of the gut to become permeable to bacteria and toxins.

Mochizuki and co-workers[20] studied early enteral feeding in burned guinea pigs to determine its effect on hypermetabolism. Animals received a gastrostomy and after recovery were subjected to a 30% dorsal flame burn under anesthesia. They were then randomly assigned to one of three groups: the first group had feeding begun immediately after the injury and were maintained on 175 kcal/kg/day; a second group had the feedings delayed for 72 hours consistent with standard clinical practice followed by infusion at the same rate; a third group had a 72-hour delay but were then given infusions of 200 kcal/kg/day in an attempt to compensate for the caloric intake differences caused by the 3-day delay. The animals were weighed daily and metabolic rates determined. Animals that were fed within 2 hours of injury lost only 5% of body weight in contrast to a 15% weight loss in both groups that were delayed in their feeding. Although feeding at a higher rate reversed the weight loss to some extent (Fig. 14–1), it was not as low as in the early-fed guinea pigs. Figure 14–2 represents the

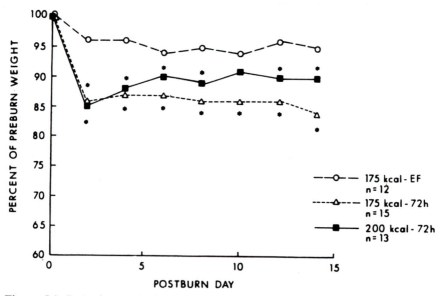

Figure 14–1. Body weight following burn. The early-fed animals maintained mass. (Modified from Mochizuki H, Trocki O, Dominioni L, et al: Mechanism of postburn hypermetabolism and catabolism by early enteral feeding, *Ann Surg* 200:297–310, 1984.)

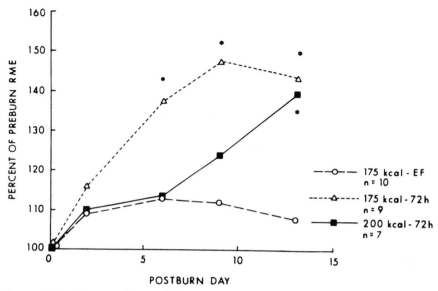

Figure 14–2. Increase in metabolic rate after surgery. Early enteral support blunts hypermetabolism. (Mochizuki H, Trocki O, Dominioni L, et al: Mechanism of postburn hypermetabolism and catabolism by early enteral feeding, *Ann Surg* 200:297–310, 1984.)

metabolic responses of these animals. The hypermetabolic response decreased significantly in animals fed early. The examination of urinary levels of vanillyl-mandelic acid, the catecholamine metabolite, as well as serum levels of cortisol and glucagon, showed amelioration of the normal rises seen after injury. Gut mucosal weight was preserved in animals fed early, consistent with increases in blood flow. This initial work confirms the importance of the gut and the role of nutritional support in the mediation of the metabolic response to injury. By preservation of lean body mass and blunting of the hypercatabolic response, improvements in respiratory function and healing can be expected. This response is not simply calorie dependent. The immediate postinjury infusion of parenteral nutrients does not elicit the same benefits. The gut is an active metabolic organ and is dependent on nutrient flow. It may well be one of the central mediators of the stress response.

FROM HYPERMETABOLISM TO RECOVERY

If the patient is appropriately resuscitated and his or her nutritional needs are met during the hypermetabolic phase, healing eventually ensues. This is evidenced by a continued diuresis of resuscitation fluids and gradual increase in body weight. Transient renal dysfunction resolves. Hepatic protein synthesis shifts from acute-phase proteins, and nutritional indicators such as prealbumin begin to rise. The patient's appetite and energy return, and if nitrogen balance studies are carried out, a decrease in nitrogen excretion is noted. Although these patients are anabolic, they may take many months to recover from the initial insult.[21] In the stressed adult for example, nitrogen losses may exceed 12 g/day. A gram of nitrogen is equivalent to 6.25 g of protein or approximately 1 ounce of lean body mass. Restoration takes place at a much slower pace of 2 to 4 g of nitrogen per day. This reemphasizes the importance of early nutritional support during the hypermetabolic phase. While moving the patient into positive nitrogen balance may not be possible, certainly the amelioration of catabolism will lead to a shorter recovery.

REFERENCES

1. Dudrick SJ, Vars HM, Raunsley HM, Rhoads JE: Total intravenous feeding and growth in puppies, *Fed Proc* 25:481, 1966.
2. Wilmore DW, Dudrick SJ: Growth and development of an infant receiving all nutrients exclusively by vein, *JAMA* 203:860, 1968.
3. Gratz RR: Accidental injury in childhood: a literature review on pediatric trauma, *J Trauma* 19:551–555, 1979.
4. Manheimer DI, Dewey J, Mellinger GD, et al: 50,000 child-years of accidental injuries, *Public Health Rep* 81:519–533, 1966.
5. Deitch EA: Does the gut protect or injure patients in the ICU? *Perspect Crit Care* 1:1–31, 1988.
6. Andrassy RJ, Dubos T: Modified injury Severity Scale and concurrent steroid therapy: independent correlates of negative nitrogen balance in pediatric trauma, *J Pediatr Surg* 20:799, 1985.
7. Hume DM, Egdahl RH: The importance of the brain in the neuroendocrine response to injury, *Ann Surg* 150:697, 1959.
8. Hume DM, Bell CL, Bartter FC: Direct measurement of adrenal secretion during operative trauma and convalescence, *Surgery* 52:174, 1962.
9. Cuthbertson DP: Observations on the disturbance of metabolism produced by injury to the limbs, *Q J Med* 1:233–246, 1932.
10. Bereiter DA, Plotsky PM, Gann DS: Tooth pulp stimulation potentiates the ACTH response to hemorrhage in cats, *Endocrinology* 111:1127, 1982.
11. Gann DS, Bereiter DA, Carlson DE, Thrivikraman KV: Neural interaction in control of adrenocorticotropin, *Fed Proc* 44:1612, 1985.
12. Blessing WW: Central neurotransmitter pathways for baroreceptor-initiated secretion of vasopressin, *NIPS* 1:90, 1986.
13. Ali M, Vedeckis WV: The glucocorticoid receptor protein binds to transfer RNA, *Science* 235:467, 1987.
14. Greengard P: Phosphorylated proteins as physiological effectors, *Science* 199:146, 1978.
15. Jensen EV: Interaction of steroid hormones with the nucleus, *Pharmacol Rev* 30:477, 1979.
16. Becker RA, Wilmore DW, Goodwin CW Jr, et al: Free T_4, free T_3 and reverse T_3 in critically ill, terminally injured patients, *J Trauma* 20:713, 1980.

17. Aun F, Medeiros-Neto GA, Younes RN, et al: The effect of major trauma on the pathways of thyroid hormone metabolism, *J Trauma* 23:104, 1983.
18. Krummel TM, Lloyd DA, Rowe MI: The postoperative response of the term and preterm newborn infant to sodium administration, *J Pediatr Surg* 20:803–809, 1985.
19. Wilmore DW, Aulick LH, Mason AD Jr, et al: The influence of the burn wound on local and systemic responses to injury, *Ann Surg* 186:444–456, 1977.
20. Mochizuki H, Trocki O, Dominioni L, et al: Mechanism of prevention of post-burn hypermetabolism and catabolism by early enteral feeding, *Ann Surg* 200:297–310, 1984.
21. Wilmore DW: The metabolic management of the critically ill, New York, 1977, Plenum Medical.

Nutritional Support

Carol Mary Medins
Edward G. Ford

Traumatic injury increases nutritional needs in both children and adults, as explained in Chapter 12. In most cases trauma victims are well nourished before injury. However, without timely nutrition support, malnutrition may ensue. Stressed children are particularly prone to rapid onset of protein-calorie malnutrition because of their limited nutrient stores. Aggressive nutritional support of the injured pediatric patient follows the initial stabilization of traumatic injuries and is a major component of overall medical care.

In general, nutritional support should be instituted following successful resuscitation, when the patient has entered Cuthbertson's "flow" phase of injury. The phase begins 2 to 3 days after injury and is characterized by a generalized catabolic response lasting from days to weeks. During this time, initiation of nutrition support is critical to minimize nitrogen losses and to attempt repletion of wasted nutritional stores.[1] Development of the initial nutritional support regimen involves the following[2]:

- Establishing projected energy requirements
- Determining protein needs based on the estimated amount of nitrogen needed for protein accretion (positive nitrogen balance)
- Establishing a safe and effective method of administering nutrients

The total energy requirement of the injured patient is the sum of the energies required by the basal metabolic rate (BMR) (Table 15–1), the specific dynamic action of ingested food substances (SDA), energy expenditure resulting from activity, and the effective energy of the injury itself.[3,4] Metabolic rate in a traumatized child is often referred to as the resting energy expenditure (RME). The RME describes the energy required for maintenance of BMR plus the energy required for nutrient assimilation and baseline physical activity. The RME should be used as a guideline for initiation of nutrition support, but it may of limited use in critically ill patients whose requirements may change daily with convalescence or the development of complications.[5] Indirect calorimetry pro-

Table 15–1. Standard Basal Metabolic Rates

Weight (kg)	Kcal/24 hr	
	Male	Female
3	140	140
5	270	270
7	400	400
9	500	500
11	600	600
13	650	650
15	710	710
17	780	780
19	830	830
21	880	880
25	1020	960
29	1120	1040
33	1210	1120
37	1300	1190
41	1350	1260
45	1410	1320
49	1470	1380
53	1530	1440
57	1590	1500
61	1640	1560

Modified from Forbes GB, ed: *Pediatric nutrition handbook,* ed 2, Elk Grove Village, Ill, 1985, American Academy of Pediatrics.
Energy requirements will change proportionally 12% per degree celcius.

vides information on minute-by-minute fuel utilization and may prove more accurate in predicting caloric needs in the critically ill.[6]

Once energy needs have been estimated, nitrogen requirements can be determined. Factors influencing nitrogen balance include the quantity of nitrogen in the diet, the patient's metabolic rate, and the quantity and quality of nonprotein energy provided. Initially the traumatically injured patient's ability to utilize protein is relatively inefficient. A pediatric patient requires significantly more dietary protein than a similarly injured adult to achieve protein accretion. In such hypermetabolic children, protein metabolism contributes up to 20% of the total energy expenditure. The nonprotein calorie/nitrogen ration needed to achieve maximal nitrogen retention is approximately 150:1. The provision of more nitrogen via large protein loads may improve nitrogen balance but is often complicated by a rise in the blood urea nitrogen (BUN) concentration.[7] Increases in BUN are particularly undesirable in patients with compromised renal or hepatic function. Initial nonprotein calories should be provided as carbohydrate.

Research indicates that nutritional support with carbohydrate during a hyper-metabolic disease has a greater impact on nitrogen retention than an equal caloric quantity of fat.[8]

Whereas Chapter 14 provided the biochemical rationale needed to understand the metabolic responses to injury, this chapter provides the guidelines required to assess nutrition support needs and to determine the most effective method of nutrient administration.

Nutritional therapy should be directed toward achieving specific goals:

- Identifying the unique metabolic and nutritional needs of each injured child
- Maintaining body weight and protein stores in the immediate postinjury catabolic state
- Providing adequate fuels by an effective delivery method
- Assessing the effectiveness of the nutritional program and adjusting it as needed on a daily basis
- Increasing body weight and protein mass in the convalescent phase

These objectives must be integrated into the overall patient care plan and should receive special consideration when fluid restriction, organ failure (kidney, lung, or liver), septicemia, mechanical ventilation, or other supportive therapy complicates the provision of optimal nutritional support.

Anabolism and positive nitrogen balance are difficult, if not impossible, to achieve in a critically ill hypermetabolic patient. The provision of adequate calories and protein lessens the profound catabolism but does not ensure maintenance of somatic protein. In fact, even weight maintenance does not ensure sparing of lean body mass. Hildreth and co-workers[9-11] demonstrated that in survivors of major trauma or burns, weight maintenance was associated with peripheral muscle wasting and truncal obesity. Since overfeeding during the postinjury hypermetabolic state may complicate patient management via over-hydration, increased energy requirements, accelerated hepatic steatosis, increased carbon dioxide production, and increased respiratory quotient, nutritional management should be designed to provide adequate calories and protein to minimize the profound catabolism and promote wound healing.

With resolution of the acute disease process, protein synthesis will occur and muscle mass will return to preillness level. The patient who is able to ambulate and effectively use major muscle groups will soon achieve positive nitrogen balance and skeletal muscle anabolism. Spontaneous conversion from a catabolic to an anabolic state is usually not observed in severely injured patients until wound or burn closure has been accomplished, with autograft if necessary. An increased requirement for exogenous calories is likely to exist for many weeks after injury if wound closure is not promptly achieved.

NUTRITIONAL ASSESSMENT

On admission the nutritional status of the critically injured child must be established so that appropriate nutritional support can be provided. These parameters are continually assessed as the patient moves from the catabolic to the anabolic state.

Nutrition History

Diet and social history includes usual food intake, food allergies, cultural or religious food preferences, and chewing or swallowing difficulties. Such information gives an idea of the nutritional problems that may be encountered during treatment and recovery. The history plays an important part in the approach to improving nutritional status through the use of accustomed and preferred foods and the identification of factors that might interfere with the nutritional support plan.

Nutrient Intake Analysis

Nutrient intake is measured daily to assess the adequacy of the diet in meeting estimated nutritional requirements. Intake includes all nutrients received via enteral and parenteral routes and the oral diet (calorie count). Graphs are used to depict the sources of calories (carbohydrate, fat, and protein) received. Daily monitoring may identify nutritional deficits before weight and laboratory values reveal losses.

Anthropometry

Admission height and weight of the injured child are measured to determine appropriateness for age (growth charts). Such screening may reveal a deficit in preinjury nutritional status. Anthropometric measurements are also a useful method of monitoring body composition during convalescence.

Weight monitoring during the hospital course provides a means of assessing adequacy of nutritional support. In a traumatized child, weight loss can provide an early indication of nutritional inadequacy but may also be the result of fluid losses, multiple surgical procedures, amputations, or the changing of bulky dressings. A weight loss of greater than 10% of the preinjury weight is frequently associated with metabolic complications.[12-15] Death often results when acute weight loss exceeds 30% of preinjury levels. The endogenous caloric reserves of a child are limited by body size. Weight loss should not be allowed to exceed 5% of the estimated usual weight in children with an injury. A daily weight graph in combination with the protein-calorie graph provides a visual means of monitoring weight status and identifying trends toward weight deficits.

Confirmatory Laboratory Tests

Biochemical data are used to identify deficiencies in visceral proteins. Concentrations of circulating serum proteins are used as indicators of visceral protein status. Visceral proteins are essential for host defenses, wound healing, substrate transport, oncotic pressure, and enzyme function. Serial measurements of these proteins provide an objective means of determining adequacy and response to nutritional support. In the burned child, deficits of serum protein concentrations occur rapidly as a result of nitrogen losses through the wound and an altered protein metabolism.[16,17] Repletion of these proteins occurs when energy and protein demands are satisfied and adequate substrate supply is provided. Circulating proteins commonly used to represent visceral protein status include serum albumin, transferrin, retinol-binding protein, and thyroxin-binding prealbumin.

Serum albumin has a relatively long half-life, which makes it a poor marker for monitoring acute changes in visceral protein status. Levels of serum albumin rise when supplemental intravenous infusions of albumin are given to maintain oncotic pressure. Accurately correlating changes in serum albumin with nutritional support may be difficult. Low serum albumin concentrations lead to changes in Starling forces, which have been implicated in lowered gastrointestinal tolerance to enteral feedings.[18] Attempts at correcting serum albumin without providing an adequate calorie source result in the patient's using the albumin as fuel. The albumin deficit is calculated by the formula:

$$\text{Albumin replacement} = (3.5 \text{ g/dl} - \text{Serum albumin in g/dl}) \times (\text{wt kg} \times 3)$$

This formula assumes a distribution of albumin in 30% of the body by weight as estimated by radioisotope dilution curves.[18] Thirty percent is used as an arbitrary replacement value based on our experience. The deficit is replaced with concentrated salt-poor albumin in four equally divided daily increments. Calories are provided via the parenteral or enteral route as the albumin level is corrected. With the provision of full calories in conjunction with albumin correction, the serum albumin concentration remains in the normal range for up to 1 week.[19,20]

Serum retinol-binding protein and thyroxin-binding prealbumin have half-lives of 10 hours and 2 days, respectively. Changes in these proteins rapidly reflect changes in nutritional status; unfortunately, circulating levels may be a reflection of the acute metabolic response to the stress of injury, as well as to malnutrition. Serum transferrin may be the most cost-effective indicator of visceral protein status, since it is easy to obtain and has a relatively short half-life (8 to 10 days). Serum transferrin values are independent of albumin infusions.[12] Low serum transferrin concentrations significantly correlate with incidence of infections and complications, indicating a relationship between visceral protein status and immunocompetence. Transferrin values are measured every 7 to 10 days. Hydration status affects the measurement of all the circulating proteins and should be considered when laboratory results are interpreted.

Nitrogen Balance Measurements

The body's protein mass is in constant flux as cells are catabolized and replaced by newly synthesized cells. Nitrogen (N) balance estimations are used to reflect the overall rates of body protein synthesis and breakdown. The following formula is commonly employed:

$$N \text{ balance} = (N \text{ in}) - (N \text{ out})$$

Intake of nitrogen is generally in the form of ingested protein or intravenously infused amino acids. Losses of nitrogen occur primarily in urine, stool, and skin.

A reasonable estimation of urine urea nitrogen is obtained from 24-hour urine collections. Urine collections are difficult to obtain in children. Some articles suggest that nitrogen losses may be extrapolated from 4- to 8-hour urine collections. We have shown that these extrapolated values may misrepresent measured losses by 7% to 149%; thus they should not be used in place of full 24-hour accurate urine collections. A correction of 2 to 4 g is added to the measured daily urine urea nitrogen loss to cover insensible nitrogen losses in the stool and through the skin. One gram of nitrogen is equivalent to 6.25 g of protein. Therefore a negative nitrogen balance of -8.2 g of nitrogen represents a protein loss of 51.2 g.[21]

The healthy individual is in nitrogen equilibrium (intake equals losses). Catabolic disorders, such as a major burn or traumatic injury, accelerate nitrogen loss and therefore result in loss of lean body mass.[3,22] One of the major goals of nutrition support is to convert these hypercatabolic patients from negative to positive nitrogen balance, signaling new protein synthesis. A reasonable goal of $+2$ g/day nitrogen balance supports anabolism without overfeeding the patient.[22–24]

When used in conjunction with other measures of nutritional assessment, the 24-hour urine urea nitrogen can provide an effective method of determining the adequacy of nutritional therapy.

The laboratory monitoring of a critically ill child is outlined in Table 15–2.

Table 15–2. Monitoring the Critically Ill Child

Daily laboratory studies*:
  Electrolytes
  Blood urea nitrogen
  Creatinine
  Glucose
For recognition of deficiency trends, observe on initiation and monitor the following:
  Twice weekly:
    Total protein
    Prealbumin
    Albumin
    Bilirubin
    Transaminase
    Alkaline phosphatase
    Triglycerides
    Cholesterol
    Creatine
    Bicarbonate
    Phosphorus
    Hemoglobin
    Hematocrit
    Red blood cell indices
  Weekly:
    Zinc
    Copper
    Magnesium
    Manganese
    Transferrin
    24-Hour urine urea nitrogen

---

*These are particularly important in patients with multiple-system organ failure.

IDENTIFYING NUTRITIONAL NEEDS
Estimation of Calorie Requirements in Children

The hypermetabolism associated with major injury generally subsides when the majority of the wounds are stabilized or closed.[25,26] Until then the body provides precursors to the visceral organs for gluconeogenesis and the synthesis of acute-phase proteins, resulting in accelerated muscle proteolysis. In children the endogenous energy stores are limited by body size; acquired malnutrition occurs rapidly, since children must meet the metabolic needs of the catabolic response to trauma and the cost of growth and maturation.[27]

Kilocalorie requirements for the growth and maintenance of normal children are identified by the Recommended Dietary Allowances (RDA).[28] Resting energy expenditure (REE) is expressed in terms of body surface area rather than age or weight. In children, energy requirements are partitioned among maintenance, muscular activity, and growth. Following major surgical trauma, children do not have significant increases in REE.[5,9,29] In addition, children have stable RQ values, indicating that a shift to noncarbohydrate metabolism does not occur, possibly because of the administration of dextrose-containing solutions. Groner and associates[5] hypothesized that in the catabolic milieu of postoperative stress, counterregulatory hormones diminish or arrest growth. Thus the increased energy expenditure following trauma would be offset by a decreased energy expenditure requirement for growth. In practical terms, caloric needs of the injured child should be estimated by use of the RDA for age.[5,22,29]

Protein Requirement

In contrast to calorie needs, protein requirements are significantly elevated in the injured child. After injury the rate of lean body mass catabolism increases along with the rate of protein synthesis.[30] When caloric intake is adequate, the amino acids provided may be used to spare lean body mass. If protein or calorie intake is not sufficient to meet the patient's need, somatic (muscle tissue) and visceral proteins become autocatabolized and depleted. Nutritional support of the injured child should provide approximately 20% of total calories as protein, for a nonprotein calorie/nitrogen ration of 150:1.[7,8,31]

Vitamin and Mineral Requirements

The optimal vitamin and mineral requirements of injured children remain to be determined. Individual nutrient needs depend on preinjury stores, absorption, ongoing losses (i.e., through the kidneys or fistulas), increased needs owing to stressed state, and extent of injury.[32]

The vitamins thiamin (B_1), riboflavin (B_2), niacin, and pyridoxine (B_6) are components of essential enzymes and coenzymes used to metabolize carbohydrates, protein, and fat.[28,33] In an injured child, requirements for these vitamins increase along with the energy requirements. Animal studies suggest that deficiencies in vitamins A and D, ascorbic acid, thiamin, riboflavin, pyridoxine, niacin, pantothenic acid, and folic acid may reduce host resistance to infection.[34–39] Vitamin K, vitamin B_{12}, and iron are not present in parenteral solutions and must be given intramuscularly or in a bolus.

The minerals known to play an essential role in human nutrition are divided into two categories, those present in large quantities (sodium, potassium, calcium, magnesium, and phosphorus) and those present in only trace amounts (iron, zinc, copper, iodine, molybdenum, cobalt, selenium, fluoride, manganese, and chromium).

Sodium and potassium are discussed in the section on fluid and electrolyte balance.

Calcium. Hypocalcemia is generally found in conjunction with hypoalbuminemia, hypomagnesemia, and vitamin D deficiency. Hypercalciuria is common during TPN because of high levels of phosphate administration. So that total body calcium stores are maintained, periods of immobilization of the patient should be limited and adequate calcium supplements for age should be provided.[40]

Magnesium. Hypomagnesemia is seen with excessive gastrointestinal or renal losses and in patients entering the anabolic phase of injury (tissue synthesis). Symptoms include apathy, muscular weakness, tetany, convulsions, nausea, vomiting, hypokalemia, and hypocalcemia.[33,40]

Phosphorus. Hypophosphatemia is seen in patients with extensive injuries during the "corticoid withdrawal" or "flow" phase of injury when phosphorus is excreted along with salt and water and when the body is involved in the synthesis of high-energy triple-phosphate bonds (adenosine triphosphate). During the anabolic phase, phosphorus is taken up by body cells, which contributes to the development of hypophosphatemia. The consequences of severe hypophosphatemia include erythrocyte and leukocyte dysfunction, central nervous system dysfunction, rhabdomyolysis, and, if not corrected, respiratory failure.[32,41]

Hypophosphatemia must be corrected cautiously because the administration of phosphorus salts may result in hyperphosphatemia. The subsequent deposition of calcium phosphate leads to hypocalcemia and hyperkalemia. Milk is a balanced solution of 1 g phosphorus to 1 g calcium and

Table 15–3. Recommended Dietary Allowances of Vitamins in Infants and Children by Age Group

	Age (Yr)	Weight (kg)	Weight (lb)	Height (cm)	Height (in)	Fat-Soluble Vitamins A (µg RE)	Fat-Soluble Vitamins D (µg)
Infants	0–0.5	6	13	60	24	375	7.5
	0.5–1	9	20	71	28	375	10
Children	1–3	13	29	90	35	400	10
	4–6	20	44	112	44	500	10
	7–10	28	62	132	52	700	10
Males	11–14	45	99	157	62	1000	10
	15–18	66	145	176	69	1000	10
	19–24	70	154	177	70	1000	5
Females	11–14	46	101	157	62	800	10
	15–18	55	120	163	64	800	10
	19–24	55	120	163	64	800	5

RE, retinol equivalents; TE, tocopherol equivalents; NE, niacin equivalents.

is a safe method of phosphorus administration for children who can tolerate lactose.

Trace elements. Deficiencies in trace elements can also have a negative impact on patient recovery. Iron deficiency may result in hypochromic microcytic anemia, with subsequent impaired cellular immunity.[42] Inadequate zinc administration has been associated with impaired cellular immunity, poor wound healing, impaired protein synthesis, anorexia, and altered sense of taste and smell.[23,43-48] Both zinc and copper are lost in patients with excessive gastrointestinal output.

Copper deficiency may lead to depigmentation, ataxia, leukopenia, skeletal demineralization, hypochromic microcytic anemia, and neutropenia.[14,33] Iodine, although not added to TPN solutions, is essential for thyroid function. Since iodine is present in many ointments, cutaneous absorption should be adequate to meet the patient's needs.[32] Molybdenum is involved in various metabolic reactions; a molybdenum deficiency may result in amino acid intolerance, fatigue, and somnolence.[32]

Selenium is a cofactor in erythrocyte glutathione peroxidase; acting as a proton donor, selenium protects cells from peroxide-induced damage. Manganese participates in energy metabolism. Prolonged TPN infrequently causes manganese deficiency with subsequent delayed clotting time, hypocholesterolemia, and change in hair color. Chromium deficiency is associated with glucose intolerance in children receiving TPN.[32,40,49]

RDAs (Tables 15-3 and 15-4) are available for vitamins and minerals.

Fat-Soluble Vitamins		Water-Soluble Vitamins						
E (mg TE)	K (mg)	C (mg)	B_1 (mg)	B_2 (mg)	Niacin (mg NE)	B_6 (mg)	B_{12} (µg)	Folic acid (µg)
3	5	30	0.3	0.4	5	0.3	0.3	25
4	10	35	0.4	0.5	6	0.6	0.5	35
5	15	40	0.7	0.8	9	1.0	0.7	50
6	20	45	0.9	1.1	12	1.1	1.0	75
7	30	45	1.0	1.2	13	1.4	1.4	100
10	45	50	1.3	1.5	17	1.7	2.0	150
10	65	60	1.5	1.8	20	2.0	2.0	200
10	70	60	1.5	1.7	15	2.0	2.0	200
8	45	50	1.1	1.3	15	1.4	2.0	150
8	55	60	1.1	1.3	15	1.5	2.0	180
8	60	60	1.1	1.3	15	1.6	2.0	180

Table 15–4. Recommended Daily Requirements of Minerals in Infants and Children by Age Group

	Age (yr)	Weight (kg)	Weight (lb)	Height (cm)	Height (in)	Ca (mg)	PO$_4$ (mg)	Mg (mg)	Fe (mg)	Zn (mg)	I (μg)
Infants	0–0.5	6	13	60	24	400	300	40	6	5	40
	0.5– 1	9	20	71	28	600	500	60	10	5	50
Children	1– 3	13	29	90	35	800	800	80	10	10	70
	4– 6	20	44	112	44	800	800	120	10	10	90
	7– 10	28	62	132	52	800	800	170	10	10	120
Males	11– 14	45	99	157	62	1200	1200	270	12	15	150
	15– 18	66	145	176	69	1200	1200	400	12	15	150
	19– 24	70	154	177	70	1200	1200	350	10	15	150
Females	11– 14	46	101	157	62	1200	1200	280	15	12	150
	15– 18	55	120	163	64	1200	1200	300	15	12	150
	19– 24	55	120	163	64	1200	1200	280	15	12	150

Safe levels of intake (Table 15–5) have been established for trace elements. Guidelines for parenteral use of trace elements have been established by the American Medical Association (Table 15–6).[28,50,51]

Until more information is available regarding the administration of vitamins and minerals to the traumatized child, supplementation should not exceed the established guidelines for healthy individuals unless a deficiency is documented. We recommend weekly determinations of serum copper, zinc, and magnesium levels.[52]

Environmental Factors

Every effort should be made to minimize energy demands as influenced by external stresses. Pain, anxiety, fear, and cold stimulate the release of catecholamines and raise energy requirements.[9,17,53,54] Narcotics and tranquilizers should be used to reduce anxiety and pain.[14] Our narcotic of preference is morphine.

Table 15–5. Recommended Daily Requirements of Trace Elements and Electrolytes in Infants, Children, and Adolescents

	Zn (mg)	Cu (mg)	Mn (mg)	Se (mg)	Cr (mg)	Cu	Mb (mg)
Infants	3–5	0.5–1	0.5–1	0.01–0.06	0.01–0.04	N/A	0.03–0.08
Children and adolescents	10–15	1–3	1–5	0.02–0.2	0.02–0.2	N/A	0.05–0.3

Modified from Forbes GB, ed: *Pediatric nutrition handbook,* ed 2, Elk Grove Village, Ill, 1985, American Academy of Pediatrics.

Table 15–6. Guidelines for Parenteral Use of Trace Elements

1. Trace elements should be provided immediately on instituting nutritional support. Follow-up is based on blood levels. Consider that normal blood levels may not indicate normal tissue levels.
2. Trace element requirements vary with age, clinical and metabolic status, and degree of losses via the gastrointestinal tract.
3. Zinc levels are aggressively supplemented in patients with acute catabolic stress or high losses of gastrointestinal fluids.
4. Pediatric requirements are based on body weight.
5. Intravenous administration of trace elements circumvents normal intestinal regulatory absorptive mechanisms. Metabolism and excretion are via the renal route. Supplementation must be modified in the patient with renal dysfunction. Copper and manganese are excreted primarily via the biliary system. Patients with biliary obstruction, hepatitis, biliary atresia, or inspissated bile syndrome must have restriction of copper and manganese as determined by blood levels.
6. Trace element levels in the very low birth weight infant are poorly understood. Observations include routinely low levels of serum copper and ceruloplasmin. Hepatic copper concentrations are high. Serum zinc levels are usually similar to maternal levels at birth and decline during the first weeks of life.
7. Intravenous supplementation of trace elements should be accomplished only in hospitals in which laboratory determinations of blood levels are available.

Adapted from American Medical Association, Department of Foods and Nutrition: *JAMA* 241:2051–2054, 1979. Copyright 1979, American Medical Association.

We use a dose of 0.01 mg/kg every 3 to 4 hours and achieve excellent pain relief. External heating devices are used to control cold stress. During operative procedures and tubing and dressing changes, attention should be given to maintaining a warm environment.

Fluid and Electrolyte Balance

Fluid and electrolyte needs are directly related to metabolic rate. Hypermetabolism leads to an increased rate of endogenous water production from the oxidation of carbohydrate, fat, and protein; increased water losses through the urine owing to increased urinary solute excretion; and increased fluid loss in sweat.

Once caloric expenditure has been established, maintenance requirements for fluids and electrolytes can be determined. For every 100 kcal expended, 115 ml of water, 3.2 mEq of sodium, and 2.4 mEq of potassium is required. Fluid requirements are decreased in patients with anuria or extreme oliguria, in which urine output is negligible. In these cases underestimation of fluid needs is preferable to avoid fluid overload.[33,55]

BURNS

Burn patients are the most metabolically stressed of injured patients and require vigorous nutritional support. However, these patients must not be overfed because the provision of too many nutrients is associated with increased morbidity.[13,53] The nutritional regimen should have the following goals[51]:

- Minimize the metabolic response by controlling environmental temperature and pain, maintaining fluid and electrolyte balance, and covering wounds
- Meet nutritional needs by providing adequate calories to prevent weight loss and to maintain or replete visceral protein stores
- Prevent Curling's ulcer through the use of antacids or continuous enteral feedings.

Calorie Needs

The metabolic rate of the burn patient is affected by several factors, including ambient temperature, severity of burn, method of dressing care, and caloric intake.[9,17,56-58] Several formulas are available to predict the burn patient's caloric needs.[22,52,59-61] These computations are based on admission weight or body surface area (BSA) plus a factor determined by using percent of BSA burned (Table 15–7).[62] Two popular formulas for estimating caloric needs are the Curreri formula and the Shriners' formula:

Curreri formula: 25 kcal kg body weight + 40 Cal × % TBSA
Shriners' formula: 1800 kcal/m² BSA + 2200 kcal/m² BSA × % TBSA

Table 15–7. Percent Body Surface Area Burned for Children

Body Part Affected	Percent Burned (By Age Group in Years)				
	0–1	1–4	5–9	10–14	15+
One half of head	9½	8½	6½	5½	4½
One half of neck	1	1	1	1	1
One half of trunk	13	13	13	13	13
One side of upper arm	2	2	2	2	2
One side of lower arm	1½	1½	1½	1½	1½
One side of hand	1½	1½	1½	1½	1½
Buttock	2½	2½	2½	2½	2½
One half of one thigh	2¾	3¼	4	4¼	4½
One half of one lower leg	2½	2½	2¾	3	3¼
One half of foot	1¾	1¾	1¾	1¾	1¾

Modified from Blumer JL, ed: *A practical guide to pediatric intensive care*, St Louis, 1990, Mosby.

Recent research indicates that total energy expenditure in burned children is lower than had been estimated and actually consists of mainly predicted RME with a stress factor between 1.2 and 1.55.[9,22,58,63] Once calorie needs are established, particular care should be used in determining the source of energy.

Protein

The exact protein needs of the burn patient are unknown. Because of the increased demand for wound healing and increased nitrogen losses via the wound and urine, protein needs are postulated to be greater than the RDA.[64] Generally, nonprotein calorie/nitrogen ratios between 100:1 and 150:1, with 20% to 25% of total calories provided as protein, should be adequate to promote anabolism.[16,51,52] Some researchers suggest providing protein at 2.5 to 3 g/kg body weight[22]; however, the ability of the pediatric burn patient to tolerate such large nitrogen loads depends on the patient's renal function and fluid balance.

The adequacy of protein intake can be assessed by evaluation of wound healing, graft take, and basic nutritional assessment parameters. Nitrogen balance studies may provide an estimate of protein needs in the burn patient but cannot account for wound losses. Nitrogen excretion decreases as wounds heal or are covered. Serum proteins with short half-lives may be useful in monitoring visceral protein status; these include prealbumin, transferrin, and retinol-binding protein.

Carbohydrate

Carbohydrate should be the chief energy source for burn patients.[8,11,22,55,65] However, high glucose infusion rates may increase stress on the pulmonary system through increased carbon dioxide production, RQ greater than 1 (indicating that some glucose is in the process of being converted to fat), and hepatomegaly from fat deposition in the liver.[22] A maximum glucose load of 4.7 to 7 mg/kg/min appears to be optimal, which equates to 45% to 55% of total calories as carbohydrate.* Although most research on carbohydrate tolerance has been performed on patients being fed parenterally, it would be prudent to use the same guidelines for those being fed enterally.

Lipid

The use of lipids in nutrition support of burn patients is important because fats are a concentrated source of calories and the only source of essential fatty acids. In the past, large amounts of lipids infused with TPN over 6 to 8 hours have been found to be immunosuppressive.[66] The same immunologic response

---

*References 8, 11, 22, 55, 65, 66.

has not been seen with enteral feedings, possibly because of slow infusion rates and fat composition (medium-chain triglycerides and omega-3 fatty acids versus long-chain triglycerides). To ensure fat tolerance, the initial lipid infusion should be limited to 15% of nonprotein calories and indicators of immune function and serum triglyceride levels should be monitored.[51] If parenteral nutrition is provided, 3 in 1 admixtures may be beneficial, since lipid administration is stretched over 24 hours.[67]

Vitamins and Minerals

The vitamin and mineral needs of burn patients are generally believed to exceed the RDA; for specific supplementation guidelines see Table 15–8. For patients taking oral feeding, supplementation may be needed; however, patients receiving hyperalimentation are generally receiving greater than the RDA because of their high calorie needs. Care must be taken when administering the fat-soluble vitamins and trace elements, since these can be toxic.[68–70] Burn patients may benefit from supplementation of vitamins and minerals known to be beneficial in wound healing (ascorbic acid and zinc) and vitamins lost through wounds or in urine (water-soluble vitamins).[22,52,71]

Fluid

Fluid losses are proportional to the size of the burn wound (3750 ml $\times$ m^2 burn per day) (Table 15–9) and caloric needs.

Nutritional Support

The method of nutritional support should be determined on an individual basis. The needs of patients with burns less than 20% TBSA can generally be met with a regular diet and oral supplementation as needed. Patients with

Table 15–8. Vitamin and Mineral Requirements of the Burned Child

Nutrient	Guidelines for Use
Sodium and potassium	Provided based on fluid needs, as well as serum and electrolyte data
Other minerals	RDA
Fat-soluble vitamins (A, D, E, K)	RDA
Water-soluble vitamins (B complex, folate, biotin, B$_{12}$)	2 $\times$ RDA
Vitamin C	5–10 $\times$ RDA
Zinc	2 $\times$ RDA
Trace elements	RDA

Modified from Blumer JL, ed: *A practical guide to pediatric intensive care,* St Louis, 1990, Mosby. *RDA,* Recommended Daily Allowance.

Table 15—9. Fluid and Electrolyte Requirements of the Burned Child

---

Fluid Requirements

First burn day: lactated Ringer's solution
  Maintenance 2000 ml/m²/day
  Evaporative losses 5000 ml/m² burn/day
  (half of the volume is administered during the first 8 hours, the second half during
    the subsequent 16 hours)
Second and subsequent burn days: D₅W and plasmanate (5% albumin)
  Maintenance 1500 ml/m²/day
  Evaporative losses 3750 ml/m² burn/day

Maintenance Electrolyte Requirements for Infants and Children

Sodium	2–4 (mEq/kg)
Potassium	2–3 (mEq/kg)
Chloride	2–3 (mEq/kg)
Lactate	20 mEq/L
Glucose	5%
Albumin	1.25 g/dl

Modified from Blumer JL, ed: *A practical guide to pediatric intensive care,* St Louis, 1990, Mosby.
Modified from Young SL: Pediatric parenteral nutrition. In DiPiro JT, et al (eds): *Pharmacotherapy: a pathophysiologic approach,* Norwalk, Conn, 1988, Appleton & Lange.

extensive burns and subsequent hypermetabolism and anorexia may require tube feedings or total parenteral nutrition (TPN). The enteral route is the preferred feeding method, but TPN may be required for patients during early burn treatment to avoid frequent interruption of feedings and for patients having persistent ileus with poor tube-feeding tolerance. Patients with 40% to 50% TBSA burned generally have a nonfunctional gastrointestinal tract and therefore require TPN.[22,25,40,51]

NUTRITIONAL SUPPORT OF THE INJURED CHILD

Although the usual hospital (regular) diet is easy to prepare, nutritious, and capable of providing adequate calories, protein, vitamins, and minerals, the injured child rarely consumes sufficient quantities to sustain metabolic efforts. Such children are often anorectic and may have a nasogastric or an endotracheal tube in place. In addition, a dysfunctional gastrointestinal (GI) tract may inhibit proper use of nutrients. In patients with a functioning GI tract, providing oral supplements between meals and encouraging good working relationships among the dietitian, nurse, patient, and parents may increase nutrient intake. Hyperalimentation may be instituted by enteral or parenteral means when volitional methods fail or nutrient absorption is impaired.

Gastrointestinal alimentation should be used whenever possible. The advantages of the enteral route for nutrient administration include the positive physiologic effects (digestion, absorption, substrate-hormone interaction, mucosal integrity), convenience, safety, and cost effectiveness. The relative contraindications to enteral alimentation of the critically ill child include persistent unresolving diarrhea, severe ileus, intestinal obstruction, upper GI bleeding, large volume high-output intestinal processes (such as fistula), and shock.[2,22,40,51]

For patients who can tolerate oral feedings, a standard infant formula, homogenized cow's milk, or a regular diet can be initiated depending on age. Infants less than 1 year of age should be given their usual formula supplemented with a protein module, if needed. Infants less than 1 year of age should never be given cow's milk because of the risk of allergy and occult GI bleeding.[51,72,73]

Initially toddlers can be fed with homogenized cow's milk. Milk is the preferred feeding for children in this age group because it is palatable and familiar and contains the recommended 20% of calories as protein. Children with a history of milk allergy or intolerance may be fed with an isotonic lactose-free formula, such as Pediasure by Ross.

Cow's milk (20 kcal/ounce) can be mixed with a formula of higher caloric concentration when a nutrient-dense formula is needed because of restricted fluid allowance. In our experience enteral formulas are tolerated best when caloric concentrations are advanced slowly to a maximum of 30 kcal/ounce or 1 kcal/ml. Greater caloric concentrations usually are poorly tolerated by children; small gains in caloric intake are frequently offset by bouts of abdominal distention, vomiting, and diarrhea.

Older children may be given a regular diet supplemented with high-calorie, high-protein snacks. A calorie count helps in determining the adequacy of a patient's oral intake and indicates if supplementation is needed.

For patients who are unable or unwilling to take oral feedings, milk or formula can be administered via a feeding tube with an infusion pump set to deliver the estimated fluid requirement.[61,74] Small, soft nasoenteric feeding tubes are well tolerated by patients. The larger, stiff, adult feeding tubes may cause duodenal perforation in children. Nasoenteric feeding tubes are preferred for short-term (less than 4 weeks) enteral support, since they are easily inserted, cost less than ostomies, and are temporary.[40,51] Transpyloric placement of the feeding tube is indicated for patients at risk for aspiration. For long-term tube feedings (longer than 1 month), enterostomies are indicated for patient convenience and comfort. Ostomies are also required for patients with facial trauma or esophageal blockage. Since the percutaneous endoscopic gastrostomy (PEG) does not require general anesthesia, it is the least expensive ostomy. A variety of tube feeding formulas are available (Table 15–10), including those designed for patients with renal or hepatic insufficiency. Carbohydrates are the main energy source and determine the relative sweetness and osmolarity of the tube feeding formula.

Since the stomach of a traumatized child empties slowly, the feeding tube

Table 15–10. Representative Enteral Formulas

Product	Constituents	CHO (g/100 ml)	Prot (g/100 ml)	Fat (g/100 ml)	Osm	NPC:N	Comments
Breast milk	Lactose, whey (70%), casein (30%), human milk fat	7.2	1.05	3.9	290	595:1	
Pregestimil	Corn syrup, solids, modified corn starch, hydrolyzed casein, corn oil (57%), MCT (42%), lecithin (1%)	7	1.9	3.8	350	329:1	For patients less than 1 yr, semielemental
Pediasure (Ross) 1 cal/ml	Corn syrup solids, sucrose sodium casein, safflower oil (50%), corn/soy oil (50%)	11	3	5	325	185:1	Contains taurine and carnitine, for patients 1-6 yr
Osmolite (Ross) 1 cal/ml	Sodium and calcium caseinates, soy protein isolate, glucose polymers, MCT (50%), corn/soy oil (50%)	13.7	3.5	3.6	300	153:1	Polymeric, lactose free
Peptamen (Clintec) 1 cal/ml	Maltodextrin, starch, hydrolyzed whey, MCT (70%), sunflower oil, and lecithin (30%)	12.7	4	4	270	131:1	Semielemental, well tolerated with fat malabsorption
ImmunAid (McGaw) 1 cal/ml	Maltodextrin, lactalbumin, supplemental amino acids, MCT (50%), canola oil (50%)	12.0	8	2.2	460	53:1	Very high nitrogen, elemental diet, well tolerated, omega-3 fatty acids, ideal protein load for severely stressed catabolic children

is advanced into the small intestine. Duodenal and jejunal feedings present less risk for abdominal distention, diarrhea, aspiration, and fluid-electrolyte abnormalities.[40] In children who are more sensitive to an osmolar load the feeding tip should remain in the stomach so that the pyloric sphincter can regulate the flow of formula into the small intestine. For patients receiving nasogastric feedings the head of the bed should be elevated to protect against aspiration.

Tube feedings should be initiated at half strength at a volume half the desired 24-hour total volume. As the GI tract adapts to the liquid diet, the volume of the solution is increased. Feedings are usually given on a continuous basis to minimize the likelihood of emesis, aspiration, bloating, and diarrhea.[40,55] The rate of infusion is gradually increased every 4 to 6 hours until the estimated fluid requirements are met. The rate of intravenous fluid infusion is simultaneously decreased so that the calculated hourly fluid requirements are not exceeded.

The concentration of enteral solution is then advanced until full caloric requirements are satisfied. Residual volumes should be checked frequently. Patients requiring long-term nasoenteric feeding may be changed from continuous to bolus feedings. Usually one fourth of the required tube feeding volume is instilled through the enteric tube every 6 hours.

For patients requiring frequent procedures such as burn scrubs, debridement, and grafting, a low-residue (lactose-free) enteral formula may be used. Tube feedings should be withheld for 4 to 6 hours before a medical procedure and reinitiated immediately afterward to minimize the fasting period.

A standard high-calorie, high-protein diet can be initiated when the pediatric patient demonstrates an ability to consume solid foods. Fluids are restricted to the prescribed milk or formula to prevent decreased food consumption resulting from a feeling of fullness associated with fluid intake. Oral intake is supplemented with the amount of milk or formula needed to meet anabolic nutrient requirements. Once a patient demonstrates the ability to consume an adequate diet as determined by a calorie count, he or she is weaned from the nasoenteric feeding tube.

PARENTERAL NUTRITION

Parenteral nutrition is indicated when the GI tract cannot be used. High-output proximal fistulas, severe diarrhea, and significant hypermetabolism in the injured child may necessitate parenteral nutritional support to provide adequate calories and protein.

Peripheral Parenteral Nutrition

Peripheral parenteral nutrition (PPN) may be used for short-term nutritional support, for example, when supplementation to enteral feedings is needed or when enteral intake is expected to resume within 5 to 7 days. Peripheral nutritional support permits a maximum 10% dextrose solution owing to the slow blood flow through peripheral veins. Parenteral nutrition solutions with concentrations greater than 10% dextrose may lead to phlebitis and infiltration at the catheter site.[32,51]

Isotonic solutions consisting of carbohydrate, protein, and fat are limited in use by the large volumes required to meet the patient's nutrient needs. Since the dextrose in a parenteral solution largely determines the osmolarity, fat should supply 50% to 60% of nonprotein calories. Intravenous lipids are an efficient fuel source, providing more than twice the energy per gram of carbohydrate and protein and therefore aiding in fluid restriction. Antibiotics, medications, and blood or blood products may be infused through the PPN catheter, but the venotomy site should be changed every other day.

Total Parenteral Nutrition

TPN becomes necessary in hypercatabolic patients with short bowel syndrome, proximal fistulas, obstruction, or hypermetabolic states in which the GI tract is completely or partly unusable. TPN can meet the increased calorie and protein needs of burn patients whose GI tract may be unusable because of multiple surgeries, sepsis-induced ileus, or organ failure.

Because of the high osmolarity of TPN solutions, a central vein must be used for administration. In neonates, acceptable venous access can be achieved with an internal jugular vein cut-down; in older children a percutaneous subclavian catheterization is preferable. However, when more cranial routes have been exhausted, a percutaneous femoral catheterization may be used. Unlike peripheral lines, TPN lines should be reserved for nutritional support, since multiple openings of these lines for blood drawing or medication administration predispose the patient to infection. Percutaneous lines should be exchanged over wires every 2 weeks to minimize the risk of colonization and infection. Children with bacteremia from colonized indwelling lines may be treated with parenteral antibiotics.[1]

Carbohydrates. Carbohydrates are available for TPN solutions in different concentrations, including D_{50} and D_{70}, depending on fluid needs. Carbohydrates should provide 45% to 55% of calories, depending on the patient's ventilatory and fluid status.

Lipids. Lipids are an efficient fuel source and are needed to supply essential fatty acids. Linoleic acid cannot be synthesized in the body and is therefore an essential nutrient. At least 2% to 4% of total calories should be supplied as fat to prevent essential fatty acid deficiency. Normally 25% to 35% of calories is supplied by fat, with a maximum of 60% of total calories.[67]

The provision of lipids in TPN helps prevent TPN-induced changes in liver function tests, cholestasis, and fatty liver. Complications from fat emulsions include phlebitis, minor disorders of platelet adhesiveness, febrile reactions, hypertriglyceridemia, and abnormalities of pulmonary function.[51]

Lipids may be administered separately from the rest of the TPN or may be included in a three in one admixture. We prefer the triple mix for convenience and longer lipid infusion.[67]

Protein. Protein in the TPN solution is provided by crystalline amino acids. Various amino acid solutions (5.5%, 8.5%, and 10%) are available for use, depending on the patient's specific disease state and fluid needs. For example, Nephramine contains only the essential amino acids and is designed for patients with renal disease.

To promote anabolism and limit the amount of protein used for energy, adequate nonprotein calories must be provided. The currently accepted nonprotein calorie/nitrogen ratio is 150:1.[7,8]

The essential amino acids include isoleucine, leucine, lysine, methionine, phenylalanine, threonine, tryptophan, and valine. In neonates and young infants, cysteine, taurine, tyrosine, and histidine may also be essential because of insufficient cystathionase activity. Specific intravenous protein formulas (Trophamine, FreAmine III) have been developed to provide these conditionally essential amino acids, but the superiority of these formulas is not yet determined.[40,74]

SUMMARY

Provision of medical care to the traumatized child is a complex process requiring a multidisciplinary approach. Although the child is usually well nourished before injury, his or her status may deteriorate quickly without aggressive nutritional support. Such aggressive care requires dedicated attention by each of the involved subspecialties (intensivists, surgeons, dietitians, and nursing staff). Chapter 14 outlines the complex nature of the metabolic response to stress and injury. This chapter presents an organized method for the evaluation, nutritional repletion, and nutritional support of the injured child.

REFERENCES

1. Clark-Christoff N, Watters VA, Sparks W, et al: Use of triple lumen subclavian catheters for administration of total parenteral nutrition, *JPEN* 16:403–407, 1992.
2. DeChicco R, Matarese LE: Selection of nutrition support regimens, *Nutr Clin Prac* 7:239–245, 1992.
3. Cuthbertson DP: Observations on the disturbance of metabolism produced by injury to the limbs, *Q J Med* 1:233–246, 1932.
4. Wilmore DW: *The metabolic management of the critically ill,* New York, 1977, Plenum Medical.

5. Groner JI, Brown MF, Stalings VA, et al: REE in children following major operative procedures, *J Pediatr Surg* 24:825–828, 1989.

6. McClave SA, Snider HL: Use of indirect calorimetry in clinical nutrition, *Nutr Clin Prac* 7:207–221, 1992.

7. Greigh PD, Elwyn DH, Askanazi J, et al: Parenteral nutrition in septic patients: effect of increasing nitrogen intake, *Am J Clin Nutr* 46:1040–1047, 1987.

8. Jeevanandam M, Leland D, Shamos RF, et al: Glucose infusion improves endogenous protein synthesis efficiency in multiple trauma victims, *Metabolism* 40:1199–1206, 1991.

9. Hildreth M, Herndon DN, Desai MH, Broemeling LD: Current treatment reduces calories required to maintain weight in pediatric burn patients, *J Burn Care Rehabil* 11:405–409, 1990.

10. McClave SA, Mitoraj TE, Thielmeier KA, Greenburg RA: Differentiating subtypes (hypoalbuminemic versus marasmic) of protein calorie malnutrition: incidence and clinical significance in a university hospital setting, *JPEN* 16:337–342, 1992.

11. Wolfe RR, Burke JF, Mullany J, et al: Glucose requirements following burn injury: parameters of optimal glucose infusion and possible hepatic and respiratory abnormalities following excessive glucose intake, *Ann Surg* 190:274–285, 1979.

12. Cohn KG, Blackburn GL: Nutritional assessment: clinical and biometric measurements of hospital patients at risk, *J Med Assoc Ga* 71:27–35, 1982.

13. Jensen TG, Long JM, Dudrick SJ, et al: Nutritional assessments indications of postburn complications, *J Am Diet Assoc* 85:68–72, 1985.

14. Luterman A, Adams M, Curreri PW: Nutritional management of the burn patient, *Crit Care Q* 7:34–42, 1984.

15. Mason AD: Weight loss in burned patients, *J Trauma* 19:902–903, 1979.

16. Soroff HS, Pearson E, Artz CP: An estimation of the nitrogen requirements for equilibrium in burn patients, *Surg Gynecol Obstet* 112:159–172, 1961.

17. Wilmore DW: Nutrition and metabolism following thermal injury, *Clin Plast Surg* 1:603–619, 1974.

18. Rothschild MA, Oratz M, Schreiber SS: Albumin synthesis, *N Engl J Med* 286:748–757, 1972.

19. Ford EG, Jennings LM, Andrassy RJ: Serum albumin (oncotic pressure) correlates with enteral feeding tolerance in the pediatric surgical patients, *J Pediatr Surg* 22(7):597–599, 1987.

20. Hardin TC, Page CP: Rapid replacement and maintenance of serum albumin in patients receiving total parenteral nutrition, *JPEN* 8:97, 1984.

21. Grant A, Deltoog S: *Nutritional assessment and support,* ed 3, Seattle, 1985, Grant & Deltoog.

22. Bell SJ, Wyatt J: Nutrition guidelines for burned patients, *J Am Diet Assoc* 86:648–653, 1986.

23. Arakawa T, Tamura T, Igarashi Y, et al: Zinc deficiency in two infants during total parenteral alimentation for diarrhea, *Am J Clin Nutr* 29:197–204, 1976.

24. Konstantinides FN: Nitrogen balance studies in clinical nutrition, *Nutr Clin Prac* 7:231–238, 1992.

25. Rudowski WJ: The treatment of burns—summing up, *Burns* 4:67–71, 1978.

26. Suarez A, Hess D, Hunt J: Early tangential excision of a deep dermal burn with immediate mesh homograft coverage, *J Burn Care Rehabil* 1:36, 1980.

27. Wilmore DW, Long JM, Mason AD, et al: Catecholamines: mediator of hypermetabolic response to thermal injury, *Ann Surg* 180:653–669, 1974.

28. Committee on Dietary Allowances: *Recomended dietary allowances,* ed 10, Washington, DC, 1989, National Academy of Sciences.

29. Shanbhogue RLK, Lloyd DA: Absence of hypermetabolism after operation in the newborn infant, *JPEN* 16:333–336, 1992.

30. Kien CL, Young VR, Rohrbaugh DK, et al: Increased rates of whole body protein synthesis and breakdown in children recovering from burns, *Ann Surg* 187:383–391, 1978.

31. Souba WW, Long JM, Dudrick SJ: Energy intake and stress as determinants of nitrogen excretion in rats, *Surg Forum* 29:76–77, 1978.

32. Skipper A, ed: *Dietitian's handbook of enteral and parenteral nutrition,* Rockville, Md, 1989, Aspen.

33. Behrman RE: *Nelson's textbook of pediatrics,* Philadelphia, 1992, WB Saunders.

34. Barbul A, Thysen B, Rettura G, et al: White cell involvement in the inflammatory, wound healing and immune actions of vitamin A, *JPEN* 2:129–138, 1978.

35. Hermann JB, Woodward SC: Stimulation of fibroplasia by vitamin A, *Surg Forum* 20:500–501, 1969.

36. Hughes RE: Nonscorbutic effects of vitamin C: biochemical aspects, *Proc R Soc Med* 70:86–89, 1977.

37. Levenson SM, Green RW, Taylor FHL, et al: Ascorbic acid, riboflavin, thiamine and nicotinic acid in relation to severe injury hemorrhage and infection in the human, *Ann Surg* 124:840–856, 1946.

38. Seifter E, Crowley LV, Rettura G, et al: Influence of vitamin A on wound healing in rats with femoral fracture, *Ann Surg* 181:836–841, 1975.

39. Stratford F, Seifter E, Rettura G, et al: Impaired wound healing due to cyclophosphamide alleviated by supplemental vitamin A, *Surg Forum* 31:224–225, 1980.

40. Blumer JL, ed: *A practical guide to pediatric intensive care,* St Louis, 1990, Mosby.

41. Knochel JP: The pathophysiology and clinical characteristics of severe hypophosphatemia, *Arch Intern Med* 137:203–220, 1977.

42. Chandra RK: Iron and immunocompetence, *Nutr Rev* 34:129–132, 1976.

43. Fosmire GJ, Sandstead HH: Effects of zinc deficiency on compositional development and protein synthesis in liver, heart and kidney of the suckling rat, *Proc Soc Exp Biol Med* 154:351–355, 1977.

44. Henkin RI, Patten BM, Re PK, et al: A syndrome of acute zinc loss: cerebellar dysfunction, mental changes, anorexia, and taste and smell dysfunction, *Arch Neurol* 32:745–751, 1975.

45. Peck MD, Alexander JW: Interaction of protein and zinc malnutrition with the murine response to infection, *JPEN* 16:232–235, 1992.

46. Pekarek RS, Powanda MC: Protein synthesis in zinc deficient rats during tularemia, *J Nutr* 106:905–912, 1976.

47. Pekarek RS, Sandstead JJ, Jacob RA, et al: Abnormal cellular immune responses during acquired zinc deficiency, *Am J Clin Nutr* 32:1466–1471, 1979.

48. Sandstead JJ, Lanier VC, Shephard GH, et al: Zinc and wound healing: effects of zinc deficiency and zinc supplementation, *Am J Clin Nutr* 23:514–519, 1970.

49. JeeJeebhoy KN, Chu RC, Marliss EB, et al: Chromium deficiency, glucose intolerance and neuropathy reversed by chromium supplementation in a patient receiving long term total parenteral nutrition, *Am J Clin Nutr* 30:531–538, 1977.

50. American Medical Association, Department of Foods and Nutrition: Guidelines for essential trace element: preparations for parenteral use, *JAMA* 241:2051–2054, 1979.

51. Mahan KL, Arlin M: *Krause's food, nutrition and diet therapy,* ed 8, Philadelphia, 1992, WB Saunders.
52. Sutherland AB, Batchelor ADR: Nitrogen balance in burned children, *Ann NY Acad Sci* 150:700–710, 1968.
53. Pruitt BA: Metabolic changes and nutrition in burn patients, *Ann Chir Plast Esthet* 24:21–25, 1979.
54. Wilmore DW, Aulick LH, Mason AD, et al: Influence of the burn wound on local and systemic responses to injury, *Ann Surg* 186:444–458, 1977.
55. Moore EE, ed: *Early care of the injured patient,* Toronto, 1990, BC Decker.
56. Carvajal HF: Management of severely burned patients: sorting out the controversies, *Emerg Med Rep* 6:89–96, 1985.
57. Dominioni L, Trocki O, Fang C, et al: Enteral feeding in burn hypermetabolism: nutritional and metabolic effects of different levels of caloric and protein intake, *JPEN* 9:269–279, 1985.
58. Gore DC, Rutan RL, Hildreth M, et al: Comparison of resting energy expenditures and caloric intake in children with severe burns, *J Burn Care Rehabil* 11:400–404, 1990.
59. Curreri P: Nutritional replacement modalities, *J Trauma* 19(suppl):906–908, 1979.
60. Pleban WE: Nutritional support of burn patients: Bridgeport Hospital Burn Unit, *Conn Med* 43:767–768, 1969.
61. Parks DH, Carvajal HF, Larson DL: Management of burns, *Surg Clin North Am* 57:875–894, 1977.
62. Hildreth M, Carvajal JF: Caloric requirements in burned children: a simple formula to estimate daily caloric requirements, *J Burn Care Rehabil* 3:78–84, 1982.
63. Goran ME, Peters EJ, Herndon DN, Wolfe RR: Total energy expenditure in burned children using the doubly labeled water technique, *Am J Physiol* 259:E576–E585, 1990.
64. Alexander JW, MacMillan BG, Stinnett JD, et al: Beneficial effects of aggressive protein feeding in severely burned children, *Ann Surg* 192:505–516, 1980.
65. Jeevanandam M, Shamos RF, Petersen SR: Substrate efficacy in early nutrition support of critically ill multiple trauma victims, *JPEN* 16:511–520, 1992.
66. Gottschlich MM, Jenkins M, Warden GD, et al: Differential effects of three enteral dietary regimens on selected outcome variables in burn patients, *JPEN* 14:225–236, 1990.
67. Vitamin C toxicity, *Nutr Rev* 34:236–237, 1976.
68. Barness LA: Safety considerations with high ascorbic acid dosage, *Ann NY Acad Sci* 258:523–527, 1975.
69. DiPalma JR, Ritchie DM: Vitamin toxicity, *Annu Rev Pharmacol Toxicol* 17:133–148, 1977.
70. Herbert V, Jacob B: Destruction of vitamin B_{12} by ascorbic acid, *JAMA* 230:241–242, 1974.
71. Lund CC, Levenson SM, Green RW, et al: Ascorbic acid, thiamine, riboflavin and nicotinic acid in relation to acute burns in man, *Arch Surg* 55:557–582, 1947.
72. American Academy of Pediatrics, Committee on Nutrition: The use of whole cow's milk in infancy, *Pediatrics* 72:253–255, 1983.
73. Oski FA: Is bovine milk a health hazard? *Pediatrics* 75:182–186, 1985.
74. Lifshitz F, ed: Nutrition for special needs in infancy, New York, 1985, Marcel Dekker.

Index

Note: Page numbers in italics refer to illustrations; page numbers followed by t refer to tables.